COMPARATIVE IMMUNOGLOBULIN GENETICS

COMPARATIVE IMMUNOGLOBULIN GENETICS

Edited by

Azad K. Kaushik, DVM, DSc (Paris), and Yfke Pasman, PharmD, MSc

University of Guelph, Guelph, Ontario Canada

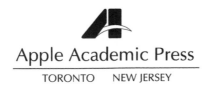

Apple Academic Press

TORONTO   NEW JERSEY

CRC Press
Taylor & Francis Group
6000 Broken Sound Parkway NW, Suite 300
Boca Raton, FL 33487-2742

Apple Academic Press, Inc
3333 Mistwell Crescent
Oakville, ON L6L 0A2
Canada

© 2014 by Apple Academic Press, Inc.

First issued in paperback 2021

Exclusive worldwide distribution by CRC Press an imprint of Taylor & Francis Group, an Informa business

No claim to original U.S. Government works

Version Date: 20140527

ISBN 13: 978-1-77463-334-2 (pbk)
ISBN 13: 978-1-77188-014-5 (hbk)

Visit the Taylor & Francis Web site at
http://www.taylorandfrancis.com

and the CRC Press Web site at
http://www.crcpress.com

For information about Apple Academic Press product
http://www.appleacademicpress.com

ABOUT THE EDITORS

Azad K. Kaushik, DVM, DSc (Paris)

Azad K. Kaushik, DSc, is Associate Professor of Immunology at the University of Guelph, Guelph, Ontario, Canada. He has published over eighty articles and book chapters as well as co-edited a book titled *Molecular Immunobiology of Self-Reactivity*, a major advance in understanding of the systemic autoimmune diseases in the context of natural autoimmunity. He is on the editorial boards of several immunology journals and is a consultant to various international organizations, including the US Veterinary Immune Reagent Network and Comparative Immunoglobulin Workshop in the USA and IMGT (International ImMunoGeneTics Information System), France. He was recognized as The Esther Z. Greenberg Honors Chair in Biomedical Research, and Visiting Professor, Oklahoma Medical Research Foundation, USA, in 1998. He received BVSc&AH (Honors) in 1976 and MVSc (1978) from the Faculty of Veterinary Science, Hisar, Haryana, India, followed by Docteur es Science in Immunology (1987) from the Pasteur Institute (University of Paris VII), Paris, France.

Yfke Pasman, PharmD, MSc

Yfke Pasman received a BA in veterinary management (1988) and a MSc in pharmacology (1994) in the Netherlands and worked for several years as a pharmacist. She received an MSc in Immunology in 2010, which involved engineering of therapeutic antibodies. Currently, she is a PhD candidate in the laboratory of Dr. Azad Kaushik, working on a project involving bovine antibody genetics and its application in therapeutics and immunodiagnosis. She is a member of American Association of Immunologists and Canadian Society of Immunology.

'*Out of Brahma, which is the Higher Self, came space; out of space, air; out of air, fire; out of fire, water; out of water, earth; out of earth, vegetation; out of vegetation, food; out of food, the body of all humanity.*'

—Taittriya Upnishad

CONTENTS

LIST OF CONTRIBUTORS

Michelle L. Baker
CSIRO Animal Food and Health Sciences, Australian Animal Health Laboratory, Geelong, Vic 3220, Australia. E-mail: Michelle.Baker@csiro.au, Tel.: +61 3 5227 5052

Nicolaas A. Bos
Department of Rheumatology and Clinical Immunology University of Groningen, University Medical Center Groningen, AA21, PO Box 30.001, 9700 RB Groningen, The Netherlands, E-mail: n.a.bos@umcg.nl

John E. Butler
Department of Microbiology, Carver College of Medicine, University of Iowa, Iowa City, IA, USA

Justin T. H. Chan
Department of Immunology, University of Toronto, Toronto, Ontario, Canada

Peter M. Dammers
Institute for Life Science and Technology, Hanze University Groningen, Zernikeplein 11, 9747 AS Groningen, The Netherlands, E-mail: p.m.dammers@pl.hanze.nl

Götz R. A. Ehrhardt
Department of Immunology, Medical Sciences Building, University of Toronto, Toronto, ON M5S 1A8, Canada, E-mail: goetz.ehrhardt@utoronto.ca, Tel.: +1 (416) 978 4427, Fax: +1 (416) 978 1938

Victoria L. Hansen
Center for Evolutionary and Theoretical Immunology, Department of Biology, University of New Mexico, Albuquerque, NM USA 87110, USA

Helena Hazanov
The Mina and Everard Goodman Faculty of Life Sciences, Building 212, Box 61, Bar-Ilan University, Ramat-Gan 5290002, Israel, E-mail: lena1907@gmail.com, Tel.: +972-3-531-7243, Fax: +972-3-736-2560

Jacobus Hendricks
Discipline of Physiology, Westville Campus, University of KwaZulu-Natal, Private Bag, X54001, Durban 4000, South Africa

Azad K. Kaushik
Department of Molecular and cellular Biology, University of Guelph, Guelph, Ontario N1G 2W1, Canada, E-mail: akaushik@uoguelph.ca, Tel.: +1 519 760 2297, FAX: +1 519 837 1802

Katherine L. Knight
Department of Microbiology and Immunology, Loyola University Chicago, 2160 S. First Ave., Maywood, IL 60153, USA, E-mail: kknight@lumc.edu

Frans G. M. Kroese
Department of Rheumatology and Clinical Immunology, University of Groningen, University Medical Center Groningen, AA21, PO Box 30.001, 9700 RB Groningen, The Netherlands, E-mail: f.g.m.kroese@umcg.nl

Ramit Mehr
The Mina and Everard Goodman Faculty of Life Sciences, Building 212, Box 61, Bar-Ilan University, Ramat-Gan 5290002, Israel, E-mail: Ramit.Mehr@biu.ac.il, Tel.: +972-3-531-7990, Fax: +972-3-736-2560.

Miri Michaeli
The Mina and Everard Goodman Faculty of Life Sciences, Building 212, Box 61, Bar-Ilan University, Ramat-Gan 5290002, Israel, E-mail: mc_miri@walla.com, Tel.: +972-3-531-7243, Fax: +972-3-736-2560.

Robert D. Miller
Department of Biology, 167 Castetter Hall MSC03 2020 1, University of New Mexico, Albuquerque, NM 87131-0001, USA, E-mail: rdmiller@unm.edu

Marion J. Parsons
Department of Immunology, University of Toronto, Toronto, Ontario, Canada

Yfke Pasman
Department of Molecular and Cellular Biology, University of Guelph, Guelph Ontario N1G 2W1 Canada

Kari M. Severson
Department of Microbiology and Immunology, Loyola University Chicago, 2160 S. First Ave., Maywood, IL 60153, USA

Gitit Lavy-Shahaf
The Mina and Everard Goodman Faculty of Life Sciences, Building 212, Box 61, Bar-Ilan University, Ramat-Gan 5290002, Israel, E-mail: gitita@gmail.com, Tel.: +972-3-531-7243, Fax: +972-3-736-2560

Heng Sun
Department of Immunology, University of Toronto, Toronto, Ontario, Canada

Yi Sun
College of Animal Science and Veterinary Medicine, Shandong Agricultural University, Taian 271018, P. R. China

Peter Terpstra
Department of Epidemiology, Unit of Genetic Epidemiology and Bioinformatics, University of Groningen, University Medical Center Groningen, AA21, PO Box 30.001, 9700 RB Groningen, The Netherlands

Nancy Wertz
Department of Microbiology, Carver College of Medicine, University of Iowa, Iowa City, IA, USA

Yaofeng Zhao
State Key Laboratory of Agrobiotechnology, College of Biological Sciences, China Agricultural University, Beijing 100193, P. R. China. Tel.: 0086-10-62734945, Fax: 0086-10-62733904, Email: yaofengzhao@cau.edu.cn

LIST OF ABBREVIATIONS

AID	activation-induced cytidine deaminase
BAC	bacterial artificial chromosomes
BCR	B-cell antigen receptors
BN	Brown Norway
CP	connecting peptide
CSNS	conserved short nucleotide sequence
CSR	class switch recombination
DG	days of gestation
ERV	endogenous retrovirus
FAE	follicle-associated epithelium
FDCs	follicular dendritic cells
FR	framework regions
GALT	gut-associated lymphoid tissues
GF	germfree
HCAbs	heavy-chain-only antibodies
HCDR3/CDR3H	Heavy Chain Complementarity-Determining Region 3
HEL	hen egg lysozyme
HIV	human immunodeficiency virus
HTS	high throughput sequencing
IELs	intraepithelial lymphocytes
IG	immunoglobulin
IPP	Ileal Peyer's patches
ITIM	Immunoreceptor Tyrosine-based Inhibitory Motifs
LRR	Leucine-rich repeat
LRRCT	C-terminal LRR
LRRNT	N-terminal LRR
LRRv	variable number of diverse LRR modules
MAMPs	Microbial-Associated Molecular Patterns
MHC	major histocompatibility complex
MID	molecular identification

MSC	mesenchymal stem cells
ORF	open reading frame
PCR	polymerase chain reaction
PHA	phytohaemagglutinin
RDA	representational difference analysis
RSS	recombination signal sequence
sGC	somatic gene conversion
SHM	somatic hypermutation
SP	signal peptide
TCR	T-cell antigen receptors
TCRL	T-cell receptor-like
UNG	uracil-DNA glycosylase
VLR	variable lymphocyte receptor
WNS	white nose syndrome

PREFACE

Antibodies are nature's most wonderful molecules and one of the most studied proteins that have found application in therapeutics, clinical diagnosis, and immunodiagnostics. The development of somatic cell fusion hybridoma technology, followed by a revolution in recombinant DNA techniques, has helped advance knowledge of antibody structure and function. Once immunogenetics of antibody unfolded, it broke the widely prevalent dogma of "one gene one protein" of the time. Given whole genome sequencing assembly of vertebrates and its annotation, including humans, it would permit development of desired tailor-made specific antibody-based drugs, vaccines, and antibody drug conjugates for a patient-specific therapy and new measures for disease prevention.

Initially, most of the studies focused on mouse immunoglobulin genetics from which inferences drawn were generalized. But as studies emerged from a variety of other species, from sea lamprey to man, novel perspectives originated that provided new schools of thought and opened new opportunities for a fast developing area of antibody design and engineering strategies. The current volume is an attempt to focus on this newly developed knowledge and the emerging concepts from comparative immunoglobulin genetics perspectives, from species other than mice and humans.

The evolutionary distant jawless vertebrates have developed an adaptive immune repertoire, parallel to jawed vertebrates, that reflects convergent evolution (Chapter 1). These antigen receptors have distinct architecture when compared to the immunoglobulin-based recombining antigen receptors of jawed vertebrates but are capable of similar functions. Study of immunoglobulin genetics in tetrapods has added new knowledge that could not be derived from studies in mice and humans (Chapter 2). For example, new antibody classes have been discovered in tetrapods that differ from those conventionally described from human and rodent studies. The insectivorous little brown bat (*Myotis lucifugus*) seem to depend essentially on combinatorial diversity, given considerable variable region gene sequence divergence, rather than somatic hypermutations in contrast to humans (Chapter 3). Interestingly, marsupials rely on light chain complexity for generating diverse antibody repertoire rather than heavy chain isotypes and variable region diversity. Monotremes share characteristics with reptile-like ancestors, as evidenced by a novel heavy chain class in platypus with characteristics common to both IgG and IgY (Chapter 4). It is thus obvious that different strategies are used across phylogeny to generate an immune antibody repertoire for adequate host protection.

The IGH locus in rats that belongs to the largest mammalian order, *Rodentia*, resembles to that of mice, given its genomic organization and extensive germline encoded combinatorial diversity (Chapter 5). By contrast, little combinatorial antibody diversity can be generated in rabbits due to single predominant *IGHV* gene (Chapter 6). Hence, most antibody diversification and maintenance of peripheral B-cell populations occurs in gut-associated lymphoid tissue by intestinal microbiota induced mutations and gene conversion. In domestic swine, only single *IGHJ* gene exists and only few genes encode most of the antibody repertoire (Chapter 7).

The distribution of light chains varies considerably across species. The studies from mice earlier suggested that kappa light chain rearrangement occurred before lambda light chain during B-lymphocyte ontogeny. This is in contrast to pigs where lambda light chain rearranges before kappa light chains leading to several questions that need to be answered. Cattle compensate limited germline encoded combinatorial diversity via generating an exceptionally long CDR3 (up to 66 codons) of the heavy variable region (Chapter 8). Such a CDR3H is rich in multiple cysteines that form intra-CDR3H disulfide bridges creating a novel type of antigen-combining site, yet to be reported in another species. In addition, cattle amplify the developing preimmune repertoire via antigen-independent somatic mutations in the variable region.

These novel perspectives from across species are likely to provide enough food for thought to develop new antibody based designer drugs to cure those diseases or conditions like cancer and autoimmune disease where conventional therapies fail. The development of antibody-based designer drugs would require new bioinformatics tools in this age of high throughput deep sequencing. The last chapter is devoted to the important informatics tools (Chapter 9) that aim to address the unique characteristics of immunoglobulin in the context of novel antibody engineering strategies. Knowledge gained from comparative immunoglobulin genetics direct us towards fulfilling the dream of patient-centered bedside medicine using antibody-based drugs.

— **Azad K. Kaushik, DVM, DSc (Paris), and**
Yfke Pasman, PharmD, MSc

CHAPTER 1

VARIABLE LYMPHOCYTE RECEPTOR-BASED ADAPTIVE IMMUNITY IN THE AGNATHAN SEA LAMPREY

MARION J. PARSONS, JUSTIN T. H. CHAN, HENG SUN, and
GÖTZ R. A. EHRHARDT

CONTENTS

ABSTRACT

The ability of organisms to respond to pathogenic challenge with a highly specific immune response was considered, until recently, to have emerged after the divergence of jawed from jawless vertebrates. It has now become clear that jawless vertebrates developed an adaptive immune system with an antigen receptor repertoire that rivals that of jawed vertebrates in magnitude. Investigations of the jawless vertebrate adaptive immune system have revealed an unexpected example of convergent evolution in which antigen receptors with fundamental structural differences when compared to the immunoglobulin-based recombining antigen receptors of jawed vertebrates fulfill similar functions. Despite the use of distinct receptor architecture, the basic operating principles of adaptive immunity, including somatic receptor diversification and differentiation into humoral and cellular lineages, are remarkably conserved between jawed and jawless vertebrates over a large evolutionary distance.

1.1   INTRODUCTION

Highly specific adaptive immune responses to a plethora of pathogens are a key characteristic of the immune systems of jawed vertebrates, ranging from humans to the most ancient representatives, the cartilaginous fish. The ability to mount antigen specific immune responses required the development of specialized hematopoietic cell lineages capable of generating a vast repertoire of clonally expressed anticipatory immune receptors. Beginning with early studies including Paul Ehrlich's description of antitoxins and his formulation of the sidechain theory (Die Seitenkettentheorie der Immunität, 1902), research efforts spanning over 100 years have delineated the characteristics of the adaptive immune systems of jawed vertebrates (gnathostomes) on the cellular and molecular level. In contrast, detailed information on the components of the adaptive immune system of jawless vertebrates (agnathans) was gained only over the last decade. Lampreys and hagfish are the only extant members of the agnathan taxon, which diverged from jawed vertebrates approximately 500 million years ago (Cooper and Alder, 2006). Studies conducted in the 1960s demonstrated the induction of circulating agglutinins, delayed type hypersensitivity reactions, and accelerated allograft rejection in sea lampreys, indicative of humoral and cellular adaptive immune responses (Finstad and Good, 1964; Marchalonis and Edelman, 1968; Perey, 1968; Litman et al., 1970; Pollara, 1970). However, efforts failed to identify orthologs of key players of gnathostome adaptive immune systems, including the recombining B cell and T cell antigen receptors (BCR and TCR, respectively), the major histocompatibility complex (MHC), or recombinase activating genes *(RAG 1/2)*. In a surprising finding, Cooper and colleagues discovered the first example of a recombining, structurally distinct anticipatory antigen receptor system in the sea lamprey *Petromyzon marinus* (Pancer, 2004). Subsequent reports shed light on an expanding family of agnathan antigen receptors and the cellular components acting in concert with these proteins. Here we review current knowledge on the molecular and cellular characteristics of the adaptive immune system of jawless vertebrates.

1.2   RECOMBINING ANTIGEN RECEPTORS IN JAWLESS VERTEBRATES

1.2.1   IMMUNE-RELATED GENES IN LAMPREY LYMPHOCYTE-LIKE CELLS

The ability of the adaptive immune system to respond to antigenic stimulation with specific humoral and cellular responses is a defining characteristic of all jawed vertebrates (Litman, 1999). However, jawless vertebrates also respond to antigenic challenge with responses suggestive of a cellular and humoral adaptive immune system. Lamprey shave circulating cells with lymphocyte-like physical characteristics as assessed by flow cytometry, light microscopy, and electron microscopy (Mayer et al., 2002). Characterization of transcripts expressed by these cells uncovered homologs of multiple genes involved in the development and regulation of adaptive immune responses of higher vertebrates, including the transcription factors *Spi* and *Ikaros*, the transmembrane phosphatase *CD45*, and the adaptor protein *BCAP* (Uinuk-Ool et al., 2002, 2003; Pancer et al., 2004; Yu et al., 2009). Interestingly, EST-libraries prepared from these cells also provided evidence of agnathan orthologs of the CD4 co-receptor and of a T cell receptor-like (*TCRL*) gene (Kasamatsu et al., 2010). The TCRL molecule contains extracellular IgV- and IgC-type domains and an intracellular domain with two canonical immunoreceptor tyrosine-based inhibitory motifs (ITIM), which proved functional when examined in a murine memory B cell line (Pancer et al, 2005). However, since the *TCRL* gene occurs as a single copy, it cannot provide receptor diversity and its function remains unknown. Although the presence of recombining immunoglobulin-based antigen receptor systems was anticipated, no studies have provided evidence for their existence in agnathans.

1.2.2 IDENTIFICATION OF RECOMBINING VARIABLE LYMPHOCYTE RECEPTOR (VLR) GENES

Interrogation of the transcriptome of activated lamprey lymphocytes discovered a highly diverse family of anticipatory receptors that are expressed in monoallelic fashion. These were named variable lymphocyte receptors (Pancer, 2004). Following the initial discovery of the lamprey *VLRB* gene and its equivalent in hagfish, two additional recombining VLR genes, *VLRA* and *VLRC,* were each discovered in lampreys and in hagfish (Das et al., 2013; Kasamatsu et al., 2007; Nagawa et al., 2007; Rogozin et al., 2007). Unlike the generation of the mammalian antibody repertoire, in which RAG1/2-mediated V(D)J rearrangement leads to the generation of a vast repertoire of immunoglobulin domain-containing antigen receptors, the VLR antigen receptors of jawless vertebrates use the β-sheet-forming leucine-rich repeat (LRR) as basic structural unit.

On the genomic level, an incomplete VLR gene consists of N-terminal and C-terminal partial capping units and invariant stalk regions that surround non-coding intervening DNA sequences (illustrated in Fig. 1). This immature gene is flanked by a large number of LRR template cassettes; the *VLRB*, *VLRA*, and *VLRC* loci contain 454, 393, and 182 cassettes, respectively (Das et al., 2013; Alder, et al., 2005). The mature VLR gene consists of the signal peptide, a capping N-terminal LRR unit, a short LRR1 unit, variable numbers of highly diverse LRRv units, a connecting peptide, a capping C-terminal LRR unit, and the invariant stalk region (Fig. 1).

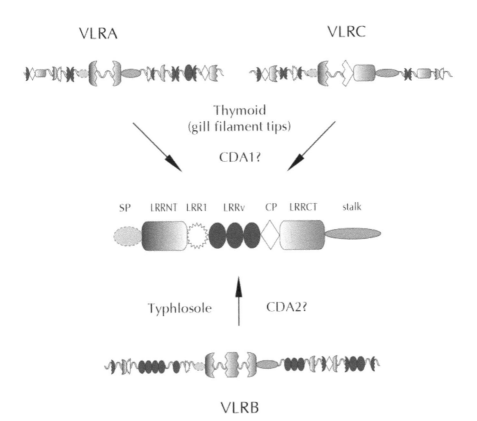

FIGURE 1 Common modular structure of *VLRA*, *VLRB*, and *VLRC* (Incomplete VLR genes in germline configuration are flanked by multiple LRR cassettes. A gene conversion-like process leads to the assembly of the mature VLR gene, consisting of signal peptide (SP), N-terminal LRR (LRRNT), LRR1, a variable number of diverse LRR modules (LRRv), connecting peptide (CP), C-terminal LRR (LRRCT), and stalk region).

The arrays of donor cassettes are located both upstream and downstream of the germline gene, and their coding strands can be in sense or antisense orientation relative to the gene. Individual cassettes do not always directly correspond to individual LRR modules of the final assembled genes; a cassette may include the sequence for an incomplete single module or may span portions of two or three modules (Das et al., 2013). In fact, none of the cassettes flanking lamprey *VLRC,* and only a small minority of the cassettes flanking lamprey *VLRA*, cover a complete LRRv module (Das et al., 2013; Alder, et al., 2005); in consequence, all or most of the modules in mature *VLRC* and *VLRA,* respectively, are chimeras generated by two or more cassette insertions. Cassettes that contain complete or partial sequences for LRRv modules are the most numerous; however, the donor cassettes are also responsible for templating the 3' end of the LR-RNT, the LRR1, the CP, and the 5' end of the LRRCT (Das et al., 2013). DNA sequencing of the modules in mature hagfish *VLRA* and *VLRB* genes has shown that the donor cassettes copied into each are mutually exclusive; despite being situated on the same chromosome, each locus is an independent recombination unit (Barreto and Magor, 2011). Similarly, the lamprey VLR genes do not share donor cassettes.

1.2.3   RECOMBINING VLR GENES: GENERATION OF REPERTOIRE DIVERSITY

Mechanistically, the generation of VLR antibody diversity is likely achieved via a series of gene conversion steps. The insertion of a donor cassette sequence into the germline locus requires a region of homology between the donor sequence and the germline sequence (or the previously copied donor cassette); these homologous stretches are 10 to 30 nucleotides in length and do not require perfect identity (Smith et al., 2013). Dependence on homologous stretches is consistent with either a homologous recombination or gene conversion model for the donor sequence insertion. However, the recombination model is not consistent with other data that have emerged from lamprey studies: this model predicts that a reciprocal coding joint would be found in the flanking region following recombination, but no such coding joints have been identified outside of the arranged VLR loci (Smith et al., 2013). Furthermore, the size of the homologous regions is smaller than that normally required for homologous recombination. The current model for VLR gene assembly is a series of gene conversion steps in which a broken DNA strand anneals to a homologous sequence elsewhere along the chromosome to reinitiate DNA replication, thus copying the donor sequence into the receptor locus (Das et al., 2013; Guo et al., 2009). The requirement for homologous regions may account for the fact that selection of donor cassettes appears to be biased rather than random. For example, the lamprey *VLRC* locus has been found to contain 182 potential donor cassettes, but in a sample of 60 mature *VLRC* genes, only 88 cassettes had contributed sequences (Alder et al., 2005). Sequencing of partially rearranged intermediates of lamprey *VLRA, VLRB* (Smith et al., 2013) and *VLRC* genes (Alder et al., 2005) reveals that serial gene conversion steps may begin at either the 5' or 3' end of the noncoding intervening DNA contained within the germline locus. However, no intermediates were found in any lineage that showed simultaneous gene conversion at both ends; once a first donor cassette is copied into the locus, the remaining cassettes are sequentially added from the same direction (Alder et al., 2005; Smith et al., 2013).

V(D)J rearrangement of antigen receptors in mammals is mediated by the RAG1/2 recombinases. In addition, activation-induced cytidine deaminase (AID) plays a key role in the B lineage cells of jawed vertebrates subsequent to antigen exposure. As an inducer of point mutations, it enables affinity maturation by means of somatic hypermutation; as an inducer of double-stranded DNA breaks, it enables class-switch recombination between immunoglobulin isotypes (Herrin et al., 2008). Furthermore, AID has been shown to catalyze primary V(D)J rearrangement in developing chicken B cells in a pathway that involves single-stranded nicking and gene conversion (Herrin et al., 2008). Thus far, sequencing of the lamprey genome has not revealed the presence of orthologs of the *RAG1/2* or *AICDA* genes in lampreys (Kim et al., 2007). However, two members of the cytidine deaminase family, CDA1 and CDA2, are expressed in lamprey VLRA⁺ and VLRB⁺ cells, respectively (Das et al., 2013). These enzymes are most closely related to the AID-APOBEC subfamily (Herrin et al., 2008). While no direct evidence exists as of yet to establish the role of CDA1 and CDA2 in lamprey VLR gene assembly, it is hypothesized that these enzymes mediate gene conversion by triggering the DNA strand breaks that lead to a free 3' end priming DNA replication at a homologous stretch in the donor cassette region based on:

(i) A role of the homologous enzyme AID in mediating gene conversion in chicken immunoglobulin (Herrin et al., 2008) setting a precedent for cytidine deaminases contributing to primary diversification.

(ii) The lineage-specific co-regulation of CDA1 and VLRA expression, and of CDA2 and VLRB expression, suggests that these enzymes may be involved in the development of VLR antigen receptors (Das et al., 2013).

(iii)   An observed 20-fold increase in the frequency of intragenic recombination in yeast expressing CDA1 in the presence of uracil-DNA glycosylase (UNG). This suggests that CDA1 may be capable of generating DNA strand breaks and thus has the potential to initiate gene conversion (Das et al., 2013).

The VLR repertoire has been estimated to exceed 10^{14} based on the number of LRRv modules in the assembled gene, the order in which the LRRv modules appear, and the identity of the donor cassettes used as templates. There is no evidence for the incorporation of n-nucleotides and consequently junctional diversity does not contribute to the VLR repertoire. However, as discussed above, the donor cassettes do not have a one-on-one correspondence with the LRR modules that they are ultimately responsible for encoding (Das et al., 2013; Alder, et al., 2005), and most LRR modules in mature genes are derived from the fusion of donor cassettes. Frequently, the cassettes contain more than one potential double-strand break site (Alder et al., 2005) and more than one sequence which can function as a homologous region to the sequence of other cassettes (Smith et al., 2013). As a result, the point of fusion between two given donor cassettes is variable, adding an additional layer of positional diversity, which contributes to the overall VLR repertoire (Alder et al., 2005).

1.3   STRUCTURAL CHARACTERISTICS OF VLR ANTIBODIES

Unlike conventional antibodies, which use the immunoglobulin-fold as basic structural unit and are heterodimers consisting of heavy and light chain segments, sea lamprey VLRs are single chain proteins that are expressed as GPI-anchored receptors on the cell surface (Pancer, 2004; Han et al., 2008). VLRB proteins (but not VLRA or VLRC molecules) can also be secreted as decamers linked by disulfide bonds located in the invariant proline/threonine-rich stalk region (Kirchdoerfer et al., 2012). Initial, structural analyses of recombinant monomeric hagfish VLRA and VLRB proteins with deleted stalk regions determined that the receptors adopted a solenoid shape (Velikovsky et al., 2009). The capping N-terminal and C-terminal LRR units contain each two intramolecular disulfide bonds that support structural integrity. Each 24-amino acid LRR unit follows the consensus sequence $xLxxL_5xxL_8xL_{10}xxxxLxxLPxxxFx$ and forms a β-sheet at the inner concave surface and a loop on the convex surface. The leucine residues at positions 5, 8, and 10 located at the inner concave surface align in rows parallel to the corresponding regions of adjacent LRR units, forming the hydrophobic core of the antigen receptor (Velikovsky et al., 2009). Highly variable residues make up the exposed inner concave surface of the solenoid VLR.

The structures of three monoclonal VLR antibodies co-crystallized with their respective antigens confirmed the predicted antigen binding at the inner concave surface and highlight the distinctive mode of interaction between agnathan antigen receptors and antigen (Cohen et al., 2005; Tasumi et al., 2009; Yu et al., 2012). These antibody-antigen complexes draw attention to a unique feature of VLRA and VLRB receptors, namely a loop structure that is variable in length and sequence and protrudes from the C-terminal capping LRR. This protruding loop is conserved in a mammalian protein, the gp1bα von Willebrand factor receptor (Cohen et al., 2005), and may thus be a clue to the evolutionary origins of the VLR anticipatory receptor system. A study by Han et al. on a monoclonal VLRB antibody specific for the comparatively small erythrocyte H-trisaccharide determined that the VLR protein forms a pocket for the antigen

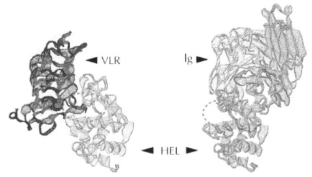

FIGURE 2 Structures of a monomeric antigen-binding unit of a monoclonal *VLRB* antibody and a mouse monoclonal Fab fragment bound to a protein antigen, HEL. HEL, VLR and Fab protein positions are indicated by arrowheads. Note that the VLR antibody extends the flexible C-terminal loop into the active site of the enzyme (indicated by a dotted circle) whereas the murine monoclonal antibody detects a planar epitope on the opposite side of the protein. Structures were modified from PDB accession numbers 3G3A and 1YQV (Cohen et al., 2005; Holliger and Hudson, 2005).

between residues located at the inner concave surface of the VLR and the C-terminal variable loop (Tasumi et al., 2009). On the other hand, a monoclonal VLRB antibody specific for hen egg lysozyme (HEL) utilizes the C-terminal variable loop structure to interact with an epitope located in the active site of the enzyme (Fig. 2) (Cohen et al., 2005). This is in contrast to conventional antibodies, which tend to interact with epitopes situated on planar surfaces (Cooper et al., 1965).VLR antibodies isolated from immunized sea lamprey to date indicate that the affinity of the individual VLR unit to antigen tends to be of low affinity (Alder et al., 2008; Kirchdoerfer et al., 2012; Rumfelt et al., 2001) indicating an avidity-based binding mechanism. No definitive evidence for in vivo affinity maturation has been demonstrated as yet. However, in vitro affinity maturation systems allow the generation of VLR antibodies with picomolar affinities, indicating that the LRR-based structural units form no impediment to high affinity antibody-antigen interactions (Alder et al., 2008).

1.4   LYMPHOID CELL LINEAGES IN THE SEA LAMPREY

1.4.1   VLR SURFACE EXPRESSION CHARACTERIZES DISTINCT LINEAGES OF LAMPREY LYMPHOCYTES

The delineation of the adaptive immune system into separate cell lineages mediating humoral and cellular immune responses is a paradigm underlying the organization of the immune system of all jawed vertebrates (Miracle et al., 2001). Similarly, recent findings indicate that this dichotomy is preserved in jawless vertebrates with B- and T-like lymphocytes that differ in their gene expression profiles, their sites of development, and their responses to antigenic stimulation. Using antibodies specific for VLRA or VLRB, Guo et al. demonstrated a mutually exclusive pattern of expression of these antigen receptors on the cell surface of lamprey lymphocytes. The preferential expression of orthologs of the *Notch1, Bcl11b, CCR9, IL-8R,* and *IL-17* genes as well as the *GATA3* transcription factor are consistent with a T cell-like function of VLRA[+] cells (Han et al., 2008). VLRA[+] cells also respond to stimulation with the T cell mitogen phytohaemagglutinin (PHA), do not secrete their antigen receptors, and do not recognize native antigen, thereby raising the possibility that antigen recognition by VLRA requires prior antigen processing. These features further support a function for these cells similar to αβ T cells of jawed vertebrates. In contrast, VLRB⁺ lamprey lymphocytes express several Toll-like receptor orthologs in addition to genes related to the *IL-17R* and *IL-8* genes, which are suggestive of reciprocal interactions with VLRA⁺ cells (Han et al., 2008). Unlike cells expressing VLRA, VLRB⁺ cells bind native antigen. Increased numbers of antigen-binding cells can be detected in response to *B. anthracis* exosporium immunization, presumably as the result of clonal expansion, and elevated VLRB antibody titres to this antigen can be detected in serum after repeated immunizations (Boehm and Bleul, 2007). The hypothesis of VLRB⁺ clonal expansion is supported by unpublished experiments in our laboratory in which we cloned VLRB antigen receptors by single cell RT-PCR from individual lamprey lymphocytes that bound fluorescently labeled antigen. Sequence analysis of 15 monoclonal VLR antibodies that gave positive signals in ELISA validation assays showed that one receptor clone was independently amplified from five individually sorted cells (Fig. 3). These features indicate that VLRB-bearing lamprey lymphocytes perform functions akin to those of B lineage cells of jawed vertebrates.

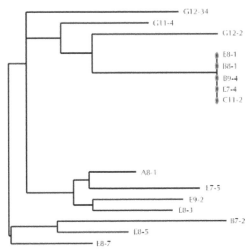

FIGURE 3 Phylogenetic analysis of gp130 (IL-6R) specific monoclonal *VLRB* antibodies. Lamprey larvae lymphocytes from a single immunized animal were stained with fluorescently labeled antigen (gp130) and individual *VLRB* clones were amplified by single cell RT-PCR. Binding specificity was verified by ELISA. Note that out of 15 sequences five from individual cells were identical, suggestive of clonal expansion.

As mentioned above, VLRC molecules are more similar to VLRA than to VLRB and they lack the prominent variable loop structure protruding from the capping C-terminal LRR. Interestingly, a comparative analysis of these cells suggests that VLRA- and VLRC-expressing cells represent two independent T cell-like lymphocytic lineages (Ardavin and Zapata, 1988).

1.4.2 DEVELOPMENTAL ORIGINS OF LAMPREY LYMPHOCYTES

The development of distinct lymphocytic lineages in separate anatomical locations is a hallmark of the gnathostome adaptive immune system. Defined sites for B lymphopoiesis have been described even in the most basal jawed verterbrates: the epigonal and Leydig organs in cartilaginous fish are equivalents to mammalian bone marrow (Bajoghli et al., 2011; Haruta et al., 2006). Published observations are consistent with a role of the typhlosole, a hematopoietic tissue formed by invagination of the intestinal wall, as the anatomical location for the generation of VLRB-expressing lymphocytes (Boehm and Bleul, 2007). Unlike B lymphopoiesis, which occurs in different anatomical locations in various gnathostome species, all jawed vertebrates including cartilaginous fish have a defined thymus (Takaba et al., 2013). In contrast, a definitive identification of thymic structures could not be established in jawless vertebrates (Herrin and Cooper, 2010), despite the presence of T cell-equivalent VLRA-bearing cells. In an elegant series of experiments, Bajoghli et al. investigated lamprey tissues for co-expression of transcripts encoding VLRA and an ortholog of Foxn1, a transcription factor that marks the thymopoietic microenvironment in jawed vertebrates (Hong et al., 2013). Anatomical sites meeting these criteria were found at the tips of the gill filaments. In addition, transcripts encoding the *CDA1* gene, which is postulated to be involved in generating the diverse *VLRA* repertoire, were detected at these sites. Importantly, sequence analysis of *VLRA* transcripts from the thymoid structures of the gill filaments revealed a high frequency of non-functional *VLRA* rearrangements, indicating an ongoing selection process, whereas *VLRA* transcripts from other locations were functionally rearranged. These studies suggest that a common ancestor of jawed and jawless vertebrates not only had defined lymphocytic lineages for humoral and cellular immune responses but also had separate anatomical locations that allowed for the development and selection of these cells.

1.5 CONCLUSIONS

Investigations directed towards the elucidation of the adaptive immune system of the evolutionarily distant jawless vertebrates revealed the existence of a structurally distinct, highly diversified antigen receptor recognition system accommodated in immune cells with conserved features. Despite this rapid progress, many questions remain to be answered. Jawed vertebrates developed elaborate mechanisms to maintain central and peripheral tolerance. Given the vast predicted VLR repertoire, similar mechanisms would be expected to exist in jawless vertebrates but have yet to be elucidated. Published observations suggest that VLRA$^+$ cells do not recognize native antigen, which raises questions concerning the possibility of processed antigen recognition, the presentation of such processed antigens, and the mechanism of allograft rejection. Initial observations in hagfish indicate involvement of NICIR3, a polymorphic transmembrane receptor with similarity to the lamprey TCRL (Haruta et al., 2006), as an allogenic leukocyte antigen recognized by VLRB proteins (Takaba et al., 2013). In addition to insights into the evolutionary origins of the adaptive immune system, VLR antibodies also offer tremendous potential in biomedical research and clinical applications (Kirchdoerfer et al., 2012; Rumfelt et al., 2012; Herrin and Cooper, 2010; Hong et al., 2013). The distinct protein architecture and unique evolutionary origins suggest that monoclonal VLR antibodies may recognize antigens that may not be readily recognized by conventional antibodies for structural or tolerogenic reasons. In this context, VLR antibodies represent a new class of reagents that complement existing panels of conventional antibodies.

KEYWORDS

- adaptive immunity
- antigen receptors
- diversification
- evolution
- jawless vertebrates
- Leucine-rich repeat
- variable lymphocyte receptors

REFERENCES

"Die Seitenkettentheorie der Immunität" in Anleitung zu hygienischen Untersuchungen, 3rd edition, München, Rieger, (1902): 381–388.

Alder, M.N., Herrin, B.R., Sadlonova, A., Stockard, C.R., Grizzle, W.E., Gartland, L.A., et al. *Nat Immunol* 9, (2008): 319–327.

Alder, M.N., Rogozin, I.B., Iyer, L.M., Glazko, G.V., Cooper, M.D., Pancer, Z. *Science* 310, (2005): 1970–1973.

Ardavin, C.F., Zapata, A. *Thymus* 11, (1988): 59–65.

Bajoghli, B., Guo, P., Aghaallaei, N., Hirano, M., Strohmeier, C., McCurley, N., et al. *Nature* 470, (2011): 90–94.

Barreto, V.M., Magor, B.G. *Dev Comp Immunol* 35, (2011): 991–1007.

Boehm, T., Bleul, C.C. *Nat Immunol* 8, (2007): 131–135.

Cohen, G.H., Silverton, E.W., Padlan, E.A., Dyda, F., Wibbenmeyer, J.A., Willson, R.C., et al. *Acta Crystallogr D Biol Crystallogr* 61, (2005): 628–633.

Cooper, M.D., Alder, M.N. *Cell* 124, (2006): 815–822.

Cooper, M.D., Peterson, R.D., Good, R.A. *Nature* 205, (1965): 143–146.

Das, S., Hirano, M., Aghaallaei, N., Bajoghli, B., Boehm, T., Cooper, M.D. *Proc Natl Acad Sci USA* 110, (2013): 6043–6048.

Finstad, J., Good, R.A. *J Exp Med* 120, (1964): 1151–1168.

Guo, P., Hirano, M., Herrin, B.R., Li, J., Yu, C., Sadlonova, A., et al. *Nature* 459, (2009): 796–801.

Han, B.W., Herrin, B.R., Cooper, M.D., Wilson, I.A. *Science* 321, (2008): 1834–1837.

Haruta, C., Suzuki, T., Kasahara, M. *Immunogenetics* 58, (2006): 216–225.

Herrin, B. R., Cooper, M. D. *J Immunol* 185, (2010): 1367–1374.

Herrin, B.R., Alder, M.N., Roux, K.H., Sina, C., Ehrhardt, G.R., Boydston, J.A., et al. *Proc Natl Acad Sci USA* 105, (2008): 2040–2045.

Holliger, P., Hudson, P.J. *Nat Biotechnol* 23, (2005): 1126–1136.

Hong, X., Ma, M.Z., Gildersleeve, J.C., Chowdhury, S., Barchi, J.J., Jr., Mariuzza, R.A., et al. *ACS Chem Biol* 8, (2013): 152–160.

Kasamatsu, J., Sutoh, Y., Fugo, K., Otsuka, N., Iwabuchi, K., Kasahara, M. *Proc Natl Acad Sci USA* 107, (2010): 14304–14308.

Kasamatsu, J., Suzuki, T., Ishijima, J., Matsuda, Y., Kasahara, M. *Immunogenetics* 59, (2007): 329–331.

Kim, H.M., Oh, S.C., Lim, K.J., Kasamatsu, J., Heo, J.Y., Park, B.S., et al. *J Biol Chem* 282, (2007): 6726–6732.

Kirchdoerfer, R.N., Herrin, B.R., Han, B.W., Turnbough, C.L., Jr., Cooper, M.D., Wilson, I.A. *Structure* 20, (2012): 479–486.

Litman, G.W., Anderson, M.K., Rast, J.P. *Annu Rev Immunol* 17, (1999): 109–147.

Litman, G.W., Finstad, F.J., Howell, J., Pollara, B.W., Good, R.A. *J Immunol* 105, (1970): 1278–1285.

Marchalonis, J.J., Edelman, G.M. *J Exp Med* 127, (1968): 891–914.

Mayer, W.E., Uinuk-Ool, T., Tichy, H., Gartland, L.A., Klein, J., Cooper, M.D. *Proc Natl Acad Sci USA* 99, (2002): 14350–14355.

Miracle, A.L., Anderson, M.K., Litman, R.T., Walsh, C.J., Luer, C.A., Rothenberg, E.V., et al. *Int Immunol* 13, (2001): 567–580.

Nagawa, F., Kishishita, N., Shimizu, K., Hirose, S., Miyoshi, M., Nezu, J., et al. *Nat Immunol* 8, (2007): 206–213.

Pancer, Z., Amemiya, C.T., Ehrhardt, G.R., Ceitlin, J., Gartland, G.L., Cooper, M.D. *Nature* 430, (2004): 174–180.

Pancer, Z., Mayer, W.E., Klein, J., Cooper, M.D. *Proc Natl Acad Sci USA* 101, (2004): 13273–13278.

Pancer, Z., Saha, N.R., Kasamatsu, J., Suzuki, T., Amemiya, C.T., Kasahara, M., Cooper, M.D. *Proc Natl Acad Sci USA* 102, (2005): 9224–9229.

Perey, D.Y., Finstad, J., Pollara, B., Good, R.A. *Lab Invest* 19, (1968): 591–597.

Pollara, B., Litman, G.W., Finstad, J., Howell, J., Good, R.A. *J Immunol* 105, (1970): 738–745.

Rogozin, I.B., Iyer, L.M., Liang, L., Glazko, G.V., Liston, V.G., Pavlov, Y.I., et al. *Nat Immunol* 8, (2007): 647–656.

Rumfelt, L.L., Avila, D., Diaz, M., Bartl, S., McKinney, E.C., Flajnik, M.F. *Proc Natl Acad Sci USA* 98, (2001): 1775–1780.

Smith, J.J., Kuraku, S., Holt, C., Sauka-Spengler, T., Jiang, N., Campbell, M.S., et al. *Nat Genet* 45, (2013): 415–421, 421e411–412.

Takaba, H., Imai, T., Miki, S., Morishita, Y., Miyashita, A., Ishikawa, N., et al. *Sci Rep* 3, (2013): 1716.

Tasumi, S., Velikovsky, C.A., Xu, G., Gai, S.A., Wittrup, K.D., Flajnik, M.F., *Proc Natl Acad Sci USA* 106, (2009): 12891–12896.

Uinuk-Ool, T.S., Mayer, W.E., Sato, A., Dongak, R., Cooper, M.D., Klein, J. *Proc Natl Acad Sci USA* 99, (2002): 14356–14361.

Uinuk-Ool, T.S., Mayer, W.E., Sato, A., Takezaki, N., Benyon, L., Cooper, M.D., Klein, J. *Immunogenetics* 55, (2003): 38–48.

Velikovsky, C.A., Deng, L., Tasumi, S., Iyer, L.M., Kerzic, M.C., et al. *Nat Struct Mol Biol* 16, (2009): 725–730.

Yu, C., Ali, S., St-Germain, J., Liu, Y., Yu, X., Jaye, D.L., et al. *J Immunol Methods* 386, (2012): 43–49.

Yu, C., Ehrhardt, G.R., Alder, M.N., Cooper, M.D., Xu, A. *Eur J Immunol* 39, (2009): 571–579.

CHAPTER 2

IMMUNOGLOBULIN GENES IN TETRAPODS

YI SUN and YAOFENG ZHAO

CONTENTS

ABSTRACT

Over the past several decades, comparative examinations of the immuno-globulin (Ig) genes of various tetrapod species have provided interesting knowledge that is unavailable from conventional mouse and human models. This chapter summarizes the progress of research on Ig gene organization and repertoire diversification in tetrapods, highlighting the evolutionary relationships among different Ig isotypes. A number of distinct Ig heavy chain (H) isotypes, such as IgM, IgD, IgG, IgA, IgE, IgY, IgX, IgF, and IgO, have been discovered in different tetrapod species. IgM and IgD are two primordial Ig isotypes that are expressed in almost all vertebrate species. Unlike IgM, IgD shows a high degree of variation in the number of δC_H exons and alternative RNA splicing patterns. IgY is the major low-molecular-weight serum Ig encoded by the υ gene in non-mammalian tetrapods and is thought to be the evolutionary precursor of mammalian IgG and IgE. IgA and its analog IgX, which play important roles in mucosal immunity, are also present in the majority of tetrapods (except for some reptiles) and are generated via the genetic combination of the IgM and IgY genes. Some species possess unique Ig isotypes such as IgO in platypus, IgF in *Xenopus*, and IgY (ΔFc) in duck and turtle. Regarding the light (L) chains, both Igκ and Igλ are expressed in tetrapods, but the frequency of expression of these two light chains differs greatly among species. A third IgL isotype, Igσ, is expressed only in amphibians and lower vertebrates (teleosts and cartilaginous fishes). Due to the translocon configuration of the IgH and IgL loci in tetrapods, V(D)J recombination is the major mechanism for generation of Ig diversity in most tetrapod species. However, two post-recombinatorial mechanisms, that is, somatic gene conversion (sGC) and somatic hypermutation (SHM), are used by some species to further expand their Ig repertoires when V(D) J-recombinational diversity alone is insufficient.

2.1 INTRODUCTION

Immunoglobulin (Ig), which first emerged approximately 500 million years ago (MYA) in jawed fishes, is a fundamental molecule upon which adaptive immunity depends. It is generated by a unique recombination of variable (V), diversity (D), and joining (J) gene segments (Flajnik and

Kasahara, 2010). The organization of the Ig genes varied from cluster to translocon configuration during the evolution of jawed vertebrates (Flajnik, 2002). In cartilaginous fishes, the Ig genes are arranged in a cluster configuration. Each cluster is composed of a single V, a single J, and a single constant (C) gene, as well as one or more D segments encoding the heavy chain (IgH). V(D)J rearrangement occurs exclusively within a cluster, and some clusters carry partially (V_HD–D–J_H and V_HDD–J_H) and fully (V_HDDJ_H or $V_L J_L$) germline-rearranged V regions. Diversity among the Ig genes in cartilaginous fishes is generated primarily by junctional diversity and somatic hypermutation (SHM) after B cell activation by antigens (Dooley and Flajnik, 2006; Flajnik and Kasahara, 2010). The translocon configuration, in which multiple tandemly arranged V genes are located upstream of many similarly arranged D, J, and C genes, first occurred in the IgH gene of teleost fishes. However, the IgH locus in teleosts is not a classical version of the translocon organization because its Cζ/τ gene is located either between the V_H and D genes or within the V_H gene region (Flajnik, 2002; Hikima et al., 2011). Furthermore, unlike cartilaginous fishes, both cluster and translocon organizations have been found in teleost light chain (IgL) loci (Hikima et al., 2011). In tetrapods, including amphibians, reptiles, birds, and mammals, all Ig genes occur in the classical translocon configuration, which greatly increases the combinational diversity by a quasi-random usage of the V, (D), and J segments and facilitates the further modification of the variable region repertoire by somatic gene conversion (sGC) in some species (Flajnik and Kasahara, 2010; Reynaud et al., 1987; Knight, and Becker, 1990).

During the evolution of the jawed vertebrates, the IgH isotypes became more complex. IgM and IgD are found in nearly all vertebrate taxa and are thus considered to be the most ancient Ig isotypes (Flajnik and Kasahara, 2010). IgM has a highly conserved structure and function in all jawed vertebrates. In contrast, IgD, which is also known as IgW in cartilaginous and some teleost fishes, displays remarkable plasticity in structure over evolution and is even lost in some species (Flajnik and Kasahara, 2010; Dooley and Flajnik, 2006; Ohta and Flajnik, 2006; Zhao et al., 2000; Lundqvist et al., 2001; Lanning et al., 2003; Wang et al., 2009). In addition to IgM and IgD, a number of other IgH isotypes with distinctive functional properties have been discovered in different vertebrates, such as IgNAR in cartilaginous fish (Dooley and Flajnik, 2006), IgZ(T) in teleost fish (Hikima et al.,

2011; Hansen, et al., 2005; Danilova et al., 2005), IgY, IgX, and IgF in amphibians (Du Pasquier et al., 2000; Zhao et al., 2006), IgY and IgA in reptiles and aves (Zhao et al, 2000; Lundqvist et al., 2001; Warr et al., 1995; Cheng et al., 2013), and IgG, IgF, IgA, and IgO in mammals (Flajnik and Kasahara, 2010; Zhao et al., 2009). All of the other IgH isotypes appear to have evolved from IgM and IgD through various mechanisms, such as gene duplication or sGC; logically, IgH isotypes could have been generated through a class switch recombination (CSR) process while maintaining the same antigen-binding specificity (Du Pasquier et al., 2000; Cheng et al., 2013).

In recent decades, some insightful ideas regarding IgH evolution have been proposed based on comparative studies. For example, IgY is accepted as the evolutionary ancestor of mammalian IgG and IgE (Warr et al., 1995). Furthermore, IgX and IgA, a pair of orthologs that are involved in mucosal immunity, appear to have been generated from genetic combination of IgM and IgY, and the latter is missing in some reptiles (Mussmann et al., 1996; Deza et al., 2007; Wei et al., 2009). In contrast to IgH, the IgL isotypes gradually diminished over evolutionary time. λ and κ are found in all vertebrate groups except aves, which have lost κ. Amphibians, teleosts, and cartilaginous fishes possess σ, and a fourth isotype, σ-cart, is exclusively expressed in cartilaginous fishes (Lundqvist et al., 2001; Edholm et al., 2011; Ratcliffe, 2006). This chapter discusses the features of Ig genes in tetrapods, with primary emphasis on amphibians and reptiles.

2.2 AMPHIBIANS

Modern amphibians consist of three living orders, with distinctive body plans, reproductive specialization, and life histories: Gymnophiona (caecilians), Caudata (salamanders), and Anura (frogs). One species of frog in the Pipidae family, *Xenopus laevis*, is frequently used as an ectothemic vertebrate model for immunological studies (Robert and Ohta, 2009). With respect to B-cell and T-cell diversification, *X. laevis* have some features that are useful for fundamental studies. First, the development of antibody (or TCR) repertoire in its larvae is rapid and free of extrinsic effects. Second, compared with mammals, *X. laevis* contains few lymphoid organs and lymphocytes. Third, the self-tolerance established during metamorphosis in *X. laevis* does not exist in mammals (Du Pasquier et al., 2000).

In recent years, another *Xenopus* species, *Xenopus tropicalis*, has attracted increased attention from researchers due to its diploid genome, which has better genetic stability (Kobel and Du Pasquier, 1986). Whole-genome sequence assembly and several EST databases of *X. tropicalis* are available for discovery of new genes, and *X. tropicalis* now represents another important model, complementing that of its relative *X. laevis*.

At present, five IgH isotypes, IgM, IgY, IgX, IgD, and IgF, and three IgL isotypes, κ, λ, and σ, have been identified in *Xenopus* (Fig. 1). Complementary DNA (cDNA) sequences encoding IgM, IgY, and IgX were first cloned from *X. laevis* (*26–28*), and the genes (δ and φ) encoding the constant regions of IgD and IgF were characterized from the genome sequence of *X. tropicalis*, in which the genomic organization of the IgH locus occurs in the order 5′ V_H-D-J_H-δ-χ-υ-φ 3′ (*7, 15*) (Fig. 1). In addition, three IgH isotypes (IgM, IgY, and IgD (also termed IgP) and IgM, IgY, and IgX, respectively) were identified in two salamander species, *Pleurodeles waltl* and *Ambystoma mexicanum* (*29–32*). The following sections present detailed information about the genes coding for amphibian Ig genes concerning specific IgH and IgL isotypes, the germline and re-combinatorial diversity of variable regions, and specific properties of CSR and SHM in *Xenopus*.

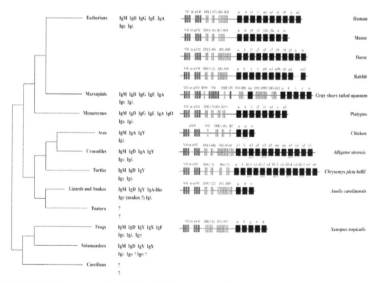

FIGURE 1   Phylogeny of the IgH and IgL isotypes in tetrapods and genomic organization of the IgH locus in different species. The arrows indicate the transcriptional orientation of the α genes in the chicken and *A. sinensis* and of the δ2 genes in *C. picta bellii*.

2.2.1   IGD(δ) GENES IN AMPHIBIANS

Although molecular analysis of the Ig genes of amphibians began as early as the 1980s, no IgH isoforms other than the well studied IgM, IgY, and IgX were found until 2006. The first δ gene identified in amphibians is from the genome sequence of *X. tropicalis*. In the IgH locus of *X. tropicalis*, the δ gene is located immediately downstream of the μ gene, as in mammals. It contains eight δC_H exons (Fig. 2); the nucleotide sequences of exons $\delta C_H 7$ and $\delta C_H 8$ show high homology to those of $\delta C_H 5$ and $\delta C_H 6$ (82% and 76%, respectively), suggesting a recent tandem duplication similar to the type frequently observed in the δ genes of teleost fishes and the ω genes of cartilaginous fishes (Ohta and Flajnik, 2006; Zhao et al., 2006).

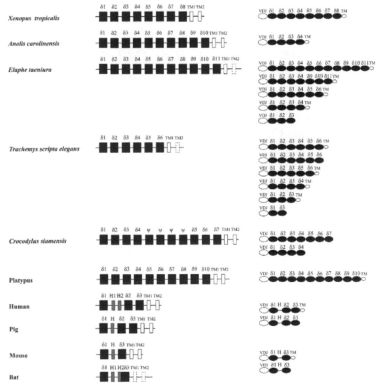

FIGURE 2   Genomic organization and RNA splicing patterns of the δ gene in different tetrapod species. The dotted boxes indicate undetermined TM exons. δ, IgD-encoded exon or domain; H, hinge exon or domain; TM, transmembrane exon or domain.

Xenopus IgD is expressed predominantly as a transmembrane form that is only detected in the spleen; therefore, similar to its ortholog in mammals, it would be a marker for mature B cells. Interestingly, in contrast with the teleost δ gene, which uses $\mu C_H 1$ instead of $\delta C_H 1$ in the mRNA, the *Xenopus* δ gene contains all eight δC_H exons in its transmembrane form (Fig. 2). Furthermore, both the $\delta C_H 1$ and δTM exons of *Xenopus* show greater homology with the corresponding regions of the mammalian genes than those of fishes, indicating that the *Xenopus* IgD is an evolutionary intermediate between the IgD (IgW) of fishes and mammals (Ohta and Flajnik, 2006; Zhao et al., 2006). Soon after the identification of *Xenopus* IgD, a four-C_H domain IgH isotype termed IgP was cloned from *P. waltl* at the cDNA level (*29*). The expression pattern and phylogenetic characteristics of the IgP gene suggest that it is most likely IgD rather than a novel Ig isotype (*33*).

2.2.2   IGX, AN ORTHOLOG OF IGA, ORIGINATED FROM RECOMBINATION BETWEEN IGM AND IGY

The cDNA sequences encoding the secreted and transmembrane forms of IgX were first isolated from *X. laevis*. Both forms of the molecule consist of four χC_H domains. The genes showed more nucleotide homology with *Xenopus* IgM than with any other vertebrate isotypes available at that time, although the homology is only 30% (Haire et al., 1989; Mussmann et al., 1996). Using specific monoclonal antibodies to IgX, Mussmann et al. (1996), demonstrated that in *Xenopus*, IgX-positive B cells resemble secretory plasma cells, are located predominantly in the gut epithelium, and are hardly detectable in the spleen and liver (Mussmann et al., 1996). More recently, a significant upregulation of IgX expression was observed in serum of *X. laevis* receiving oral immunization compared with animals receiving systemic immunization (Du et al., 2012).

These data strongly suggest that IgX in *Xenopus* is a functional analog of IgA in mammals and aves. Although both IgX and IgA have major functions in mucosal immunity, the phylogenetic relationship between IgX and other IgH isotypes was less clear until an IgA-like isotype was observed in a reptile, *Eublepharis macularius*. The IgA-like molecule contains four C_H

domains, of which $C_H 1$ and $C_H 2$ are homologous with $C_H 1$ and $C_H 2$ of IgY, while $C_H 3$ and $C_H 4$ are closer in sequence to $C_H 3$ and $C_H 4$ of IgM. Notably, a similar homology pattern can be observed in *Xenopus* IgX and avian IgA (Gambon-Deza et al., 2007). Based on these findings, it seems that IgX and IgA arose from recombination between IgM and IgY, but whether IgX and IgA arose from only one recombination event or originated from separate recombination events at different evolutionary time points is still a matter of debate.

2.2.3 IGF: THE EARLIEST IGH ISOTYPE WITH A SEPARATELY ENCODED GENETIC HINGE

The φ gene encoding the constant region of IgF was first identified from EST clones of *X. tropicalis* and then located in the 3' terminal region of the IgH locus. The φ consists of two C_H exons, $φC_H 1$ and $φC_H 2$, and an exon that encodes a hinge region between the two C_H exons. Because the hinge region in the φ, γ, and α genes is generally considered to have evolved independently after the divergence of mammals, IgF has become the earliest example of an IgH isotype with a separately encoded genetic hinge. When $φC_H 1$ and $φC_H 2$ were separately subjected to sequence analysis, $φC_H 1$ showed a high degree of homology with $C_H 1$ of *Xenopus* IgY and mammalian IgG, whereas $φC_H 2$ was similar to $C_H 4$ of *Xenopus* IgY and $C_H 3$ of mammalian IgG, indicating that the φ gene might have been generated via the duplication of the υ gene, followed by the deletion of the internal C_H exons. This idea is also supported by phylogenetic analysis, which indicates that the φ gene became linked first with the υ gene of *Xenopus* and then with the γ and ε genes of mammals. Additionally, sequence analysis of the hinge exon of the φ gene seems to favor the splice-site-incorporation model proposed by Tucker et al. (1981) to explain the origin of the hinge region (Zhao et al., 2006; Tucker et al., 1981).

2.2.4   κ, λ, AND σ LIGHT CHAINS ARE EXPRESSED IN *XENOPUS*

Before genome data for *X. tropicalis* were available, most information about the IgL isotypes expressed in amphibians was obtained using *X. laevis*. Three distinct IgL isotypes identified in *X. laevis* were designated ρ or L1, σ or L2, and type III. Based on sequence homology and phylogenetic analysis of the V and C genes and on the RSS spacer lengths, the ρ and type III genes were classified as members of the κ and λ gene families, respectively (Schwager et al., 1991; Zezza et al., 1991; Zezza et al., 1992; Haire et al., 1996; Litman et al., 1999). Orthologs of the σ isotype were subsequently identified only in fishes, suggesting that the σ isotype was lost during the evolution of higher tetrapods. Recently, the genomic organization of all three IgL gene loci has been characterized based on the genome data of *X. tropicalis*; the results of this analysis strongly support the phylogenetic relationship suggested by previous data (Qin et al., 1998).

2.2.5   GERMLINE DIVERSITY OF THE V, D, AND J GENE SEGMENTS IN IGH AND IGL LOCI OF *XENOPUS*

To date, approximately 100 V_H gene segments belonging to 11 V_H families have been found in the IgH locus of *Xenopus*. The members of most V_H families are interspersed, and all likely have the same transcriptional orientation. $V_H I$, $V_H II$, and $V_H III$ are the three major V_H families; each comprises 15 to 20 V_H segments per haploid genome identified by genomic Southern blotting (Hsu et al., 1989; Haire et al., 1990; Schwager et al., 1991; Haire et al., 1991). In *X. laevis*, more than ten putative D segments were deduced from a large number of rearranged CDR3 sequences; however, only two of these were cloned as germline sequences (Schwager et al., 1988; Hsu et al., 1989; Haire et al., 1990; Schwager et al., 1991). The D locus of *X. tropicalis* contains only five identified D segments, but some D genes are likely missing due to gaps in sequence information (Zhao et al., 2006). Eight, nine, and seven germline J_H elements were identified in *X. laevis*, *X. gilli*, and *X. tropicalis*, respectively (Zhao et al., 2006; Schwager et al., 1991).

Qin et al. (2008) provided a detailed analysis of the germline V and J segments of the three IgL loci in *X. tropicalis*. In the ρ light chain locus, nine J_ρ gene segments are located upstream of the single C_ρ gene. Of these, $J_\rho 1$, $J_\rho 3$, $J_\rho 4$, $J_\rho 5$, and $J_\rho 6$ are functional, whereas the remaining four gene segments may be pseudogenes due to their non-conserved RSSs. At least ten functional V_ρ genes belonging to one V_ρ family were identified upstream of the J_ρ cluster. Similar to the ρ locus, four J_σ gene segments were found upstream of the single C_σ gene, and all eight deduced V_σ genes were classified into one family. The genomic organization of the type III light chain locus is similar to that of the λ light chain locus in reptiles and mammals. The $C_{III}2$ and $C_{III}3$ genes are preceded by a single J_{III} segment, but three J_{III} genes have been observed upstream of $C_{III}1$. Another two J_{III} segments were found preceding $\psi V_{III}1$. A total of 17 V_{III} genes were identified upstream of the J_{III}–C_{III} clusters; these can be divided into six subfamilies according to their sequence homologies (Qin et al., 2008).

2.2.6 V SEGMENTS WERE REARRANGED IN A STEPWISE MANNER DURING THE ONTOGENY OF XENOPUS

In *Xenopus* larvae, the early development of B cells occurs in the liver in the absence of selection by external antigens (Du Pasquier et al., 2000). Rearranged IgH chains can be detected at 5–6 days after fertilization (daf), and the rearranged light chains are observed three days later (at 8 daf). B cells expressing complete B-cell receptors are not detectable until 10 daf (Mussmann et al., 1998). The various V_H families are rearranged in a step-wise manner; members of the $V_H 1$ and $V_H 3$ families undergo rearrangement earliest, at 5–6 daf, but other V_H families continue to rearrange until 9 daf. Interestingly, the earliest developing $V_H 1$ family is homologous to the mammalian $V_H III$ clan, the members of which are also preferentially expressed in the fetus of humans and mice (Mussmann et al., 1998; Wu and Paige, 1986; Jeong and Teale, 1988; Willems et al., 1992; Pascual et al., 1993). For light chains, V_ρ and V_σ rearrangements were first observed on 8 or 9 and 13 daf, respectively; however, no rearranged type III chains was detected during early ontogeny (Mussmann et al., 1998). From 12 daf, the larval spleen differentiates, and the Ig repertoire can be selected by external antigens. The usage profile of the V_H and J_H segments in larvae then becomes similar to that of adults in that rearrangements of all V_H families (except V_H11) are observed (Du Pasquier et al., 2000; Mussmann et al., 1998).

2.2.7 DIVERSITY OF HEAVY CHAIN COMPLEMENTARITY DETERMINING REGION 3 (CDR-H3) IN LARVAE AND ADULTS OF XENOPUS

The usage of D gene segments and addition of N nucleotides are two factors that determine the diversity of CDR-H3. In larvae at all stages, few or no N nucleotides are added at the V_H–D and D–J_H junctions in genomic and expressed gene rearrangements; this is the most likely reason for the presence of shorter CDR-H3 sequences in larvae than in adults. Two D segments, D1 and D10, are used in the majority of rearrangements in larvae, and the high representation of D1 persists in adults (Schwager et al., 1991; Mussmann et al., 1998). As in mammals, in which antigen receptor-based selection favors B cells expressing Igs with tyrosine- and glycine-enriched CDR-H3, the glycine-enriched reading frame I of D1 and D10 in larvae is positively selected during the later stages of B cell development (Schwager et al., 1991; Mussmann et al., 1998; Ippolito et al., 2006; Ivanov et al., 2005; Schroeder et al., 1998). An additional bias toward rearrangement that depends on the microhomology between the 3' end of D and 5' end of J_H is preferred in the expressed IgH repertoire of larvae. As in the mouse, the homology-based D1–J_H3 junctions in larvae also favor the use of reading frame I of the rearranged D1 regions. Conversely, in adults, it is common for additional D segments to contribute to the CDR-H3 diversity with some flexible patterns (including inversion, fusion, and the use of different reading frames), as well as for more N nucleotides to be incorporated at the VDJ junctions (Schwager et al., 1991; Mussmann et al., 1998; Gu et al., 1990; Feeney, 1992).

2.3 REPTILES

As the only ectothermic amniotes, reptiles occupy a key position in evolutionary history. They represent the first vertebrates to adopt a terrestrial lifestyle; in addition, they underwent physiological and ethological changes related to variable environmental temperatures. The majority of extant reptiles can be divided into two clades, Lepidosauria and Archosauria. The former consists of primitive diapsid reptiles, including tuataras, lizards, and snakes, while the latter contains more highly evolved diapsid reptiles, such as crocodiles and aves. Additionally, the living turtles (Testudunes), which were traditionally considered the only surviving species of anapsid reptiles, are currently suggested to have diapsid affinities and have been further placed as the sister group of the Archosauria clade by many molecular phylogenic studies (Platz and Conlon, 1997; Zardoya and Meyer, 1998; Cao et al., 2000; Iwabe et al., 2005).

To date, research on reptilian Ig genes has involved many species, including three crocodilian species, *Crocodylus siamensis*, *Alligator sinensis*, and *Caiman crocodylus* (Cheng et al., 2013; Litman et al., 1985), three turtle species, *Trachemys scripta elegans*, *Chrysemys picta bellii*, and *Pelodiscus sinensis* (Turchin and Hsu, 1996; Li et al., 2012; Magadan-Mompo et al., 2013; Xu et al., 2009), two lizard species, *Anolis carolinensis* and *Eublepharis macularius* (Edholm et al., 2011; Gambon-Deza et al., 2007; Gambon-Deza and Espinel, 2008; Wu et al., 2010), and eight snake species, *Elaphe taeniura*, *Python molurus bivittatus*, *Corallus hortulanus*, *Crotalus atrox*, *Python regius*, *Masticophis flagellum testaceus*, *Boa constrictor*, and *Thamnophis elegans* (Wang et al., 2012; Gambon-Deza et al., 2012). In general, the genomic organization of the IgH constant gene locus varies widely among different reptilian orders. In the lizard *A. carolinensis*, one copy of the μ, δ, and υ genes are rearranged in the order 5' μ–δ–υ 3', and no α gene has been identified (Wei et al., 2009) (Fig. 1). In two species of turtles, one copy of the μ and δ genes is located at the extreme 5' end of the IgH constant gene locus, followed by several υ and $\delta2$ genes, resulting in the order 5' μ-δ-$\delta2.1$-$\upsilon1$-$\delta2.2$-$\upsilon2$-$\psi\delta2.3$-$\upsilon3$-$\delta2.4$-$\upsilon4$-$\psi\delta2.5$-$\upsilon5$-$\upsilon6$ 3' in *C. picta bellii* and 5' μ-δ-$\delta2.1$-$\upsilon1$-$\psi\delta2.2$-$\psi\upsilon2$-$\upsilon3$-$\delta2.3$-$\upsilon4$-$\delta2.4$-$\upsilon5$-$\psi\delta2.5$-$\upsilon6$-$\delta2.6$-$\upsilon7$-$\delta2.7$-$\upsilon8$ 3' in *P. sinensis* (Magadan-Mompo et al., 2013) (Fig. 1). Moreover, the IgH constant gene locus of two crocodilian species, *C. siamensis* and *A. sinensis*, contains multiple μ, υ, and α genes, and the physical map is deduced as 5' $\mu1$-δ-$\alpha1$-$\mu2$-$\alpha3$-$\mu3$-$\psi\alpha$-$\psi\mu$-$\alpha2$-$\upsilon3$-$\upsilon2$-$\upsilon1$ 3' (Cheng et al., 2013) (Fig. 1). Compared with that of amphibians, the most interesting feature of the reptilian IgH constant gene locus is the first occurrence of subclass divergence of the μ, υ, and α genes. The following sections provide a detailed description of the subclasses of reptilian μ, δ (or δ2), υ, and α genes, as well as the IgL gene.

2.3.1   MULTIPLE COPIES OF IGM(μ) GENES CAN BE EXPRESSED THROUGH CSR IN CROCODILES

The IgH locus of *C. siamensis* and *A. sinensis* contains three functional and one pseudo μ gene, termed μ1, μ2, μ3, and ψμ. The μ1 gene is located at the extreme 5' end of the IgH constant gene locus, and the μ2, μ3, and ψμ genes are found downstream. There are several pieces of evidence that suggest that CSR is utilized to express μ2 and μ3. First, a switch (S) region and an intronic (I) exon are located upstream of each μ gene in the IgH locus of *C. siamensis*. Second, recombined $S_\mu 1$–$S_\mu 2$ and $S_\mu 1$–$S_\mu 3$ fragments, as well as the germline transcripts of three μ genes, have been identified. Third, the 5' regions of all three I_μ exons demonstrate promoter activities (Cheng et al., 2013).

Except for a short membrane-bound μ transcript ($V_H DJ_H$–$C_H 3$–$C_H 4$–TM) cloned from *A. carolinensis*, all of the reptilian germline and expressed μ genes detected to date contain four C_H domains. Secreted IgM can form polymers in the serum of *C. siamensis* and *E. taeniura*. The conserved cysteine residues that covalently polymerize IgM are also found in all other species, although there is no direct evidence that they function in this manner. Additionally, in $\mu C_H 1$, another important cysteine residue that is used to associate with light chains is conserved in turtles and crocodiles but is absent in snakes and lizards (Cheng et al., 2013; Wei et al., 2009; Li et al., 2012; Magadan-Mompo et al., 2013; Xu et al., 2009; Gambon-Deza and Espinel, 2008; Wang et al., 2012; Gambon-Deza et al., 2012).

2.3.2   MULTIPLE COPIES OF THE IGD(δ) AND IGD2(δ2) GENES ARE PRESENT IN THE TURTLE GENOME

The germline organization of the δ gene includes 11 functional C_H exons in the two lizard species *A. carolinensis* and *E. macularius* and in *C. picta bellii* and *E. taeniura*, but only seven in two species of crocodiles (another four mutated δC_H exons were identified between $\delta C_H 4$ and $\delta C_H 5$) and six in *T. scripta elegans* (Cheng et al., 2013; Wei et al., 2009; Li et al., 2012; Magadan-Mompo et al., 2013; Gambon-Deza and Espinel, 2008; Wang et al., 2012) (Fig. 2). None of the IgD genes presented here display similar C_H exons, which would presumably have been produced by recent gene duplication. The expressed IgD shows various splicing patterns in different species: zero, one, four, and four types of the membrane-bound form and two, zero, one, and two types of the secreted form have been cloned from *C. siamensis*, *A. carolinensis*, *E. taeniura*, and *T. scripta elegans*, respectively (Cheng et al., 2013; Wei et al., 2009; Li et al., 2012; Wang et al., 2012) (Fig. 2).

In all four species for which there is a clear map of the IgH constant gene locus, only one copy of the δ gene is located closely downstream of the μ gene. However, multiple copies of δ genes were detected in the genome of *T. scripta elegans* by Southern blotting using both $\delta C_H 1–3$ and $\delta C_H 1$ as probes (Li et al., 2012). Similarly, five and seven copies of another type of δ gene termed $\delta 2$ were identified in the IgH locus of *C. picta bellii* and *P. sinensis*, respectively. As a variant of the δ gene, which was first cloned from *E. macularius*, the last two C_H exons of $\delta 2$ show more similarity to the $C_H 3$ and $C_H 4$ exons of the avian α gene. In the IgH constant gene locus of two turtle species, the transcription orientation of the $\delta 2$ genes also resembles that of the avian α genes, which is opposite to that of the μ and υ genes. Furthermore, some $\delta 2$ genes contain duplicated C_H exons; these are found in the δ genes of some fishes but not in the classic δ gene described above (Danilova et al., 2005; Magadan-Mompo et al., 2013; Bengten et al., 2002; Saha et al., 2004). Looking back, the multiple copies of δ genes in *T. scripta elegans* likely include both δ and $\delta 2$ genes. Thus far, no $\delta 2$ genes from other reptiles, except *E. macularius* and turtles, have been cloned or identified.

2.3.3   DIVERSIFICATION OF IGY(υ) GENES IN TURTLES, SNAKES, AND CROCODILES

Although IgY(υ) is the most important IgH isotype in the humoral immune response of non-mammalian tetrapods, subclass divergence of υ genes has been observed in some reptilian species (including turtles, snakes, and crocodiles) but not in amphibians or aves (Cheng et al., 2013; Li et al., 2012; Magadan-Mompo et al., 2013; Wang et al., 2012; Bengten et al., 2002). Most of the υ genes in reptiles contain four $υC_H$ exons that correspond to the four IgY domains. However, multiple copies of a truncated υ gene that encodes IgY(ΔFc) without the $υC_H3$ and $υC_H4$ domains are present in the genome of *T. scripta elegans* (Li et al., 2012), and another type of υ gene that lacks the $υC_H2$ exon is found in the IgH constant region locus of *P. sinensis* and the draft genome of *P. molurus bivittatus*. The latter υ gene exhibits a genomic structure similar to that of the mammalian γ genes, although a genetic hinge exon is absent (Magadan-Mompo et al., 2013; Bengten et al., 2002). Thus, the divergence of υ genes in reptiles provides additional evidence for the hypothesis that the υ gene is the evolutionary precursor of the mammalian γ and ε genes.

Using specific mAbs, some special features of the IgY1 and IgY2 proteins of *E. taeniura* have been found. First, the IgY1 H chains are able to associate with the L chain despite lacking the cysteine residue in the N terminus of the $υC_H1$. Second, both the υ1 and υ2 genes can be expressed as truncated forms at the C terminus. Interestingly, the truncation does not result from alternative splicing or transcription termination (Wang et al., 2012).

2.3.4 CROCODILIAN IGA: A MISSING LINK BETWEEN AMPHIBIANS AND AVES

Among reptiles, an IgA-encoding gene (α gene) has only been identified in crocodiles. Three functional (four $αC_H$ exons) and one pseudo α gene (only $αC_H1$ and $αC_H2$) were found in the IgH constant gene locus of both *C. siamensis* and *A.sinensis*, indicating that subclass divergence of α genes also occurred in reptiles. In the phylogenetic analysis, crocodilian α genes are first clustered with those of aves and mammals and then with amphibian χ genes. This clustering suggests an orthologous relationship linking IgX with IgA. Furthermore, all four crocodilian α genes are placed in an inverted transcription direction with respect to the remaining genes within the locus, suggesting that the α gene inversion occurred before the divergence of crocodiles and aves. Finally, as in aves and mammals, crocodilian IgA may play a role in mucosal defense because both α1 and α2 genes are expressed at much higher levels in the intestine than in other organs (Cheng et al., 2013). It is also worth noting that strong IgM expression was detected in the intestine of some species lacking IgA, such as *A. carolinensis*, *E. taeniura*, and *T. scripta elegans*. One can deduce that IgM may substitute for IgA in the mucosal immune response in some reptiles (Wei et al., 2009; Li et al., 2012; Wang et al., 2012).

2.3.5   BOTH κ AND λ LIGHT CHAINS ARE EXPRESSED IN SOME REPTILES

Compared with the IgH genes, the IgL genes of reptiles have been less well investigated. Both κ and λ light chains are expressed in *A. carolinensis*, and the genomic organization of both gene loci is similar to that of their respective counterparts in mammals (Wu et al., 2010). However, by searching the genomes, transcriptomes, and ESTs, only C_λ genes were identified in snakes. Whether the Igκ gene is lost in snakes is currently unknown (Gambon-Deza et al., 2012).

2.4   AVES

As the most speciose class of tetrapod vertebrates, all living avian species belong to the subclass Neornithes (modern birds). According to the molecular and morphological evidence, the Neornithes can be divided into two superorders: Paleognathae and Neognathae. The former contains the tinamous and ratites, while the latter is composed of Galloanserae (galliform and anseriform aves) and Neoaves (all other birds), within which the evolutionary relationships of several orders remain controversial (Hackett et al., 2008; Pacheco et al., 2011). Thus far, three IgH isotypes (IgM, IgY, and IgA) and a single IgL isotype (λ) have been identified in chicken, duck

(*Anas platyrhynchos*), pheasant (*Phasianus colchicus*), turkey (*Meleagris gallopavo*), quail (*Coturnix japonica*), zebra finch (*Taeniopygia guttata*), and ostrich (*Struthio camelus*) (Ratcliffe, 2006; Dahan et al., 1983; Mansikka, 1992; Parvari et al., 1988; Magor et al., 1994; Magor et al., 1998; Choi et al., 2010; Huang et al., 2012; Magor et al., 1994; Das et al., 2010; Bao et al., 2012) (Fig. 1). In the IgH loci of both chickens and ducks, single μ, α, and υ genes are arranged in the order 5' μ–α–υ 3', whereas the α gene, as in its counterpart in crocodiles, is placed in an inverted transcription direction relative to the μ and υ genes (Zhao et al., 2000; Lundqvist et al., 2001) (Fig. 1). No putative IgD and κ sequences have been cloned from cDNA or genomic DNA in the above-mentioned avian species. Unlike the situation in amphibians, reptiles, and mammals, diversification of the Ig variable regions in aves depends primarily on the occurrence of sGC after V(D)J recombination (Reynaud et al., 1987; Thompson and Neiman, 1987; Reynaud et al., 1989; McCormack et al., 1990; Reynaud et al., 1991; McCormack et al., 1991). Given that the isotypes of the Ig genes and the generation of the Ig repertoire in chicken are described in detail in many reviews, we discuss only the Ig genes of other avian species here.

2.4.1   AVIAN μ GENES

The cDNAs of the μ gene in duck, pheasant, turkey, quail, and ostrich have been cloned and sequenced. Each of these μ genes encodes a conserved four-domain structure, and they share overall amino acid sequence identities of 54%, 73%, 64%, 65%, and 53% with the chicken μ gene according to the above order (Magor et al., 1998; Choi et al., 2010; Huang et al., 2012). The secretory form of the IgM heavy chain constant region in duck and ostrich contains 12 positionally conserved cysteines that are used to establish the inter- and intra-chain disulfide bonds and four potential N-linked glycosylation sites, two of which are found exclusively in aves. The μ gene is primarily expressed in the spleen in both duck and ostrich, as detected by Northern blotting (Magor et al., 1998; Huang et al., 2012).

2.4.2   AVIAN α GENES

Similar to their counterpart in crocodiles, avian α genes possess four αC_H exons and no genetic hinge exon. Compared with the chicken α gene, the overall amino acid sequence identity of the α gene in duck, pheasant, turkey, quail, and ostrich is 51%, 69%, 68%, 60%, and 44%, respectively (Magor et al., 1998; Choi et al., 2010; Huang et al., 2012). The IgA heavy chain constant region in duck and ostrich contains ten cysteines that are conserved among reptiles, aves, and mammals and another four cysteines that are found only in aves. There are four N-linked glycosylation sites in $\alpha C_H 1$, $\alpha C_H 2$, $\alpha C_H 3$, and the secretory tail, all of which are conserved in aves. Using Northern blotting analysis, strong expression of the α gene was observed in the respiratory, alimentary, and reproductive tracts of the adult duck and in the large and small intestine of the ostrich (*79, 81*). The IgA appeared to be tetrameric in bile of the duck but dimeric in intestinal secretions of the ostrich (Magor et al., 1998; Huang et al., 2012). In ostrich, another short form of the α gene derived from alternative splicing of $\alpha C_H 2$ onto the TM exon (i.e., $V_H DJ_H - \alpha C_H 1 - \alpha C_H 2 - TM$) was also expressed in the spleen and intestine at a much lower level than the full-length form (Huang et al., 2012).

2.4.3   AVIAN υ GENES

Two forms of IgY, full-length IgY and truncated IgY(ΔFc), have been cloned from the aves. The full-length IgY with all four υC_H domains has been observed in all studied aves. An alignment of the amino acid sequences encoded by the full-length υ genes from ostrich, chicken, duck, *A. carolinensis*, and *X. tropicalis* revealed nine cysteines that are conserved across all species examined and two N-linked glycosylation sites in $\alpha C_H 2$ and $\alpha C_H 3$ that are conserved in three avian species (Huang et al., 2012). The truncated IgY(ΔFc), which lacks the $\upsilon C_H 3$ and $\upsilon C_H 4$ domains, has been detected only in duck and goose to date. Unlike the turtle *T. scripta elegans*, in which the constant region of the IgY(ΔFc) is encoded by one or several separate υ gene(s), υ(ΔFc) in the duck arises from alternative splicing of the primary transcript from a single υ gene. During this process, the υC_H1 and υC_H2 exons are spliced into a short terminal exon that lies between the υC_H2 and υC_H3 exons (Magor et al., 1994). Although the mechanism that regulates the expression of IgY and IgY(ΔFc) has not been determined, it has been observed that IgY(ΔFc) is predominantly produced after repeated immunization. Because IgY(ΔFc) lacks the Fc region and therefore lacks secondary effector functions, neutralization is likely the primary function of this antibody (Grey, 1967; Humphrey et al., 2004).

2.4.4   GENOMIC ORGANIZATION OF THE λ LOCI IN TURKEY AND ZEBRA FINCH

In addition to the chicken, the genomic organization of the λ locus is currently available for turkey and zebra finch. In both of these species, as in chicken, a single set of functional V_λ, J_λ, and C_λ genes, followed by multiple pseudo-V_λ (ψV_λ) genes, are present in the λ locus, suggesting that this type of genomic organization was present before the divergence of Galloanserae and Neoaves and that it remained approximately conserved over a long evolutionary time (more than 100 Myr) (Das et al, 2010; Bao et al., 2012; Pereira and Baker, 2006; Brown et al., 2008). The arrangement of the ψV_λ genes in two transcriptional orientations is observed in chicken and turkey but not in zebra finch. This finding is in accordance with the evolutionary phylogeny of the galliform aves; the chicken and turkey diverged only 25–30 MYA (Das et al, 2010; Bao et al., 2012; McCormack et al., 1991; Griffin et al., 2008). An analysis of the recombinatorial characteristics of these genes suggested the presence of a single functional V_λ gene and multiple ψV_λ genes in other aves, such as quail, duck, pigeon (*Columbia livia*), cormorant (*Phalacrocorax olivaceous*), and hawk (*Buteogallus urubitinga*); the muscovy duck (*Cairina moschata*) is an exception in which more than one potentially functional V_λ gene was found. The vast majority of avian species may, similar to the chicken, generate light chain and heavy chain diversity by sGC in combination with SHM (McCormack et al., 1989).

2.5 MAMMALS

Extant mammals are divided into three lineages: Eutheria (cutherians), Metatheria (marsupials), and Prototheria (monotremes). Eutheria and Metatheria are very closely related to each other; both belong to Theria, which diverged from Prototheria approximately 166 MYA (Bininda-Emonds et al., 2007; van Rheede et al., 2006; Warren et al., 2008).

2.5.1 MONOTREMES

The living monotremes consist of only three species: the duck-billed platypus (*Ornithorhynchus anatinus*) and two echidnas, the short-beaked echidna (*Tachygolssus aculeatus*) and long-beaked echidna (*Zaglossus bruijni*). These three species are found only in Australia and New Guinea and represent the most primitive living mammals; they exhibit a combination of reptilian (e.g., egg laying and cloaca) and mammalian (e.g., hair and mammary glands) characteristics. The earliest studies on the monotreme lymphoid system demonstrated the presence of lymphoid nodules instead of the lymph nodes found in therian mammals and a slower and weaker anamnestic antibody response than that of eutherians (Belov and Hellman, 2003). To date, the constant-region genes of six distinct Ig isotypes, IgM, IgD, IgG, IgE, IgA, and IgO, have been identified in the genome of the platypus; they are arranged in the order 5' μ-δ-o-γ2-γ1-α1-ε-α2 3' (Zhao et al., 2009; Gambon-Deza et al., 2009) (Fig. 1). cDNA sequences encoding IgM, IgG, IgE, and IgA have also been reported in *T. aculeatus* (Belov et al., 2002a, 2002b, 2002c; Vernersson et al., 2004, 2010). All of the above genes are comparable to their counterparts in therian mammals, except the δ and o genes of the platypus, which show combined features of both the nonmammalian tetrapod and eutherian genes (Zhao et al., 2009; Gambon-Deza et al., 2009). In addition, as in reptiles and therian mammals, two light chain isotypes, κ and λ, are expressed in the monotremes (Nowak et al., 2004; Johansson et al., 2005) (Fig. 1). The following section will review the molecular genetics of the Ig genes in monotremes, focusing on the features of Ig genes that are absent in therian mammals.

2.5.1.1   IGG, IGE, AND IGA OF MONOTREMES ARE STRUCTURALLY IDENTICAL TO THOSE OF THERIAN MAMMALS

At the genomic level, two γ genes ($\gamma1$ and $\gamma2$), two α genes ($\alpha1$ and $\alpha2$), and one ε gene were characterized in both the platypus and *T. aculeatus*, but no transcripts of the $\alpha1$ gene were detected in *T. aculeatus*, indicating that this gene is most likely functionally inactivated. The genomic structures of the monotreme γ, ε, and α genes are similar to those of their therian counterparts, especially the γ and α genes, each of which encodes three C_H domains plus a hinge region. Additionally, similar to therian mammals, a separate hinge-encoding exon is present in the platypus in two γ genes but absent from two α genes. Phylogenetic analyses of the amino acid sequences encoded by the γ, ε, and α genes of the platypus and *T. aculeatus* with those encoded by the υ, γ, ε, and α genes of various tetrapods demonstrated that although the monotreme γ, ε, and α genes each form a separate branch, they still show higher homology with their therian counterparts than with the υ or α genes of the aves. All of the above observations suggest that the structure of the modern post-switch Ig isotypes was established before the divergence of monotremes from therian mammals (Belov et al., 2002b, 2002c; Vernersson et al., 2002, 2004, 2010). It is worth noting that the amino acid sequences encoded by the platypus $\gamma1$ and $\gamma2$ genes display a remarkably high degree of divergence compared with the γ subclasses of therian species; a similar situation has been observed for the platypus $\alpha1$ and $\alpha2$ genes, indicating that the duplication event of the platypus γ and α genes appears to have occurred prior to the evolutionary separation of eutherians and marsupials (Vernersson et al., 2002, 2010).

2.5.1.2   THE δ GENE OF PLATYPUS: THE FIRST LONG FORM OF THE δ GENE IDENTIFIED IN MAMMALS

In platypus, a 10 C_H domain-encoding δ gene was first identified in the genomic DNA sequence and further amplified from spleen total RNA, strongly suggesting that the platypus δ gene shares significant similarity with the δ genes of nonmammalian vertebrates (Fig. 2). A domain-to-domain phylogenetic analysis showed that the 10 δC_H domains of the platypus are successively orthologous with the $\delta C_H 1$–$\delta C_H 4$ and $\delta C_H 6$–$\delta C_H 11$ domains of two reptilian species, *A. carolinensis* and *E. macularius*. Another clear homologous relationship exists between the $\delta C_H 1$, $\delta C_H 6$, and $\delta C_H 7$ domains of the platypus and the $\delta C_H 1$, $\delta C_H 2$, and $\delta C_H 3$ domains, respectively, of eutherian mammals, indicating that a selective loss of C_H domains occurred during IgD evolution. Similar to the situation in non-mammalian vertebrates, no hinge region is encoded by the δ gene of the platypus, suggesting that the IgD hinge arose after the evolutionary separation of monotremes and therians (Zhao et al., 2009; Gambon-Deza et al., 2009).

2.5.1.3 THE *o* GENE OF PLATYPUS: AN EVOLUTIONARY INTERMEDIATE BETWEEN *υ* AND γ

The o gene encodes a distinct IgH constant region that includes four C_H domains and a hinge region. Phylogenetic analysis of the relationship of IgO with other Ig isotypes of tetrapods showed that IgO is closely related to IgG. There are clear correspondences between the $\gamma C_H 1$, $\gamma C_H 2$, and $\gamma C_H 3$ domains and the $o/\upsilon/\varepsilon C_H 1$, $o/\upsilon/\varepsilon C_H 2$, and $o/\upsilon/\varepsilon C_H 4$ domains, respectively, indicating that IgO represents an evolutionary intermediate between IgY and IgG. The finding of a hinge region attached to the N-terminal of the $oC_H 2$ domain suggests that development of the hinge occurred earlier than the loss of C_H domains. The 3' end of the hinge-encoding sequence exhibits features of a 3' splice site, and the adjacent downstream sequence possesses a functional 5' splice site. All of the above observations support the splice site incorporation model proposed by Tucker et al. to explain the origin of the hinge region (Zhao et al., 2009; Tucker et al., 1981).

2.5.1.4 THE GERMLINE AND RECOMBINATORIAL DIVERSITY OF IGH CHAINS IN MONOTREMES

Based on the genome sequence, 45 germline V_H gene segments, including 36 potentially functional segments and nine pseudogenes, were identified in the platypus. The majority of the V_H genes (28/45) form one separate group (Group I) that further belongs to the mammalian V_H clan III, and the remainder are organized into two other groups (Groups II and III) that cluster with V_H genes from reptiles (Gambon-Deza et al., 2009). Although the germline V_H repertoire is not limited, all of the expressed V_H regions identified to date are from Group I, indicating that the earlier V_H groups (Groups II and III) were gradually eliminated with the evolution of mammals. However, long and highly diversified D and N nucleotides were observed in the CDR-H3, thus well compensating for the usage of a single V_H group. In addition, the platypus J_H locus consists of ten potentially functional J_H gene segments, at least five of which seem to participate in gene rearrangement (Johansson et al., 2002). Compared with the platypus, *T. aculeatus* may utilize alternative mechanisms to generate heavy chain diversity. Although only a few V_H sequences have been obtained from *T. aculeatus*, they belong to all three mammalian V_H clans, suggesting that relatively diverse germline V_H families are used to create the expressed V_H repertoire in *T. aculeatus*. The divergence of the V_H repertoire in the platypus and *T. aculeatus* may be due to their different living environments (Belov et al., 2002; Vernersson et al., 2004; Belov and Hellman, 2003).

2.5.1.5 λ CHAIN USAGE IS MUCH HIGHER THAN κ CHAIN USAGE IN THE PLATYPUS

In platypus, the λ locus contains multiple V_λ and three (or possibly four) C_λ genes. The C_λ genes are located in tandem with one or several J_λ segments positioned upstream of each C_λ gene. To date, all V_λ gene segments cloned from platypus and *T. aculeatus* form a separate branch on the phylogenetic tree, and they can be further divided into two closely related families. Despite the limited number of V_λ families, substantial variations in both sequence and length were observed in all three CDR regions (Johansson et al., 2005). In both monotreme species, the κ locus consists of a number of V_κ genes, followed by multiple J_κ genes and a single C_κ gene. The expressed V_κ repertoire contains at least four and nine families in platypus and *T. aculeatus*, respectively. Two of the V_κ families are present in both species (Nowak et al., 2004). When the mRNA frequency of both light chain isotypes was analyzed from a platypus spleen cDNA library, the λ transcripts were found to be 10-fold as abundant as the κ transcripts. This phenomenon indicates that the presence of a highly diversified CDR repertoire has a greater effect on the total repertoire than the total number of V gene families, at least in the platypus (Johansson et al., 2005).

2.5.2 MARSUPIALS

Extant marsupials include more than 330 species. Over 70% of these species are distributed in Australasia, with the remainder spread over American continents. The most significant feature that distinguishes marsupials and eutherians is their reproductive characteristics. Marsupial infants are born in an extreme altricial state after a short gestation period. Therefore, the majority of their development, including much of the development of their immune system, is completed external to the mother (Old and Deane, 2000). To date, most studies of the marsupial Ig repertoire and postnatal B cell ontogeny come from the gray short-tailed opossum, *Monodelphis domestica*, which is a model marsupial species in basic biology and biomedically oriented research (Samollow 2006, 2008; Wang et al., 2012). By analyzing the available whole genome sequence for this species, a detailed organization of the IgH, κ, and λ loci has been established and fully annotated. One copy of each of the μ, γ, α, and ε genes but not the δ gene is present in the *M. domestica* genome, and the overall structures of these genes are identical to those of their eutherian counterparts (Aveskogh and Hellman, 1998; Aveskogh et al., 1999) (Fig. 1). Analysis of the diversity of the variable region demonstrated a limited V_H repertoire but a diverse V_L repertoire, which was also observed in the Australian brushtail possum (*Trichosurus vulpecula*) (Aveskogh et al., 1999; Miller et al., 1998, 1999; Lucero et al., 1998; Baker et al., 2005). Further details regarding marsupial Igs can be found in the chapter titled "Marsupial and Monotreme Immunoglobulin Genetics."

2.5.3 EUTHERIANS

Most of the knowledge about the structure and diversity of the Ig genes acquired to date is based on studies of eutherian mammals, especially humans and mice. Most of the eutherians that have been examined express five Ig isotypes: IgM, IgD, IgG, IgA, and IgE; exceptions are the rabbit, the African elephant (*Loxodonta Africana*), the guinea pig (*Cavia porcellus*), and some camelids, in which the δ gene is absent or pseudogenized (Ros et al., 2004; Guo et al., 2011, 2012; De Genst et al., 2006). Compared with their homologs in other tetrapods, the majority of the δ genes present in eutherians have been considerably shortened to only three δC_H domains; in addition, most have developed genetic hinge exons. Even in the mouse, rat, and little brown bat (*Myotis lucifugus*), the δ genes have only two C_H exons (Tucker et al., 1980; Zhao and Hammarstr, 2003; Butler et al., 2011) (Fig. 2). It is also interesting that in many eutherian mammals (but not in some closely related mammals such as cattle and sheep), multiple copies of the γ or α genes have been generated by relatively recent gene duplication occurring after speciation. These distinct γ or α gene copies may encode distinct IgG or IgA subclasses that exert diverse effector functions. Human, mouse, horse, pig, and elephant have four, four, seven, six, and eight γ genes from a single haplotype, respectively, and the rabbit has 13 α genes (Guo et al., 2011; Schroeder et al., 2006; Wagner et al., 2004; Eguchi-Ogawa et al., 2012; Burnett et al., 1989) (Fig. 1).

The diversity of the germline V_H locus and how it is utilized to generate the heavy chain repertoire varies between eutherian mammals. The genomic V_H locus of humans and mice is composed of a relatively large number of functional V_H genes. These are grouped into multiple V_H families and distributed across all three mammalian V_H clans (Schroeder et al., 2006; de Bono et al., 2004; Johnston et al., 2006; Schroeder et al., 1990). In contrast, some domestic animals, such as pig, horse, cow, and sheep, may possess <30 functional germline V_H genes, and among these, a single V_H family belonging to either clan II (e.g., in horse, cattle, and sheep) or clan III (e.g., in pig) is predominantly utilized in the expressed V_H repertoire (Eguchi-Ogawa et al., 2010; Sun et al., 1994, 2010; Almagro et al., 2006; Niku et al., 2012; Lopez et al., 1998; Dufour et al., 1996). The rabbit is an extreme example. Despite the presence of approximately 200 V_H genes, more than 80% of the rearrangements are derived from the D-proximal $V_H 1$ gene segment (Ros et al., 2004; Gallarda et al., 1985; Currier et al., 1988). The preferential usage of a single V_H family (or even a single V_H gene) may make VDJ rearrangement alone insufficient to produce the required immunological diversity. Therefore, in these species, the primary antibody repertoire is further diversified by one or both of two post-rearrangement mechanisms, sGC and SHM (Becker and Knight 1990; Short et al., 1991; Weinstein et al., 1994; Parng et al., 1996; Lucier et al., 1998; Reynaud et al., 1995; Butler et al., 2011).

With respect to the immunoglobulin light chains, both the κ and λ isotypes are expressed in most eutherians. However, their relative contributions to the light chain repertoire vary substantially between different species. κ is the predominant light chain isotype in the mouse and rabbit, while the λ isotype is preferentially utilized in horses, cattle, and sheep. In humans and pigs, the two isotypes are relatively equal in abundance (Butler, 1997). In some cases, a light chain is not necessary to create a functional Ig molecule. For example, IgG2 and IgG3 are expressed as heavy-chain-only antibodies (HCAbs) in the serum of camelids (De Genst et al., 2006).

In other chapters, the genetics of the immunoglobulins of five eutherians, including rat, cow, pig, rabbit, and bat, will be discussed in more detail.

KEYWORDS

- **diversity**
- **immunoglobulin**
- **isotype**
- **repertoire**
- **tetrapod**

REFERENCES

Almagro, J.C., Martinez, L., Smith, S.L., Alagon, A., Estevez, J., Paniagua, J., Analysis of the horse V(H) repertoire and comparison with the human IGHV germline genes, and sheep, cattle and pig V(H) sequences. *Mol Immunol* 43, (2006): 1836–1845.

Amemiya, C.T., Haire, R.N., Litman, G.W., Nucleotide sequence of a cDNA encoding a third distinct Xenopus immunoglobulin heavy chain isotype. *Nucleic Acids Res* 17, (1989): 5388.

Aveskogh, M., Hellman, L., Evidence for an early appearance of modern postswitch isotypes in mammalian evolution; cloning of IgE, IgG and IgA from the marsupial Monodelphis domestica. *Eur J Immunol* 28, (1998): 2738–2750.

Aveskogh, M., Pilstrom, L., Hellman, L., Cloning and structural analysis of IgM (mu chain) and the heavy chain V region repertoire in the marsupial Monodelphis domestica. *Dev Comp Immunol* 23, (1999): 597–606.

Baker, M.L., Belov, K., Miller, R.D., Unusually similar patterns of antibody V segment diversity in distantly related marsupials. *J Immunol* 174, (2005): 5665–5671.

Bao, Y., Wu, S., Zang, Y., Wang, H., Song, X., Xu, C., et al. The immunoglobulin light chain locus of the turkey, Meleagris gallopavo. V*et Immunol Immunopathol* 147, (2012): 44–50.

Becker, R.S., Knight, K.L., Somatic diversification of immunoglobulin heavy chain VDJ genes: evidence for somatic gene conversion in rabbits. *Cell* 63, (1990): 987–997.

Belov, K., Hellman, L., Cooper, D.W., Characterization of echidna IgM provides insights into the time of divergence of extant mammals. *Dev Comp Immunol* 26, (2002): 831–839.

Belov, K., Hellman, L., Cooper, D.W., Characterization of immunoglobulin gamma 1 from a monotreme, Tachyglossus aculeatus. *Immunogenetics* 53, (2002): 1065–1071.

Belov, K., Hellman, L., Immunoglobulin genetics of Ornithorhynchus anatinus (platypus) and Tachyglossus aculeatus (short-beaked echidna). *Comp Biochem Physiol A Mol Integr Physiol* 136, (2003): 811–819.

Belov, K., Hellman, L., Platypus immunoglobulin M and the divergence of the two extant monotreme lineages. *Australian Mammalogy* 25, (2003): 87–94.

Belov, K., Zenger, K.R., Hellman, L., Cooper, D.W., Echidna IgA supports mammalian unity and traditional Therian relationship. *Mamm Genome* 13, (2002): 656–663.

Bengten, E., Quiniou, S.M., Stuge, T.B., Katagiri, T., Miller, N.W., Clem, L.W., et al. The IgH locus of the channel catfish, Ictalurus punctatus, contains multiple constant region gene sequences: different genes encode heavy chains of membrane and secreted IgD. *J Immunol* 169, (2002): 2488–2497.

Bininda-Emonds, O.R., Cardillo, M., Jones, K.E., MacPhee, R.D., Beck, R.M., Grenyer, R., et al. The delayed rise of present-day mammals. *Nature* 446, (2007): 507–512.

Brown, J.W., Rest, J.S., Garcia-Moreno, J., Sorenson, M.D., Mindell, D.P., Strong mitochondrial DNA support for a Cretaceous origin of modern avian lineages. *BMC Biol* 6, (2008): 6.

Burnett, R.C., Hanly, W.C., Zhai, S.K., Knight, K.L., The IgA heavy-chain gene family in rabbit: cloning and sequence analysis o*f* 13 C alpha genes. *EMBO J* 8, (1989): 4041–4047.

Butler, J.E. Immunoglobulin gene organization and the mechanism of repertoire development. *Scand J Immunol* 45, (1997): 455–462.

Butler, J.E., Sun, X., Wertz, N., Lager, K.M., Chaloner, K., Urban, J., Jr., et al. Antibody repertoire development in fetal and neonatal piglets XXI. Usage of most VH genes remains constant during fetal and postnatal development. *Mol Immunol* 49, (2011): 483–494.

Butler, J.E., Wertz, N., Zhao, Y., Zhang, S., Bao, Y., Bratsch, S., et al. The two suborders of chiropterans have the canonical heavy-chain immunoglobulin (Ig) gene repertoire of eutherian mammals. *Developmental and Comparative Immunology* 35, (2011): 273–284.

Cao, Y., Sorenson, M.D., Kumazawa, Y., Mindell, D.P., Hasegawa, M., Phylogenetic position of turtles among amniotes: evidence from mitochondrial and nuclear genes. *Gene* 259, (2000): 139–148.

Charlton, K.A., Moyle, S., Porter, A.J., Harris, W.J., Analysis of the diversity of a sheep antibody repertoire as revealed from a bacteriophage display library. *J Immunol* 164, (2000): 6221–6229.

Cheng, G., Gao, Y., Wang, T., Sun, Y., Wei, Z., Li, L., et al. Extensive diversification of IgH subclass-encoding genes and IgM subclass switching in crocodilians. *Nat Commun* 4, (2013): (1337):

Choi, J.W., Kim, J.K., Seo, H.W., Cho, B.W., Song, G., Han, J.Y., Molecular cloning and comparative analysis of immunoglobulin heavy chain genes from Phasianus colchicus, Meleagris gallopavo, and Coturnix japonica. V*et Immunol Immunopathol* 136, (2010): 248–256.

Currier, S.J., Gallarda, J.L., Knight, K.L., Partial molecular genetic map of the rabbit VH chromosomal region. *J Immunol* 140, (1988): 1651–1659.

Dahan, A., Reynaud, C.A., Weill, J.C., Nucleotide sequence of the constant region of a chicken mu heavy chain immunoglobulin mRNA. *Nucleic Acids Res* 11, (1983): 5381–5389.

Danilova, N., Bussmann, J., Jekosch, K., Steiner, L.A., The immunoglobulin heavy-chain locus in zebrafish: identification and expression of a previously unknown isotype, immunoglobulin Z. *Nat Immunol* 6, (2005): 295–302.

Das, S., Mohamedy, U., Hirano, M., Nei, M., Nikolaidis, N., Analysis of the immunoglobulin light chain genes in zebra finch: evolutionary implications. *Mol Biol Evol* 27, (2010): 113–120.

de Bono, B., Madera, M., Chothia, C., VH gene segments in the mouse and human genomes. *J Mol Biol* 342, (2004): 131–143.

De Genst, E., Saerens, D., Muyldermans, S., Conrath, K., Antibody repertoire development in camelids. *Dev Comp Immunol* 30, (2006): 187–198.

Deza, F.G., Espinel, C.S., Beneitez, J.V., A novel IgA-like immunoglobulin in the reptile Eublepharis macularius. *Dev Comp Immunol* 31, (2007): 596–605.

Dooley, H., Flajnik, M.F., Antibody repertoire development in cartilaginous fish. *Dev Comp Immunol* 30, (2006): 43–56.

Du Pasquier, L., Robert, J., Courtet, M., Mussmann, R., B-cell development in the amphibian Xenopus. *Immunol Rev* 175, (2000): 201–213.

Du, C.C., Mashoof, S.M., Criscitiello, M.F., Oral immunization of the African clawed frog (Xenopus laevis) upregulates the mucosal immunoglobulin IgX. V*et Immunol Immunopathol* 145, (2012): 493–498.

Dufour, V., Malinge, S., Nau, F., The sheep Ig Variable region repertoire consists of a single VH family. *J Immunol* 156, (1996): 2163–2170.

Edholm, E.S., Wilson, M., Bengten, E., Immunoglobulin light (IgL) chains in ectothermic Vertebrates. *Dev Comp Immunol* 35, (2011): 906–915.

Eguchi-Ogawa, T., Toki, D., Wertz, N., Butler, J.E., Uenishi, H., Structure of the genomic sequence comprizing the immunoglobulin heavy constant (IGHC) genes from Sus scrofa. *Mol Immunol* 52, (2012): 97–107.

Eguchi-Ogawa, T., Wertz, N., Sun, X.Z., Puimi, F., Uenishi, H., Wells, K., et al. Antibody repertoire development in fetal and neonatal piglets. XI. The relationship of Variable heavy chain gene usage and the genomic organization of the Variable heavy chain locus. *J Immunol* 184, (2010): 3734–3742.

Feeney, A.J. Predominance of VH-D-JH junctions occurring at sites of short sequence homology results in limited junctional diversity in neonatal antibodies. *J Immunol* 149, (1992): 222–229.

Fellah, J.S., Kerfourn, F., Wiles, M.V., Schwager, J., Charlemagne, J., Phylogeny of immuno-globulin heavy chain isotypes: structure of the constant region of Ambystoma mexicanum upsilon chain deduced from cDNA sequence. *Immunogenetics* 38, (1993): 311–317.

Fellah, J.S., Wiles, M.V., Charlemagne, J., Schwager, J., Evolution of Vertebrate IgM: complete amino acid sequence of the constant region of Ambystoma mexicanum mu chain deduced from cDNA sequence. *Eur J Immunol* 22, (1992): 2595–2601.

Flajnik, M.F. Comparative analyzes of immunoglobulin genes: surprises and portents. *Nat Rev Immunol* 2, (2002): 688–698.

Flajnik, M.F., Kasahara, M., Origin and evolution of the adaptive immune system: genetic events and selective pressures. *Nature Reviews Genetics* 11, (2010): 47–59.

Gallarda, J.L., Gleason, K.S., Knight, K.L., Organization of rabbit immunoglobulin genes. I. Structure and multiplicity of germline VH genes. *J Immunol* 135, (1985): 4222–4228.

Gambon-Deza, F., Espinel, C.S., Beneitez, J.V., A novel IgA-like immunoglobulin in the reptile Eublepharis macularius. *Dev Comp Immunol* 31, (2007): 596–605.

Gambon-Deza, F., Espinel, C.S., IgD in the reptile leopard gecko. *Mol Immunol* 45, (2008): 3470–3476.

Gambon-Deza, F., Sanchez-Espinel, C., Magadan-Mompo, S., The immunoglobulin heavy chain locus in the platypus (Ornithorhynchus anatinus). *Mol Immunol* 46, (2009): 2515–2523.

Gambon-Deza, F., Sanchez-Espinel, C., Mirete-Bachiller, S., Magadan-Mompo, S., Snakes antibodies. *Dev Comp Immunol* 38, (2012): 1–9.

Grey, H.M. (1967): Duck immunoglobulins. II. Biologic and immunochemical studies. *J Immunol* 98, 820–826.

Griffin, D.K., Robertson, L.B., Tempest, H.G., Vignal, A., Fillon, V., Crooijmans, R.P., Groenen, M.A., Deryusheva, S., Gaginskaya, E., Carre, W., Waddington, D., Talbot, R., Volker, M., Masabanda, J.S., Burt, D.W., Whole genome comparative studies between chicken and turkey and their implications for avian genome evolution. *BMC Genomics* 9, (2008): 168.

Gu, H., Forster, I., Rajewsky, K., Sequence homologies, N sequence insertion and JH gene utilization in VHDJH joining: implications for the joining mechanism and the ontogenetic timing of Ly1 B cell and B-CLL progenitor generation. *EMBO J* 1990, 9, 2133–2140.

Guo, Y., Bao, Y., Meng, Q., Hu, X., Meng, Q., Ren, L., et al. Immunoglobulin genomics in the guinea pig (Cavia porcellus). *PLoS One* 7, (2012): e39298.

Guo, Y., Bao, Y., Wang, H., Hu, X., Zhao, Z., Li, N., Zhao, Y., A preliminary analysis of the immunoglobulin genes in the African elephant (Loxodonta africana). *PLoS One* 6, (2011): e16889.

Hackett, S.J., Kimball, R.T., Reddy, S., Bowie, R.C., Braun, E.L., Braun, M.J., et al. A phylogenomic study of birds reveals their evolutionary history. *Science* 320, (2008): 1763–1768.

Haire, R.N., Amemiya, C.T., Suzuki, D., Litman, G.W., Eleven distinct VH gene families and additional patterns of sequence Variation suggest a high degree of immunoglobulin gene complexity in a lower Vertebrate, Xenopus laevis. *J Exp Med* 171, (1990): 1721–1737.

Haire, R.N., Ohta, Y., Litman, R.T., Amemiya, C.T., Litman, G.W., The genomic organization of immunoglobulin VH genes in Xenopus laevis shows evidence for interspersion of families. *Nucleic Acids Res* 19, (1991): 3061–3066.

Haire, R.N., Ota, T., Rast, J.P., Litman, R.T., Chan, F.Y., L.I. Zon et al. A third Ig light chain gene isotype in Xenopus laevis consists of six distinct VL families and is related to mammalian lambda genes. *J Immunol* 157, (1996): 1544–1550.

Haire, R.N., Shamblott, M.J., Amemiya, C.T., Litman, G.W., A second Xenopus immunoglobulin heavy chain constant region isotype gene. *Nucleic Acids Res* 17, (1989): 1776.

Hansen, J.D., Landis, E.D., Phillips, R.B., Discovery of a unique Ig heavy-chain isotype (IgT) in rainbow trout: Implications for a distinctive B cell developmental pathway in teleost fish. *Proc Natl Acad Sci USA* 2005, 102, 6919–6924.

Hikima, J., Jung, T.S., Aoki, T., Immunoglobulin genes and their transcriptional control in teleosts. *Dev Comp Immunol* 35, (2011): 924–936.

Hsu, E., Schwager, J., Alt, F.W., Evolution of immunoglobulin genes: VH families in the amphibian Xenopus. *Proc Natl Acad Sci USA* 1989, 86, 8010–8014.

Huang, T., Zhang, M., Wei, Z., Wang, P., Sun, Y., Hu, X., et al. Analysis of immunoglobulin transcripts in the ostrich Struthio camelus, a primitive avian species. *PLoS One* 7, (2012): e34346.

Humphrey, B.D., Calvert, C.C., Klasing, K.C., The ratio of full length IgY to truncated IgY in immune complexes affects macrophage phagocytosis and the acute phase response of mallard ducks (Anas platyrhynchos). *Dev Comp Immunol* 28, (2004): 665–672.

Ippolito, G.C., Schelonka, R.L., Zemlin, M., Ivanov, II, Kobayashi, R., Zemlin, C., et al. Forced usage of positively charged amino acids in immunoglobulin CDR-H3 impairs B cell development and antibody production. *J Exp Med* 203, (2006): 1567–1578.

Ivanov, II, Schelonka, R.L., Zhuang, Y., Gartland, G.L., Zemlin, M., Schroeder, H.W., Jr. Development of the expressed Ig CDR-H3 repertoire is marked by focusing of constraints long, amino acid use, and charge that are first established in early B cell progenitors. *J Immunol* 174, (2005): 7773–7780.

Iwabe, N., Hara, Y., Kumazawa, Y., Shibamoto, K., Saito, Y., T. Miyata et al. Sister group relationship of turtles to the bird-crocodilian clade revealed by nuclear DNA-coded proteins. *Mol Biol Evol* 22, (2005): 810–813.

Jeong, H., Teale, J.M., Comparison of the fetal and adult functional B cell repertoires by analysis of VH gene family expression. *The Journal of experimental medicine* 168, (1988): 589–603.

Johansson, J., Aveskogh, M., Munday, B., Hellman, L., Heavy chain V region diversity in the duck-billed platypus (Ornithorhynchus anatinus): long and highly Variable complementarity-determining region 3 compensates for limited germline diversity. *J Immunol* 168, (2002): 5155–5162.

Johansson, J., Salazar, J.N., Aveskogh, M., Munday, B., Miller, R.D., Hellman, L., High Variability in complementarity-determining regions compensates for a low number of V gene families in the lambda light chain locus of the platypus. *Eur J Immunol* 35, (2005): 3008–3019.

Johnston, C.M., Wood, A.L., Bolland, D.J., Corcoran, A.E., Complete sequence assembly and characterization of the C57BL/6 mouse Ig heavy chain V region. *J Immunol* 176, (2006): 4221–4234.

Knight, K.L., Becker, R.S., Molecular basis of the allelic inheritance of rabbit immunoglobulin VH allotypes: implications for the generation of antibody diversity. *Cell* 60, (1990): 963–970.

Kobel, H.R., L. Du Pasquier. Genetics of polyploid *Xenopus*. *Trends in Genetics* 2, (1986): 310–315.

Lanning, D.K., Zhai, S.K., Knight, K.L., Analysis of the 3' Cmu region of the rabbit Ig heavy chain locus. *Gene* 309, (2003): 135–144.

Li, L., Wang, T., Sun, Y., Cheng, G., Yang, H., Wei, Z., et al. Extensive diversification of IgD-, IgY-, and truncated IgY(deltaFc)-encoding genes in the red-eared turtle (Trachemys scripta elegans). *J Immunol* 189, (2012): 3995–4004.

Litman, G.W., Murphy, K., Berger, L., Litman, R., Hinds, K., Erickson, B.W., Complete nucleotide sequences of three VH genes in Caiman, a phylogenetically ancient reptile: evolutionary diversification in coding segments and Variation in the structure and organization of recombination elements. *Proc Natl Acad Sci USA* 82, (1985): 844–848.

Litman, G.W., Person, M.K., Rast, J.P., Evolution of antigen binding receptors. *Annu Rev Immunol* 17, (1999): 109–147.

Lopez, O., Perez, C., Wylie, D., A single VH family and long CDR3 s are the targets for hypermutation in bovine immunoglobulin heavy chains. *Immunol Rev* 162, (1998): 55–66.

Lucero, J.E., Rosenberg, G.H., Miller, R.D., Marsupial light chains: complexity and conservation of lambda in the opossum Monodelphis domestica. *J Immunol* 161, (1998): 6724–6732.

Lucier, M.R., Thompson, R.E., Waire, J., Lin, A.W., Osborne, B.A., Goldsby, R.A., Multiple sites of V lambda diversification in cattle. *J Immunol* 161, (1998): 5438–5444.

Lundqvist, M.L., Middleton, D.L., Hazard, S., Warr, G.W., The immunoglobulin heavy chain locus of the duck. Genomic organization and expression of D, J, and C region genes. *J Biol Chem* 276, (2001): 46729–46736.

Magadan-Mompo, S., Sanchez-Espinel, C., Gambon-Deza, F., Immunoglobulin genes of the turtles. *Immunogenetics* 65, (2013): 227–237.

Magor, K.E., Higgins, D.A., Middleton, D.L., Warr, G.W., cDNA sequence and organization of the immunoglobulin light chain gene of the duck, Anas platyrhynchos. *Dev Comp Immunol* 18, (1994): 523–531.

Magor, K.E., Higgins, D.A., Middleton, D.L., Warr, G.W., One gene encodes the heavy chains for three different forms of IgY in the duck. *J Immunol* 153, (1994): 5549–5555.

Magor, K.E., Warr, G.W., Bando, Y., Middleton, D.L., Higgins, D.A., Secretory immune system of the duck (Anas platyrhynchos). Identification and expression of the genes encoding IgA and IgM heavy chains. *Eur J Immunol* 28, (1998): 1063–1068.

Mansikka, A. Chicken IgA H chains. Implications concerning the evolution of H chain genes. *J Immunol* 149, (1992): 855–861.

McCormack, W.T., Carlson, L.M., Tjoelker, L.W., Thompson, C.B., Evolutionary comparison of the avian IgL locus: combinatorial diversity plays a role in the generation of the antibody repertoire in some avian species. *Int Immunol* 1, (1989): 332–341.

McCormack, W.T., Thompson, C.B., Chicken IgL Variable region gene conversions display pseudogene donor preference and 5' to 3' polarity. *Genes Dev* 4, (1990): 548–558.

McCormack, W.T., Tjoelker, L.W., Thompson, C.B., Avian B-cell development: generation of an immunoglobulin repertoire by gene conversion. *Annu Rev Immunol* 9, (1991): 219–241.

Miller, R.D., Bergemann, E.R., Rosenberg, G.H., Marsupial light chains: IGK with four V families in the opossum Monodelphis domestica. *Immunogenetics* 50, (1999): 329–335.

Miller, R.D., Grabe, H., Rosenberg, G.H., V(H) repertoire of a marsupial (Monodelphis domestica). *J Immunol* 160, (1998): 259–265.

Mussmann, R., Courtet, M., L. Du Pasquier. Development of the early B cell population in Xenopus. *Eur J Immunol* 28, (1998): 2947–2959.

Mussmann, R., L. Du Pasquier, and Hsu, E., Is Xenopus IgX an analog of IgA? *Eur J Immunol* 26, (1996): 2823–2830.

Mussmann, R., Wilson, M., Marcuz, A., Courtet, M., L. Du Pasquier. (1996): Membrane exon sequences of the three Xenopus Ig classes explain the evolutionary origin of mammalian isotypes. *Eur J Immunol* 26, 409–414.

Ng, P.L., Higgins, D.A., Bile immunoglobulin of the duck (Anas platyrhynchos). I. Preliminary characterization and ontogeny. *Immunology* 58, (1986): 323–327.

Niku, M., Liljavirta, J., Durkin, K., Schroderus, E., Iivanainen, A., The bovine genomic DNA sequence data reveal three IGHV subgroups, only one of which is functionally expressed. *Dev Comp Immunol* 37, (2012): 457–461.

Nowak, M.A., Parra, Z.E., Hellman, L., Miller, R.D., The complexity of expressed kappa light chains in egg-laying mammals. *Immunogenetics* 56, (2004): 555–563.

Ohta, Y., Flajnik, M., IgD, like IgM, is a primordial immunoglobulin class perpetuated in most jawed Vertebrates. *Proc Natl Acad Sci USA* 103, (2006): 10723–10728.

Old, J., Deane, E., Development of the immune system and immunological protection in marsupial pouch young. *Developmental and Comparative Immunology* 24, (2000): 445–454.

Pacheco, M.A., Battistuzzi, F.U., Lentino, M., Aguilar, R.F., Kumar, S., Escalante, A.A., Evolution of modern birds revealed by mitogenomics: Timing the radiation and origin of major orders. *Mol Biol Evol* 28, (2011): 1927–1942.

Parng, C.L., Hansal, S., Goldsby, R.A., Osborne, B.A., Gene conversion contributes to Ig light chain diversity in cattle. *J Immunol* 157, (1996): 5478–5486.

Parvari, R., Avivi, A., Lentner, F., Ziv, E., Tel-Or, S., Burstein, Y., Schechter, I., Chicken immunoglobulin gamma-heavy chains: limited VH gene repertoire, combinatorial diversification by D gene segments and evolution of the heavy chain locus. *EMBO J* 7, (1988): 739–744.

Pascual, V., Verkruyze, L., Casey, M.L., Capra, J.D., Analysis of Ig H chain gene segment utilization in human fetal liver. Revisiting the "proximal utilization hypothesis". *J Immunol* 151, (1993): 4164–4172.

Pereira, S.L., Baker, A.J., A mitogenomic timescale for birds detects Variable phylogenetic rates of molecular evolution and refutes the standard molecular clock. *Mol Biol Evol* 23, (2006): 1731–1740.

Platz, J.E., Conlon, J.M., Reptile relationships turn turtle and turn back again. *Nature* 389, (1997): 246–246.

Qin, T., Ren, L., Hu, X., Guo, Y., Fei, J., Zhu, Q., et al. Genomic organization of the immunoglobulin light chain gene loci in Xenopus tropicalis: evolutionary implications. *Dev Comp Immunol* 32, (2008): 156–165.

Ratcliffe, Antibodies, M.J., immunoglobulin genes and the bursa of Fabricius in chicken B cell development. *Dev Comp Immunol* 30, (2006): 101–118.

Reynaud, C.A., Anquez, V., Grimal, H., Weill, J.C., A hyperconversion mechanism generates the chicken light chain preimmune repertoire. *Cell* 48, (1987): 379–388.

Reynaud, C.A., Anquez, V., Weill, J.C., The chicken D locus and its contribution to the immunoglobulin heavy chain repertoire. *Eur J Immunol* 21, (1991): 2661–2670.

Reynaud, C.A., Dahan, A., Anquez, V., Weill, J.C., Somatic hyperconversion diversifies the single Vh gene of the chicken with a high incidence in the D region. *Cell* 59, (1989): 171–183.

Reynaud, C.A., Garcia, C., Hein, W.R., Weill, J.C., Hypermutation generating the sheep immunoglobulin repertoire is an antigen-independent process. *Cell* 80, (1995): 115–125.

Reynaud, C.A., Mackay, C.R., Muller, R.G., Weill, J.C., Somatic generation of diversity in a mammalian primary lymphoid organ: the sheep ileal Peyer's patches. *Cell* 64, (1991): 995–1005.

Robert, J., Ohta, Y., Comparative and developmental study of the immune system in Xenopus. *Dev Dyn* 238, (2009): 1249–1270.

50 Comparative Immunoglobulin Genetics

Ros, F., Puels, J., Reichenberger, N., W. Van Schooten, Buelow, R., Platzer, J., Sequence analysis of 0.5 Mb of the rabbit germline immunoglobulin heavy chain locus. *Gene* 330, (2004): 49–59.

Saha, N.R., Suetake, H., Kikuchi, K., Suzuki, Y., Fugu immunoglobulin D: A highly unusual gene with unprecedented duplications in its constant region. *Immunogenetics* 56, (2004): 438–447.

Samollow, P.B. Status and applications of genomic resources for the gray, short-tailed opossum, Monodelphis domestica, an American marsupial model for comparative biology. *Australian J Zoology* 54, (2006): 173–196.

Samollow, P.B. The opossum genome: insights and opportunities from an alternative mammal. *Genome research* 18, (2008): 1199–1215.

Schaerlinger, B., Bascove, M., Frippiat, J.P., A new isotype of immunoglobulin heavy chain in the urodele amphibian Pleurodeles waltl predominantly expressed in larvae. *Mol Immunol* 45, (2008): 776–786.

Schaerlinger, B., Frippiat, J.P., IgX antibodies in the urodele amphibian Ambystoma mexicanum. *Dev Comp Immunol* 32, (2008): 908–915.

Schroeder, H.W., Jr. Similarity and divergence in the development and expression of the mouse and human antibody repertoires. *Dev Comp Immunol* 30, (2006): 119–135.

Schroeder, H.W., Jr., Hillson, J.L., Perlmutter, R.M., Structure and evolution of mammalian VH families. *Int Immunol* 2, (1990): 41–50.

Schroeder, H.W., Jr., Ippolito, G.C., Shiokawa, S., Regulation of the antibody repertoire through control of HCDR3 diversity. *Vaccine* 16, (1998): 1383–1390.

Schwager, J., Burckert, N., Courtet, M., L. Du Pasquier. The ontogeny of diversification at the immunoglobulin heavy chain locus in Xenopus. *EMBO J* 10, (1991): 2461–2470.

Schwager, J., Burckert, N., Schwager, M., Wilson, M., Evolution of immunoglobulin light chain genes: analysis of Xenopus IgL isotypes and their contribution to antibody diversity. *EMBO J* 1991, 10, 505–511.

Schwager, J., Mikoryak, C.A., Steiner, L.A., Amino acid sequence of heavy chain from Xenopus laevis IgM deduced from cDNA sequence: implications for evolution of immunoglobulin domains. *Proc Natl Acad Sci USA* 1988, 85, 2245–2249.

Short, J.A., Sethupathi, P., Zhai, S.K., Knight, K.L., VDJ genes in VHa2 allotype-suppressed rabbits. Limited germline VH gene usage and accumulation of somatic mutations in D regions. *J Immunol* 147, (1991): 4014–4018.

Sun, J., Kacskovics, I., Brown, W.R., Butler, J.E., Expressed swine VH genes belong to a small VH gene family homologous to human VHIII. *J Immunol* 153, (1994): 5618–5627.

Sun, Y., Wang, C., Wang, Y., Zhang, T., Ren, L., Hu, X., et al. A comprehensive analysis of germline and expressed immunoglobulin repertoire in the horse. *Dev Comp Immunol* 34, (2010): 1009–1020.

Sun, Y., Wei, Z., Hammarstrom, L., Zhao, Y., The immunoglobulin delta gene in jawed Vertebrates: a comparative overview. *Dev Comp Immunol* 35, 975–981.

Thompson, C.B., Neiman, P.E., Somatic diversification of the chicken immunoglobulin light chain gene is limited to the rearranged Variable gene segment. *Cell* 48, (1987): 369–378.

Tucker, P.W., C.-Liu, P., Mushinski, J.F., Blattner, F.R., Mouse immunoglobulin D: messenger RNA and genomic DNA sequences. *Science* 209, (1980): 1353–1360.

Tucker, P.W., Slightom, J.L., Blattner, F.R., Mouse IgA heavy chain gene sequence: implications for evolution of immunoglobulin hinge axons. *Proc Natl Acad Sci USA* 1981, 78, 7684–7688.

Turchin, A., Hsu, E., The generation of antibody diversity in the turtle. *J Immunol* 156, (1996): 3797–3805.

van Rheede, T., Bastiaans, T., Boone, D.N., Hedges, S.B., W.W. de Jong, and Madsen, O., The platypus is in its place: Nuclear genes and indels confirm the sister group relation of monotremes and Therians. *Mol Biol Evol* 23, (2006): 587–597.

Vernersson, M., Aveskogh, M., Hellman, L., Cloning of IgE from the echidna (Tachyglossus aculeatus) and a comparative analysis of epsilon chains from all three extant mammalian lineages. *Dev Comp Immunol* 28, (2004): 61–75.

Vernersson, M., Aveskogh, M., Munday, B., Hellman, L., Evidence for an early appearance of modern postswitch immunoglobulin isotypes in mammalian evolution (II); cloning of IgE, IgG1 and IgG2 from a monotreme, the duck-billed platypus, Ornithorhynchus anatinus. *Eur J Immunol* 32, (2002): 2145–2155.

Vernersson, M., Belov, K., Aveskogh, M., Hellman, L., Cloning and structural analysis of two highly divergent IgA isotypes, IgA1 and IgA2 from the duck billed platypus, Ornithorhynchus anatinus. *Mol Immunol* 47, (2010): 785–791.

Wagner, B., Miller, D.C., Lear, T.L., Antczak, D.F., The complete map of the Ig heavy chain constant gene region reveals evidence for seven IgG isotypes and for IgD in the horse. *J Immunol* 173, (2004): 3230–3242.

Wang, T., Sun, Y., Shao, W., Cheng, G., Li, L., Cao, Z., et al. Evidence of IgY subclass diversification in snakes: evolutionary implications. *J Immunol* 189, (2012): 3557–3565.

Wang, X., Olp, J.J., Miller, R.D., On the genomics of immunoglobulins in the gray, short-tailed opossum Monodelphis domestica. *Immunogenetics* 61, (2009): 581–596.

Wang, X., Sharp, A.R., Miller, R.D., Early Postnatal B Cell Ontogeny and Antibody Repertoire Maturation in the Opossum, Monodelphis domestica. *PLoS One* 7, (2012): e45931.

Warr, G.W., Magor, K.E., Higgins, D.A., IgY: clues to the origins of modern antibodies. *Immunol Today* 16, (1995): 392–398.

Warren, W.C., Hillier, L.W., J.A. Marshall Graves, Birney, E., Ponting, C.P., Grutzner, F., et al. Genome analysis of the platypus reveals unique signatures of evolution. *Nature* 453, (2008): 175–183.

Wei, Z., Wu, Q., Ren, L., Hu, X., Guo, Y., Warr, G.W., et al. Expression of IgM, IgD, and IgY in a reptile, Anolis carolinensis. *J Immunol* 183, (2009): 3858–3864.

Weinstein, P.D.,erson, A.O., Mage, R.G., Rabbit IgH sequences in appendix germinal centers: VH diversification by gene conversion-like and hypermutation mechanisms. *Immunity* 1, (1994): 647–659.

Willems Van Dijk, K., Milner, L.A., Sasso, E.H., Milner, E.C., Chromosomal organization of the heavy chain Variable region gene segments comprizing the human fetal antibody repertoire. *Proc Natl Acad Sci USA* 89, (1992): 10430–10434.

Wu, G.E., Paige, C.J., VH gene family utilization in colonies derived from B and preB cells detected by the RNA colony blot assay. *EMBO J* 1986, 5, 3475–3481.

Wu, Q., Wei, Z., Yang, Z., Wang, T., Ren, L., Hu, X., et al. Phylogeny, genomic organization and expression of lambda and kappa immunoglobulin light chain genes in a reptile, Anolis carolinensis. *Dev Comp Immunol* 34, (2010): 579–589.

Xu, Z., Wang, G.L., Nie, P., IgM, IgD and IgY and their expression pattern in the Chinese soft-shelled turtle Pelodiscus sinensis. *Mol Immunol* 46, (2009): 2124–2132.

Zardoya, R., Meyer, A., Complete mitochondrial genome suggests diapsid affinities of turtles. *Proc Natl Acad Sci USA* 95, (1998): 14226–14231.

Zezza, D.J., Mikoryak, C.A., Schwager, J., Steiner, L.A., Sequence of C region of l chains from Xenopus laevis Ig. *J Immunol* 146, (1991): 4041–4047.

Zezza, D.J., Stewart, S.E., Steiner, L.A., Genes encoding Xenopus laevis Ig l chains. Implications for the evolution of kappa and lambda chains. *J Immunol* 149, (1992): 3968–3977.

Zhao, Y., Cui, H., Whittington, C.M., Wei, Z., Zhang, X., Zhang, Z., et al. Ornithorhynchus anatinus (platypus) links the evolution of immunoglobulin genes in eutherian mammals and nonmammalian tetrapods. *J Immunol* 183, (2009): 3285–3293.

Zhao, Y., Hammarstr, L., Cloning of the complete rat immunoglobulin delta gene: evolutionary implications. *Immunology* 108, (2003): 288–295.

Zhao, Y., Pan-Hammarstrom, Q., Yu, S., Wertz, N., Zhang, X., Li, N., Butler, J.E., Hammarstrom, L., Identification of IgF, a hinge-region-containing Ig class, and IgD in Xenopus tropicalis. *Proc Natl Acad Sci USA* 2006, 103, 12087–12092.

Zhao, Y., Rabbani, H., Shimizu, A., Hammarstrom, L., Mapping of the chicken immunoglobulin heavy-chain constant region gene locus reveals an inverted alpha gene upstream of a condensed upsilon gene. *Immunology* 101, (2000): 348–353.

CHAPTER 3

THE IMMUNOGLOBULIN GENES OF BATS*

J. E. BUTLER, NANCY WERTZ, and MICHELLE L. BAKER

CONTENTS

***Research Support:** The work described was partially supported by NSF-IOF grant 0077237 and a Future Fellowship from the Australian Research Council FT110100234.

ABSTRACT

The constant region immunoglobulin (Ig) genes in the two major suborders of bats have the canonical structure and repertoire of other eutherian mammals. Analysis of their sequences indicates that microbats and megabats arose from a common ancestor. The bat Ig sequences form a separate group distinct from other eutherian mammals, which in the case of IgD and IgG, have a distant relationship to carnivores but with no evidence they are "flying mice." Consistent with other mammals, their IgG diversified into subclasses after speciation and their IgG hinge motifs are species-specific. Studies on the variable heavy chain repertoire of especially the insectivorous little brown bat (*Myotis lucifugus*) indicate an extremely diverse repertoire. Studies reveal five to seven V_H gene families, but with some differences among suborders. In *M. lucifugus,* there are >200 V_H genes of which V_H3 is the largest family. As many as 13 J_H genes and an apparently diverse D_H repertoire is also present in this species. Preliminary data suggest that the little brown bat may depend more on combinatorial diversity and less on somatic hypermutation in the generation of its antibody repertoire.

3.1   INTRODUCTION

3.1.1   DIVERSITY, PHYLOGENY AND ECOLOGY

Among living vertebrates, bats and birds are unique in their ability to fly, and this common feature sets them apart ecologically and physiologically from other groups. Bats are in some ways the nocturnal equivalent of birds, having evolved and radiated into a diversity of forms to fill many of the same niches as birds. Bats have successfully colonized almost every continental region on earth (except Antarctica) as well as many oceanic islands and archipelagos (Kunz, 1982; Kunz and Lumsden, 2003). Of the >5,400 species of mammals, bats comprise 20%, second only to rodents (Teeling et al., 2002; Simmons, 2005). Bats impact the environment in many ways. Insectivorous microbats suppress insect populations (Cleveland et al., 2006, Kalka et al., 2008; Williams-Guillen et al., 2008; Jones et al., 2009) and plant-visiting bats serve as pollinators and disperse seeds (Fujita and Tuttle, 1991; Shilton et al., 1999; Muscarella and Fleming, 2007; Fleming et al., 2009). Insectivorous microbats like the common little brown bat (*Myotis lucifugus*) may consume their entire body weight each night in insects (Kurta et al., 1989). These bats of the Yangochiroptera, also known as microbats, are the most important predators of nocturnal insects and consume 5–10 times more insects than swallows and flycatchers. So-called "megabats" of the suborder Yinpterochiroptera are important pollinators and seed dispersers, but can be pests when they damage fruit crops. The migration of bats between camps and foraging sites provides an important mechanism of seed dispersal and pollination for plants, with some tropical plants entirely dependent on bats for the distribution of their seeds (Banack, 1998).

All bat species can be vectors for zoonotic viral diseases (Messenger et al., 2003; Calisher et al., 2006; Wibbelt et al., 2009; Lau et al., 2005; Halpin et al., 2008). More than 85 viruses which are known from bats include a number that are associated with animal and human epidemics (Calisher et al., 2006; Wong et al., 2007). These include Hendra and Nipah viruses (horse, humans and swine; Mackenzie and Field, 2004) SARS (rodents, cattle, swine, dogs, human; Dobson, 2005 Li et al., 2005; Mueller et al., 2007; Shi and Hu, 2008) Ebola (human and other primates; Swanepoel et al., 1996; Leroy et al., 2005) and West Nile viruses (horses and humans; Lau et al., 2005).

Some insectivorous bats are themselves victims of the microbes they carry, such as in the case of white nose syndrome (WNS) an epizootic that has decimated little brown bat populations in the Eastern US (Blehert et al., 2009; Gargas et al., 2009; Frick et al., 2010). WNS killed a million bats in north-eastern USA in the first two years of the epizootic and some suggest regional populations may become extinct in 16–20 years (Frick et al., 2010). WNS is caused by the fungus *Geomyces destructus,* which is a cold-loving fungus that proliferates at low hibernation temperature (Blehert, 2012). *G. destructus* is not known to be a pathogen for non-hibernating bats or other mammals. Current evidence indicates that *G. destructus* is the sole pathogen responsible for WNS (Lorch et al., 2011). The fungus infects at least six species, many of the genus *Myotis,* all of which are members of the family Vespertilionidae that includes hibernating insectivorous bats. WNS has spread into Canada, south to the Carolina and even as far west as Oklahoma (Puechmaille et al., 2011). The fungus also infects Vespertiliondae in Europe but does not appear to be pathogenic. However, the European strain is lethal for little brown bats in N. America (Warnecke et al., 2012). This raises many questions including whether European bats have developed immunity and whether there are differences between Vespertiliondae species in Europe and N. America as regards their immune systems or whether major ecological factors are involved (Puechmaillie et al., 2011).

Bats are believed to have evolved early and to have morphologically changed very little over the past 52 million years (Hill and Smith, 1984; Simmons et al., 2008). Bats are divided into 18 families that comprise two major suborders: Yinpterochiroptera ("Yin") and Yangochiroptera ("Yan"). The former suborder includes the family Pteropodidae, which comprises the so-called "megabats" while the Yan includes all other families that comprise the "microbats" (Teeling et al., 2002). Frugivorous megabats are non-echolating compared to the insectivorous microbats. The Yan includes the small insectivorous hibernators of the family Vespertiliondae that are victims of WNS. The appearance of certain megabats ("flying foxes") and neurological features of the eye and prestrinate cortex lead Pettigrew to propose that the order was diphyletic, that is, the Yin arose from a primate/lemurs stock while the Yan evolved from the Insectivora (Pettigrew, 1986). This was a fascinating hypothesis since it implied that mammalian flight evolved twice. However, advances in molecular analyzes, including what we review here, have largely laid to rest the diphylic hypothesis for the Chiropteran (Murphy et al., 2007; Teeling et al., 2005; Adkins and Honeycutt, 1991; Mindell et al., 1991).

Bats were originally considered members of the superorder Archonta, which also included primates, tree shrews and flying lemurs (Gregory, 1910; Simpson, 1945). Others have placed bats closer to ungulates, whales, horses and carnivores (Teeling et al., 2002, 2005) (a clade referred to as Laurasiatheria). Bat transcriptome and genome sequence datasets support a relationship within Laurasiatheria. Of the species from which sequence data are currently available, bats appear to be most closely related to horses (Papenfuss et al., 2012; Shaw et al., 2012; Zhang et al., 2013). Analysis of coding sequence from the whole genome sequence from *Pteropus alecto* and *M. davidii* have revealed that bats separated from the equine ancestor approximately **88** million years ago (Zhang et al., 2013). Phylogenetic relationships based on immunoglobulin (Ig) genes presented here reveal no close relationship to any other eutherian mammal. However, the comparison of certain Ig isotypes reveals a distant relationship to the Laurasiatheria.

Although bats comprise the second largest order of mammals and 20% of all mammals (Kunz, 1982; Wimstatt, 1970) little is known about their immune system, including their Igs and the manner in which they generate their antibody repertoire. This seems important to know considering their role in epizootics and in WNS. In this chapter, we review the Ig genes of representatives of the two major suborders of the Chiroptera; Yin and Yan, including several species of Pteropid megabats, two species of insectivorous microbats and one fruit bat from the Americas of the Yan suborder.

3.1.2 IMMUNOLOGICAL ADAPTATION FOR FLIGHT

The value of bats to agriculture, ecology and their roles as vectors of human disease demands that more attention be given to this large order of mammals. In addition, their adaption to flight makes them unique among mammals. Successful flight, whether an evolutionary or human engineering achievement, shares numerous principles among which are simplicity and reduction in weight. Birds evolved a weight to muscle ratio that makes flight possible and this adaptation is reflected in the less complex B cell repertoire of birds. Birds also lack lymph nodes, use somatic gene conversion instead of non-templated somatic hypermutation (SHM), lack germinal centers, deoxynucleotide transferase (Tdt) activity have only three antibody isotypes and no pre-B cell receptor. Birds have only λ-light chains while lower vertebrates use four light chains and mammals use two. Furthermore, birds simultaneously rearrange both their heavy chain and light chain loci (Ratcliffe, 2006; Reynaud et al., 1989; McCormack et al., 1991). The weighty bone marrow of mammals that is used for hematopoiesis is missing in birds and lymphogenesis and antibody repertoire diversification is limited to about 3 weeks, that is, the process is determinant compared to mice and humans that generate new B cells throughout life.

Bats may also have made adaptations associated with flight, since a recent analysis of the genomes of *P. alecto* and *M. davidii* have revealed changes in genes with links to both energy metabolism (associated with flight) and immunity (Zhang et al., 2013). However, our recent studies argue against flight induced adaptations of bat Ig genes (Butler et al., 2011; Bratsch et al., 2011). Here we review that bats display the canonical pattern of eutherian mammals with genes encoding IgM, IgD, IgE, IgA and IgG subclasses with species-specific hinges and that diversified after speciation (Figs. 1–4). Furthermore, transcriptome data generated from immune tissues and

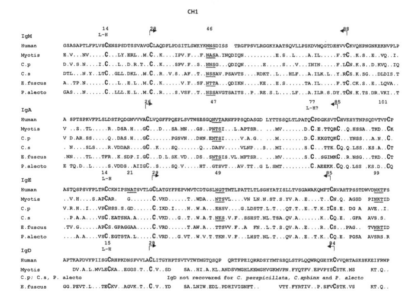

FIGURE 1   The deduced amino acid sequences of the heavy chains of IgM, IgD, IgE and IgA from five bat species fit the canonical pattern for the corresponding human Ig isotypes. P.a = *Pteropus alecto*; C.p. *Carollia perspicillata*; C.s.= *Cynoterus sphinx*, M.f. = *Myotis lucificugus*, E.f = *Eptiscus fuscus*. IgD has not been described for P.a, C.s. and C.p and IgE has not been described or *P. alecto*. Amino acid positions are numbered according to the IMGT system (Lefranc and Lefranc 2001) and those of interest are in boldface. Cysteines involved in the intradomain S-S loop are in bold with arrows indicating the loop. The cysteines involved in the covalent bond to the light chain, are also in bold and indicated as L-H. Potential N-linked glycosylation sites are in boldface. Positions in each domain start with 1 as is done in the IMGT system. The functional hinge of IgA is part of the 5′ portion of the CH 2 domain. Dots indicate that the residue is the same as for the reference human sequence. Human IgA2 was used for comparison since the extended hinge of human IgA1 is unique among mammals. Accession numbers for the sequences used are given in Table 1.

stimulated cells from *P. alecto* provides evidence for the transcription of both Igκ and Igλ light chains (Papenfuss et al., 2012) not the loss of Igκ as in birds. At this time no additional data are available on the light chains of bats such as the kappa:lambda ratio, whether lambda rearranges before kappa or visa-versa and whether B cell development involves a pre-B cell receptor bearing a surrogate light chain. Such is not present in birds and is questionable in swine (Chapter 7). The anatomical sites of B cell lymphogenesis have not been identified or whether the process is determinant or continuous throughout life. The heavy chain variable gene repertoire of bats is very diverse, complementary determining region three (CDR3) diversity is extensive and there is little evidence of somatic gene conversion that is used by birds to generate their antibody repertoire (Bratsch et al., 2011).

TABLE 1   IgM, IgA, IgE and IgD sequences used for the phylogenetic analysis shown in Fig. 2.

Species	IgM	IgA	IgE	IgD
Mouse	V00818	J00475	X01857	V00788
Panda	AY818392	AY818387	AY818389	AY818394
Opossum	AF012109	AF012110	AF035194	
Swine	U50149	U12594	U96100	AF411239
Cattle	U63637	AF109167	U63640	AF515672
Dog		L36871	L36872	DQ297185
Dolphin	AAG40853	AY621035		
Echidna	AF416952	AF416951	AY099258	
Horse	L49414	AY247966	AJ305046	AY631942
Human	X14940	J00220	J00222	BC063384.1
Platypus	AY168639	AY055778	AY055780	EU503149
Rabbit	J00666	X51647		
Rat		AJ510151.1	K02901	AY148494.1
Sheep	X59994	AF024645	M84356	AF41123
Camel	AB091831			

TABLE 1   *(Continued)*

Species	IgM	IgA	IgE	IgD
Cat	AB016712			
M. lucifugus	HM1344924	HM134924	HM134927	HM134925
E. fuscus	HM134943	HM134938	HM134941	HM134939
C. perspicillata	HM134947	HM134944	HM134945	
C. sphinx	HM134953	HM134948	HM134950	
P. alecto	GQ427150	GQ427150	SRR350710.3	

TABLE 2   IgG sequences used for the phylogenetic analysis shown in Fig. 3.

Species	IgG
Dog IGHGa	AF354264
Dog IGHGb	AF354265
Dog IGHGc	AF354266
Dog IGHGd	AF354267
Horse IGHG1	AJ302055
Horse IGHG2	AJ302056
Horse IGHG3	AJ312379
Horse IGHG4	AY445518
Horse IGHG5	AJ312380
Horse IGHG6	AJ312381
Horse IGHG7	AJ302058
Cattle IGHG1	X16701
Cattle IGHG2	M36946
Cattle IGHG3	U63638
Camel IGHG1a	AJ421266
Swine IGHG1a	U03781
Swine IGHG2a	U03779
Swine IGHG4a	U03782
Swine IGHG5a	EU372657

TABLE 2 *(Continued)*

Species	IgG
Swine IGHG6a	EU372655
Mouse IGHG1	J00453
Mouse IGHG2a	V00798
Mouse IGHG2b	V00763
Mouse IGHG2c	J00479
Mouse IGHG3	X00915
Opossum IGHG	AF035195
Possum IGHG	AF157619
Rabbit IGHG	L29172
Sheep IGHG1	X69797
Sheep IGHG2	X70983
Platypus IGHG	AY055781
Human IGHG1	J00228
Human IGHG2	J00230
Human IGHG3	X03604
Human IgHG4	K01316
P. alecto IGHG	GQ427152
C. sphinx IGHG2	HM134952
C. sphinx IGHG1	HM134951
M. lucifugus IGHG1	HM134929
M. lucifugus IGHG2	HM134931
M. lucifugus IGHG3	HM134933
M. lucifugus IGHG4	HM134934
E. fuscus IGHG	HM134942
C. perspicillata IGHG	HM134946

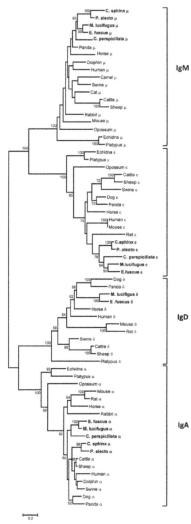

FIGURE 2   Genes encoding the heavy-chain genes of IgM, IgD, IgE and IgA of bats comprise a separate group with highest similarity with carnivores. The phylogenetic tree is based on alignment of IgA, IgE, IgD and IgM sequences from bats and representatives of other mammals. Protein sequences were aligned using the Muscle program (Edgar 2004) via the software package, MEGA v5.1 (Tamura et al., 2011), and using default parameters. Alignments were made using the CH1 and CH3 domains. Based on the protein alignments, phylogenetic trees were constructed by the maximum likelihood method using the MEGA5.1 program (Kumar et al., 2004). The numbers on the branch nodes indicate bootstrap values based on 1,000 replicates. Accession numbers for the sequences used are given in Table 1.

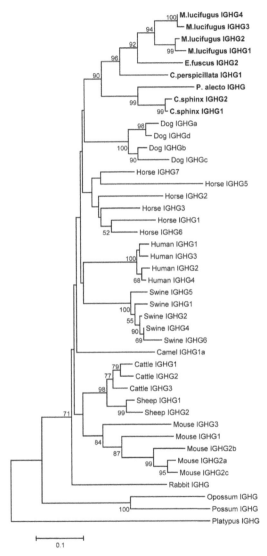

FIGURE 3 A phylogenetic tree shows that the IgG subclasses of bats diversified after speciation as in other eutherian mammals. Protein sequences were aligned using the Muscle program (Edgar, 2004) via the software package, MEGA v5.1 (Tamura et al., 2011), and using default parameters. Alignments were made using the CH1, CH2 and CH3 domains, excluding the hinge region. Based on the protein alignments, the phylogenetic tree was constructed by the nearest neighbor method using the MEGA5.1 program (Kumar et al., 2004). The numbers on the branch nodes indicate bootstrap values based on 1,000 replicates. Accession numbers for the sequences compared are given in Table 2.

Bos tarus	γ1	DPTCKPSPCDCCP
	γ2	GVSSDCSKPNNQH
	γ3−1	TARRPVPTTPKTTIPPGKPTTP
	γ3−2	KSEVEKTPCQCSKCP
Human	γ1	EPKSCDKTHTCPPCP
	γ2	ERKCCVECPPCP
	γ3−1	ELKTPLGDTTHTCPRCP
	γ3−2,−3,−4	EPKSCDTPPPCPRCP
	γ4	ESKYGPPCPSCP
European Domestic Swine	γ1ᵃ	GTKTKPPCPICPGCEVAG
	γ1ᵇ	GIHQPQTCPICPGCEVAG
	γ2ᵃ or γ2ᵇ	GTKTKPPCPICPACESPG
	γ3	DIEPPTPICPEICSCPAAEVLGA
	γ4ᵃ	GTKTKPPCPICPGCEVGP
	γ4ᵇ	GIHQPQTCPICPGCEVGP
	γ5ᵃ	GRPCPICPGCEGPG
	γ5ᵇ	GKKTKPTCPICPCCEVAG
	γ6ᵃ	GRPCPICPACEGPG
	γ6ᵇ	GRPCPICPACEGNG

M. musculus	γ1	VPRDCGCKPCICT
	γ2a	EPRGPTIKPCPPCKCP
	γ2b	EPSGPISTINPCPPCKECHKCP
	γ2c	EPRVPITQNPCPPLKECPPCA
	γ3	EPRIPKPSTPPGSSCP
M. lucifugus	γ1	PLIPGPPPTKCPPHTCPPCENPGG
	γ2	PSTPVIRPTICPPHTCPACENPGG
	γ3	PVIKEPTCPPHTCPPCENPGG
	γ4	PLFEEKPTCPPHTCPPCENPGG
E. fuscus	γ1 or γ2	PVTGGPTPPPCKCPACETLGG
C. perspicillata	γ1	PVPSEHEPNPCTCPVESSGG
C. sphinx	γ1	PTTYKCRDPDGKPRPCPPCPAPELLGG
	γ2	PTTYKCRDPDQPRPCPPCPAPELLGG
P. alecto	γ1	PTKYTCDNGGNPCPAPDLLGG

FIGURE 4 Comparison of the hinge regions of bats IgG subclasses with those for other mammals. Sequence motifs shared by the hinge regions of different subclasses within a species are underlined. The −1, −2, etc. associated with subclasses in cattle and humans indicate the use of alternative hinge exons and many reflect allotypic differences. Superscripts for swine Cγ genes denote allotypic variants. In some cases, the hinge of different allelic or subclass variants does not differ, which is indicated by "or." Noteworthy is that hinge region motifs are shared among subclasses in the same species but not among species. See Table 2 for sources of hinge sequences compared.

3.1.3   HIBERNATION AND THE IMMUNE RESPONSE

Bats include families that contain hibernators. The torpid state is known to affect local/mucosal immunity in that intraepithelial lymphocytes (IELs) are less mature and express few activation markers (Kurtz and Carey, 2007). It is generally held that hibernation is a response to the availability of food, which indirectly provides the energy for all physiological activities including immune function (Lochmilla and Deerenberg, 2000). In the most-studied hibernator, for example, ground squirrel, there are also periodic arousals, which may be stimulated by infectious agents that ramp up immune function (Luis and Hudson, 2006). This might explain arousal in WNS-infected bats that indirectly leads to their death by emaciation since arousal occurs when flying insects are not available (Veilleux, 2008). Bats that are aroused early from hibernation due to WNS have recently been demonstrated to display a immune reconstitution inflammatory syndrome, which causes tissue destruction and subsequent death (Meteyer et al., 2012). This may explain the elevated leucocyte levels in bats from WNS-infected caves (Moore et al., 2013). In any case, studies on the effect of hibernation on the immune response in any mammal, have not been pursued at the molecular and cellular level like those in mice.

3.1.4 THE ANTIBODY RESPONSE OF BATS

Some of the earliest studies on the immune response of bats examined the nature of the antibody response. Neutralizing antibodies to viruses have been detected in wild caught and experimentally infected megabats, demonstrating that bats are capable of mounting an antibody response (Halpin et al., 2000; Leroy et al., 2005; McColl et al., 2002; Middleton et al., 2007; Williamson et al., 1998; Williamson et al., 2000). However, neutralizing antibody responses have been reported to be lower in bats compared to other species (Halpin et al., 2011; Williamson et al., 1998). In addition, a delay in the development of primary and secondary antibody responses following experimental infection or vaccination has been reported in bats compared to conventional laboratory mammals (Hatten et al., 1968; Wellehan et al., 2009; Chakraborty and Chakravarty, 1984).

The role of antibodies in providing protection against subsequent infection in bats is also unclear. Evidence for the simultaneous presence of virus and antigen has been reported with speculation that this could be due to the formation of low avidity virus-antibody complexes, which dissociate readily or virus-specific antibody, which fails to neutralize infectivity (Sulkin et al., 1966). Several studies have also demonstrated that vaccinated bats are capable of clearing viral infection even in the absence of detectible neutralizing antibody suggesting a role for innate immunity (Aguilar-Setien et al., 2002, Turmelle et al., 2010b, Sétien et al., 1998, Seymour et al., 1978). Although these studies provided evidence that bats develop protective immunity following vaccination, the failure to often detect an antibody response in some bats is striking. Although this result may be a technical artifact it could indicate that the nature of protective immunity in bats differs from other mammals. Evidence for an increase in the affinity of antibodies for ϕX174 has been reported in the big brown bat, *Eptesicus fuscus,* indicating that somatic mechanisms for improving antigen specificity exist in bats (Hatten et al., 1970). Currently, our understanding of antibody diversity and antibody responses in bats requires further work and a panel of Ig-specific reagents.

3.2   THE CLASS AND SUBCLASS OF IG GENES OF BATS

3.2.1   GENOMIC COMPOSITION OF IG ISOTYPES

The major classes and subclasses of Chiropteran Ig from five species have been cloned and sequenced and compared to sequences for Ig isotypes in humans (Fig. 1). Evidence so far indicates that IgD may be unique to microbats but absent from the genomes and transcriptome datasets of the megabats (Baker et al., 2010; Bratsch et al., 2011; Papenfuss et al., 2012). Although a broader survey of megabats will be required to rule out the absence of IgD in this group, it should be remembered that IgD is not present in birds and rabbits. Thus, it may not be exceptional that megabats have lost this Ig isotype. Figure 1 shows that the gene structure for the constant regions of all bat species fit the canonical pattern for eutherian mammals using human Ig sequences for comparison. Since multiple IgG subclasses were identified, especially in *M. lucifugus,* their comparison to those of humans and other mammals are treated in subsequent figures.

IgD is present in the genome of most mammals and has a long evolutionary history dating to bony fishes and amphibians and is probably the equivalent of IgW in sharks (Solem and Stenvik, 2006; Dooley and Flajnik, 2006). In common bony fishes, the African lungfish and the African clawed frog (*Xenopus laevis*), IgD has a mutidomain structure (Ohta and Flajnik, 2006; Zhao et al., 2006, 2009; Solem and Stenvik 2006; Ota et al., 2003). While bats are believed to belong to an older mammalian order, IgD recovered from *M. lucifugus* and *E. fuscus* is more mammal-like than the IgD in sharks, bony fishes and amphibians (Fig. 5).

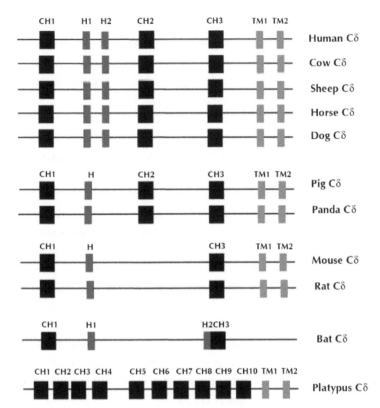

FIGURE 5 The domain structure of IgD in *M. lucifugus* is rodent-like but unique because of the fusion of the second hinge exon with the CH3 domain. The transmembrane exons were missing in the retrieved genomic sequence. IgD was only recovered from two bat species and only the genomic domain structure of *M. lucifugus* is indicated. From Butler et al. (2011).

3.2.2 PHYLOGENETIC TREES INDICATE BAT IG GENES FORM A SEPARATE GROUP

Only in Fig. 2, the sequences for the CH1 and CH3 domains were compared. The hinge or ancestral hinge was excluded from the comparisons. This was done because hinge variations among allotypes and subclasses of the same species can skew comparisons.

Figure 2 shows that bats form a separate group of eutherian mammals distinct from marsupials and monotremes. Within the bat group, the Yin and Yan suborders form separate branches. The Seba fruit bat (*Carollia perspicillata*) of the Yan suborder sometimes forms a branch with the Yan but in the case of IgE, groups with the Yin. In all cases, bat Igs do not allow them to be classified as "flying mice." Rather, IgD (Fig. 2) and IgG (Fig. 3) show a weak relationship to carnivores and bat IgA shows some relationship to IgA of ungulates (Laurasiatheria). Bat IgE shows no consistent relationship and is clearly distinct from ungulates IgE. Thus, a consistently close relationship between the Ig genes of bats and those of any other eutherian mammalian group is absent. Unfortunately, there are currently no data on the Igs of the Insectivores (shrews and moles) to which a closer relationship might be expected.

As in the case of other mammals, studies show that IgG subclasses in bats diversified after speciation (Fig. 3). Each species forms its own cluster and subclasses from a particular species group together not with IgGs from other species. The IgG from the short-tailed fruit bats *C. sphinx* and *P. alecto* of the Yin suborder form a separate branch from the one leading to the insectivorous members of the Yan suborder represented by *M. lucifugus* and *E. fuscus*. The neotropical, Seba's short-tailed fruit bat, *C. perspicillata* groups with the Yan suborder. Based on available data, IgG in *M. lucifugus* has diversified into as at least four subclasses (Butler et al., 2011). Comparing only IgG sequences provides the strongest evidence for a link between bats and carnivores (Fig. 3).

In all mammals, the hinge sequences of IgGs may be shared with the hinge of other subclasses in the same species but rarely with hinge sequences in other species. Figure 4 illustrates the hinge variations among IgG subclasses of bats, mice, domestic swine, cattle and humans A common motif is shared by IgG subclasses in humans, in swine (except for IgG3), three fifths of mouse subclasses and in the four IgG subclasses of *M. lucifugus*. Thus the analysis of the hinge of IgG subclasses in bats is consistent with the pattern seen in other eutherian mammals.

The available data on Chiropteran Igs indicates that their isotype and subisotype diversity is overwhelmingly characteristic of mammals, not that of birds or lower vertebrates. Thus, adaptation to flight in this mammal is not associated with any identifiable difference from other eutherian mammals.

3.2.3 EXPRESSION OF IG ISOTYPES

Quantitative analyses of the transcription of each of the Ig classes have been carried out in various tissues and cells from *P. alecto* (Wynne et al., 2013). IgG and IgM were most abundantly transcribed in lymph node, spleen and PBMCs while IgA was most abundantly transcribed in small intestine, lung and salivary gland. Although the expression of light chains has not been studied in detail, transcriptome data from *P. alecto* has demonstrated the transcription of the constant regions of both lambda and kappa light chains (Papenfuss et al., 2012). In addition, Ig from *P. alecto* recovered from protein γ affinity columns provide evidence for the expression of light chains at the protein level (Wynne et al., 2013).

Initial fractionation of serum from *P. giganteus* and *P. alecto* suggested that megabats possessed IgM, IgG and IgA similar to humans (Chakravarty and Sarka 1994; McMurray et al., 1982). A recent study used immobilized anti-Fab to recover Igs from megabat serum and to characterize these by SDS-PAGE. This confirmed the presence of IgG and IgM, while IgA was not recovered although a similar procedure led to the recovery of IgA from human serum (Wynne et al., 2013). 2-D electrophoresis detected multiple isoforms of IgM and IgG, most likely due to variable region charge or subclass diversity as in other mammals (Butler 1985; Butler et al., 1987). While IgA was not recovered from serum by the method employed, transcription of IgA and the polyIg receptor in mucosal tissues appeared normal. Thus bat serum IgA levels are low as in mice and most other mammals and do not resemble the very high levels seen in humans (Radl et al., 1974; Butler et al., 2013). For example, serum IgA levels in rabbits, rats and mice are only 0.01 mg/mL versus 2.91 mg/mL in humans (Butler et al., 2013). Thus bat serum IgA levels appear similar to all other eutherian mammals except human and other primates.

The availability of polyclonal anti-IgG and IgM for megabats will now make it possible to accurately quantify Ig levels and to determine the isotype of antibodies involved in viral neutralization and other antibody-dependent serological assays (Wynne et al., 2013). However, the situation for insectivorous and other microbats persists because of the volume of blood that would be needed for the type of Ig purification procedure described by Wynne et al., for megabats. Purification from microbats would require mass exsanguination, a procedure not likely to gain animal care approval. Fortunately in the last 25 years, the Ig repertoire can be characterized from their encoding genes, regardless of the size of the animals and Igs can be synthesized in vitro. These engineered Igs can be used to make mAbs and to serve as reference standards (Butler et al., 2012). Such procedures and reagents can allow the level of the major isotypes in serum or secretions of microbats or minor isotypes or IgG subclasses in megabats to be determined as well as the isotype antibody response to any antigen of interest.

3.3   THE VARIABLE IG REPERTORIE OF BATS

3.3.1   GENOMIC DIVERSITY IN M. LUCIFUGUS AND GENUS PTEROPUS

Information at this time is only available for genes encoding the heavy chain variable region genes of one insectivorous bat (*M. lucifugus*) and one genus of Asian fruit bats (*P. alecto* and *P. vampyrus*). As described below, these are highly diverse. Assignment of V_H genes to discrete families when quite different species are involved can be difficult since VH genes in some species have diversified into families that lack close homology to those from well-studies species that are used as a reference. This is true for the clade II genes that comprise the majority of VH-*x* genes in cattle, sheep and horses (Fig. 6). With the exception of families found in all three-bat species that fit into this VH-*x* category, all other bat VH families had close homology to established families in humans. Initial studies on the little brown bat (*M. lucifugus*) revealed a surprisingly diverse repertoire with orthologs of five of the seven human VH gene families belonging to all three VH clades (Bratsch et al., 2011; Fig. 6). The VH3 family was large and was grouped into six subfamilies, 3–1; 3–2; 3–3; 3–4; 3–5; and 3–6. Some VH3 subfamilies had homology to VH genes in dog, others to VH3 in mouse and others to VH3 in marsupials (Fig. 6). Based on the probability of random recovery Bratsch et al. (2011) estimated there were 236 VH3 genes in the genome. A 7X coverage of the *M. lucifugus* genome identified 220 VH genes from five families. It is possible that by filling existing gaps, the number may increase. The higher estimate by Bratsch et al. (2011) could in part be due to the recovery of different alleles of VH3 genes.

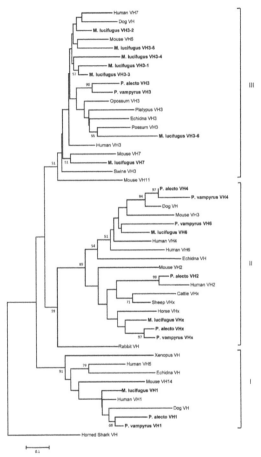

FIGURE 6 Comparison of sequences of bat V_H genes with V_H genes of other species. Comparisons are made using sequences for the major VH genes in other vertebrates Accession numbers for those used are given in Table 3. The percent sequence similarity is integrated into the dendrogram. VH-x genes of clade II comprise are not sufficiently homologous to any human clade II family. VH-x comprises the majority of VH genes in artiodactyls and the horse. Alignments were made using sequences corresponding to the framework regions (FR) 1–3 of the V domains, inclusive of complementary determining regions (CDR) 1 and 2. Based on the protein alignments, the phylogenetic tree was constructed using the neighor joining tree method using the MEGA5.1 program (Kumar et al., 2004). The numbers on the branch nodes indicate bootstrap values based on 1,000 replicates.

TABLE 3   VH sequences used for phylogenetic analysis shown in Fig. 6.

Species	Accession Number
Mouse VH3 (3660)	K01569
Mouse VH2 (Q52)	M27021
Mouse VH7 (S107)	J00538
Mouse VH14 (SM7)	M31285
Mouse VH11	Y00743
Mouse VH5 (X24)	X00163
Rabbit VH	AY359298
Cattle VH	AF015505
Sheep VH	Z49180
Pig VH	U15194
Dog VH	AC194586
Possum VH	AAL87470
Opossum VH	AF12122
Platypus VH	AF381291
Echidna VH	AAM61760
	AAM60783
	AY101439
	AY101442
	AY101445
Horned shark VH	X13449
M. lucifugus VH3–1	GQ923681
M. lucifugus VH3–2	GQ923685
M. lucifugus VH3–3	GQ923662
M. lucifugus VH3–4	GQ923672
M. lucifugus VH3–5	GQ923661
M. lucifugus VH3–6	GQ923671

TABLE 3 *(Continued)*

Species	Accession Number
P. alecto VH4	GQ427151
P. alecto VH1	GQ427152
P. alecto VH2	GQ427155
P. alecto VH3	GQ427168
P. alecto VHx	GQ427162

Human sequences were obtained from VBASE (Tomlinson et al., 1996). *M. lucifugus* sequences corresponding to other VH families were obtained from the *M. lucifugus* whole genome available in the Ensembl database. All *P. Vampyrus* VH sequences were obtained from the *P. Vampyrus* genome available in Ensembl.

Similar to *M. lucifugus*, the VH genes of the large fruit bats are also distributed in all three mammalian VH clades and a higher number of VH genes belong to clade III (which includes the VH3 family) than to clades I and II (Baker et al., 2010). The transcriptome sequence data from immune tissues and mitogen stimulated *P. alecto* cells have provided further evidence for the transcription of diverse VH gene repertoire (Papenfuss et al., 2012).

The Ig loci corresponding to the heavy and light chains are fragmented onto multiple scaffolds in the *P. vampyrus*, *P. alecto* and *M. lucifugus* genomes. However, preliminary evidence indicates that each of the genomes contain scaffolds with multiple V segments arranged in tandem. This arrangement is consistent with a translocon organization similar to other mammals. The genomic diversity of the VH segments have been examined in Pteropid bats using the *P. vampyrus* genome sequence. Thirty-three scaffolds ranging from 1.22–54.06 kB containing VH segments were identified in the *P. vampyrus* genome resulting in the identification of 74 unique VH sequences including 11 which contained stop codons and are presumably pseudogenes. Representative VH sequences were found in all three mammalian VH clades (I, II and III; see above and Fig. 6). The most complete VH sequences shared 49–99% nucleotide identity and belong to five of the seven human VH families (Baker et al., 2010). The amphibian *X. laevis* has VH segments corresponding to all three VH clans, consistent with the appearance of VH groups, I, II and III early in tetrapod evolution (Haire et al., 1990). The VH genes of rabbits, Ungulates and marsupials are mainly found in a single VH family while humans and rodents have between 7 and 14 VH families within the three VH clans (Butler, 2006). Cats and dogs also have representative VH genes in all three mammalian VH clans, but the majority of their VH genes belong to clan III and they have only limited diversity in clans I and II (cats have three clade I genes and a single clade II gene while dogs have only a single member in both clade I and II; Das et al., 2008). Thus, bats belong in the group with rodents and primates in retaining a highly diverse VH repertoire (Das et al., 2008).

3.3.2 GENOMIC LIGHT CHAIN DIVERSITY

The diversity of light chains in bats of either suborder have not been examined in detail. However, transcriptome sequencing of immune tissues and mitogen stimulated cells from *P. alecto* has provided evidence for the transcription of both kappa (Vκ) and lambda (Vλ) light chains (Papenfuss et al., 2012). The assembled *P. alecto* transcriptome dataset contained a higher number of Vλ (38) compared to Vκ (6) sequences. Preliminary analysis of the genomes of *P. alecto* and *P. vampyrus* has also provided evidence for greater complexity in the lambda than the kappa locus (unpublished data). The use of the two light chains differs between species, some preferentially using one light chain over the other. Mice and rabbits predominantly use kappa, whereas horses, sheep and cattle primarily use lambda. The use of lambda and kappa appears to correlate with the overall complexity of the loci in most species (Butler, 2006). The genomic and transcriptome data available from *P. alecto* is consistent with the possibility that *P. alecto* may use lambda in a higher proportion of its light chains than kappa, consistent with the Laurasiatherian group. However, it is not known whether lambda rearranges before kappa in bats, as in swine, and whether there is a pre-B cell receptor (Sun et al., 2012)

3.3.3 CDR3 DIVERSITY

Utilizing a VH3FR1/Cγ1 primer set allowed the CDR3 region of VDJ rearrangements involving VH3 genes in *M. lucifugus* to be analyzed. These studies showed extensive diversity, and allowed for the identification of several DH motifs and 13 putative JH segments in 62 sequences (Bratsch et al., 2011; Fig. 7A). The same strategy was applied to *P. alecto*, a fruit bat belonging to the family Pteropodidae (Baker et al., 2010). Twenty-three CDR3 sequences recovered for *P. alecto* are shown in Fig. 7B. These suggest at least five JH segments. Perhaps if 3-fold more CDR3 sequences had been obtained from *P. alecto*, more JH segments would have been recovered. Length diversity is variable in both *M. lucifugus* and *P. alecto*. The number of functional JH segments in other species ranges from only one in chickens to nine six in humans (Reynaud et al., 1989; Lefranc and Lefranc, 2001; Butler, 2006). Therefore, the number of JH segments in bats appears to be very large compared to other mammals so far examined.

A.

FR3	CDR3		FR4	J_H	Nr.	CDR3 Length
GCAACA	GGGATCGCAGCTGGTT	ACTACGGTATGGACTAC	TGGGGCCAGGGGACCCTGGTCACCGTCTCCTCA	J_H1	3	24-36
GCAACA	GGGT	ACTACGGTTTGGACTAC	TGGGGCCAGGGGACCCTGGTCACCGTCTCCTCA	J_H2	2	21
GCAACA	**GATTGGGGTCATGGCCG**	CTTCGATGTA	TGGGGCCAGGGCACCATGGTCACCGTCTCCTCA			
GCAACA	GAGATA **ACTACGGTG** GACTACTA	CTTCGATGTA	TGGGGCCAGGGCACCATGGTCACCGTCTCCTCA	J_H3	16	24-42
GCAACA	GATGAATTTACT **GACTGGGTGGGATC** TGGGCA	CTTCGATGTA	TGGGGCCAGGGCACCATGGTCACCGTCTCCTCA			
GCAACA	A **GATAGTGGCGG**	CTTTGACTAC	TGGGGCCAGGGCACCATGGTCACCGTCTCCTCA	J_H4	9	12-36
GCAACA	GAGGGGCTGGGTGTCGA	CTTCGATGTC	TGGGGCCAGGGCACCATGGTCACCGTCTCCTCA	J_H5	3	12-30
GCAACA	GAATTGATTTTTGGAGGGGCATACTT	CTTCGATGTA	TGGGGCCAGGGCACCCTGGTCACGGTCTCCTCA	J_H6	5	21-36
GCAACA	GATCTGTATACAGGAGCTACCCGCCG	CTTCGATTTA	TGGGGCCAGGGCACCCTGGTCACGGTCTCCTCA	J_H7	3	24-36
GCAACA	GAGCGGATACGGGAATTACGGGCTTA	CATGGAATAC	TGGGGCCAGGGCACCCTGGTCACGGTCTCCTCA	J_H8	3	21-36
GCAACA	**GATAGTTGGGTGGG**	CTTGGATTAC	TGGGGTCCGCGGACCCTGGTCACCGTCTCCTCA	J_H9	6	21-33
GCAACA	TATA **ACTACGGTG** ACGA	TGCTTTTGATGTG	TGGGGCCCAGGGACCCTGGTCACCGTCTCCCAA	J_H10	9	15-36
GCAACA	AGGAGCGATTGGGGTAGTGGTCA	TGCTTACTTCGAGCAC	TGGGGCCAGGGCACCCTGGTCACCGTCTCCTCA	J_H11	3	24-39
GCAACA	**CCACTTAGTAGCGGGTGGTCCTTTGG**	TTAC	TGGGGCCAGGGCACCCTGGTCACCGTCTCGTCA	J_H12	3	18-30
GCAACA	CGACT	CAAAGTC	GGAGGCCAGGGCAGCCTGGTCACCGTCCCGTCA	J_H13	2	12

The germline sequence of J_H1 and J_H2 with their RSS. Heptamer and nonamer sequences are in bold face. The underlined sequence corresponds to the expressed J_H genes.

J_H1 **CAGTTTTTG**tggggtgaggatggagattgagc**TGTTGTG**AGGACTACGGTATGGACTACTGGGGCCAGGGGACCCTGGTCACCGTCTCCTCA

J_H2 **TTTG**tggggtgaggatggagattgagc**TGTTGTG**AGGACTACGGTTTGGACTACTGGGGCCAGGGGACCCTGGTCACCGTCTCCTCA

B.

FR3	CDR3	FR4	JH	Nr	CDR3 length
TACTGT	GCACGGACGGGCCTTAAAGTGGGCTACTCGTACGTCGACGTC	TGGGGCCAGGGTTCGCCAGTCACCGTCTCCTCA	J_H1	2	36-48
TACTGT	GCGAGAGGTATAGCTGGAGATAACTTGGATTTC	TGGGGCCAGGGAACCGTGGTCACCGTCTCCTCA	J_H2	6	18-54
TACTGT	GCGGCGGCGTGGTTTGACTCC	TGGGGCCAGGGAGCCCTGGTCACCGTCTCCTCG	J_H3	9	15-51
TACTGT	GCGAGATCCTACGGATTTGATCTC	TGGGGCCAGGGAACCGTGGTCACCGTCTCCTCA	J_H4	3	18-42
CACTGT	ACCCAAGAGTCGTATGGGTGGAGCCGGAACGATCGTTTCTACGGCATGGACGTC	TGGGGTCGGGGAGTCTTGGTCAGCGTCTCCCCAG	J_H5	1	48

FIGURE 7 CDR3 diversity in *M. lucifugus* (A) and in *P. alecto* (B). The end of FR3 has been identified by the ACA codon (threonine) and FR4 by the TGG (tryptophan) codon for *M. lucifugus*. Segments derived from putative DH segments are in bold. In the case of *P. alecto*, TGT was recognized as the end of FR3. In both cases the number of different JH genes identified is indicated as well as CDR3 length.

The amino acid composition of the CDR3 sequences from *P. alecto* differs from other species by containing fewer tyrosines and a greater proportion of arginine and alanine residues (Baker et al., 2010). Tyrosine confers structural diversity and is directly involved in antigen binding through interaction through with its aromatic ring or through polar atoms in its side chain (Mian et al., 1991; Zemlin et al., 2003). Some suggest that arginine residues may lower binding site specificity and are associated with self-reactivity (Birtalan et al., 2008; Radic et al., 1993). The presence of fewer tyrosines and a higher number of arginine's in the bat CDR3 regions may have resulted in the evolution of antibodies with lower polyreactivity that form only a weak association with antigen. Such antibodies may be less promiscuous, of lower avidity and could explain observations that bats fail to produce neutralizing antibody following infection with certain viruses (Sulkin et al., 1966).

3.3.4 ESTIMATION OF SHM

Difference among 75 germline VH3 genes from *M. lucifugus* allowed the identification of putative parent germline genes for 67 unique VH3 transcripts based on their characteristic FR3 and CDR2 sequences. Based on this comparison, we calculated an overall nucleotide mutation frequency of 26 ± 12, similar to that seen in newborn piglets (Bratsch et al., 2011). This is surprising since the samples were collected from free-living conventional bats. Mutations typically accumulate in CDR regions during adaptive response. However, the frequency in *M. lucifugus* was 2–10 fold lower than in piglets exposed to environmental antigens. Parallel data for megabats and a more extensive study on somatic mutation in bats is warranted.

3.4 SUMMARY AND CONCLUSIONS

The Ig genes of representatives of the two major suborders have been analyzed; Yinpterochiroptera (Yin) and Yangochiroptera (Yan). The former includes the family Pteropodidae which comprises the so-called megabats or flying foxes. The Yangochiroptera include the insectivorous microbats and the South American fruit bat. The genes encoding the constant region of both megabats and microbats group together and are separate from other eutherian mammals. This observation rejects the hypothesis that bats are diphyletic, i.e. that Yin megabats arose from primates/lemurs and the Yan microbats arose from the Insectivora.

Microbats possess the major five Ig isotypes common to most eutherian mammals while studies on megabats are incomplete with regard to IgD. The structure of IgD in microbats is similar to that in other eutherian mammals and distinctly different from the multi-domain structure of IgD seen in lower vertebrates.

The VH genes of both suborders include members of clades I-III although clade III that includes the VH3 family seems dominant in both Yin and Yan bats. The number of VH3 genes in *M. lucifugus* using recovery statistics and genome studies indicate the number exceeds 200. Both indicate a very large VH genome in bats. Data on DH and JH diversity is incomplete but at least 13 putative JH segments were identified among 62 samples from *M. lucifugus* and five from 23 recovered from *P. alecto*. Overall, this degree of diversity places bats in the mouse/human category in which many VH genes from many families are present. This is quite distinct from mammals that use a single VH gene family.

We conclude that the available data on their Ig repertoire places both bat suborders in the same category as other eutherian mammals. Thus, their adaptation to flight does not distinguish them from other mammals as regards their Ig repertoire. However, VH and JH gene diversity is extremely large, perhaps the largest among mammals and similar to that for bony fishes. Exactly how this might influence the preimmune repertoire or adaptive antibody response is unknown. The high level of VH diversity in all bats could mean that bats rely more on combinatorial diversity rather than somatic hypermutation to generate antibody diversity. In lower vertebrates, activation-induced cytidine deaminase (AID) and Tdt appears less active than in homoeothermic higher vertebrates, forcing them to depend on combinatorial mechanisms to generate their diverse antibody repertoire. Perhaps this dependence has carried over into bats. The paucity of tyrosine residues in CDR3 of *P. alecto* are another feature that may influence the specificity of the bat antibody response. The extent to which the extraordinary variable heavy chain repertoire, the low frequency of SHM and the paucity of tyrosines in CDR3 affects the bat immune response to zoonotic viral infections, the antigens of *G. destructus* and other antigens of pathogens, needs further investigation. The loss of insectivorous bats to WNS could be ecologically devastating. Likewise, failure to understand the immunobiology of emerging disease that use bats as vectors, could compromise the health of humans.

This review of the Ig genes of bats represents a step toward achieving a greater understanding of the bat immune system and we hope it will provide a stimulus for more directed studies.

KEYWORDS

- antibody repertoire
- immunoglobulin genes
- *M. lucifugus*
- *P. alecto*
- Yin and Yan

REFERENCES

Adkins, R.M., Honeycutt, R.L., (1991): Molecular phylogeny of the superorder Archonta. *Proc. Nat'l. Acad. Sci.* 88, 10317–10321.

Aguilar-Setien, A., Leon, Y., Tesoro, E., Kretschmer, R., Brochier B., Pastoret, P., (2002): Vaccination of vampire bats using recombinant vaccinia-rabies virus. *J Wildl Dis*, 38, 539–544.

Baker, M., Tachedjian, M., Wang, L.-F., (2010): Immunoglobulin heavy chain diversity in Pteropid bats: evidence for a diverse and highly specific antigen binding repertoire. *Immunogenetics* 62, 173–184.

Banack, S. A., (1998): Diet selection and resource use by flying foxes (Genus Pteropus). *Ecology* 79(6), 1949–1967.

Birtalan, S., Zhang, Y., Fellouse, F.A., Shao, L., Schaefer, G., Sidhu, S.S., (2008): The intrinsic contributions of tyrosine, serine, glycine and arginine to the affinity and specificity of antibodies. *J. Mol. Biol.* 377, 1518–1528.

Blehert, D.S., Hicks, A.C., Behr, M., Meteyer, C.U., Berlowski-Zier, B.M., Buckles, E.L., Coleman, J.T.H., Darling, S.R., Gargas, A., Niver, R., Okoniewski, J.C., Rudd, R.J., Stone, W.B., (2009): Bat White-Nose Syndrome: An Emerging Fungal Pathogen? *Science* 323, 227.

Blehert, D.S., 2012 Fungal disease and the developing story of bat white-nose syndrome. PLoS Pathog. 8(7):e1002779. doi: 0.1371/journal.ppat.1002779. Epub 2012 Jul 19.

Bratsch, S., Wertz, N., Chaloner, K., Kunz, T.H., Butler, J.E., (2011): The little brown bat displays a highly diverse VH, DH and JH repertoire but little evidence of somatic hypermutation. *Dev. Com. Immunol.* 35, 421–430.

Butler, J.E., (1985): Biochemistry and biology of ruminant immunoglobulins. Prog. Vet. Microbiol. Immun. Vol. 2, pp. 1–53 (R. Pandey, Ed.), Karger, Basel.

Butler, J.E., Wertz, N., Zhao, Y., Kunz, T.H., Bratsch, S., Whitaker, J., Schountz, T., (2011): Two suborders of bats have the canonical isotypes repertoire of other eutherian mammals. *Dev. Com. Immunol.* 35, 272–284.

Butler, J.E., Wertz, N., Sun, X-Z, Lunney, J.K., Muyldermanns, S., (2012): Resolution of an immunodiagnostic dilemma: Heavy chain chimeric antibodies for species in which plasmacytomas are unknown. *Mol. Immunol.* 53, 140–148.

Butler, J.E., (2006): Preface: Why I agreed to do this. In: J.E.Butler, Guest Ed. Antibody Repertoire Development. *Dev. Com. Immunol.* Special Edition 30, 1–17.

Butler, J. E., Borca, M. V. Heyermann. H. Dillender, M. Bielecka, M., (1987): The heterogeneity of bovine IgG2. III. The basis of the ion-exchange heterogeneity of bovine IgG2a is the result of V_H-region Variation. *Mol. Immunol.* 24:1317–1326.

Butler, J.E., Rainard, P., Lippolis, J., Salmon, H., Kacskovics, I. 2013. The mammary gland in mucosal and regional immunity. In. Mucosal Immunology (M. Russell, J. Mestecky, et al., ed.) Academic Press (in press).

Calisher, C.H., Childs, J.E., Field, H.E., Homes, K.V., Schountz, T., (2006): Bats: Important reservoir host of emerging viruses. *Clin. Microbial. Reviews* 19, 531–545.

Chakraborty, A.K., Chakravarty, A.K., (1984): Antibody-mediated response in the bat, *Pteropus giganteus*. *Dev. Com. Immunol.* 8, 415–423.

Chakravarty, A., Sarkar, S., (1994): Immunofluorescence analysis of immunoglobulin bearing lymphocytes in the Indian fruit bat: *Pteropus giganteus*. *Lymphology* 27, 97–104.

Cleveland, C.J., Frank, J.D., Federico, P., Gomez, I., Hallam, T.G., Horn, J., Lopez, J., Mc-Cracken, G.F., Medellin, R.A., Moreno-Valdez, A., Sansone, C., Westbrook, J. K., Kunz, T.H., (2006): Economic value of the pest control service provided by Brazilian free-tailed bat in south-central Texas. *Front. Ecol. Environ.* 4, 238–243.

Das, S., Nozawa, M., Klein, J., Nei, M., (2008): Evolutionary dynamics of the immunoglobulin heavy chain variable region genes in vertebrates. *Immunogenetics* 60, 47–55.

Dobson, A.P., (2005): What links bats to emerging infectious diseases? *Science* 310, 628–629.

Dooley, H., Flajnik, M.F., (2006): Antibody repertoire development in cartilagenous fish. *Dev. Com. Immunol.* 30, 43–56.

Edgar, R.C., (2004): MUSCLE: multiple sequence alignment with high accuracy and high throughput. *Nucleic Acids Res.* 32.1792–1797.

Fleming, T.H., Geiselman, C., Kress, W.J., (2009): The evolution of bat pollination: a phylogenetic perspective. *Annals of Botany* 104, 1017–1043.

Frick, W.F., Pollock, J.F., Hicks, A., Langwig, K., Reynolds, D.S., Turner, G., Butchowski, C., Kunz, T.H., (2010): A common bat faces rapid extinction in the north-eastern United States from fungal pathogen. *Science* 328, 679–682.

Fujita, M.S., Tuttle, M.D., (1991): Flying foxes (Chiroptera: *Pteropodidae*): threatened animals of key ecological and economic importance. *Conservation Biology* 5, 455–463.

Gargas, A., Trest, M.T., Christensen, M., Volk, T.J., Blehert, D.S., (2009): *Geomyces destructans* sp. associated with bat white-nose syndrome. *Mycotaxon* 108, 147–154.

Gregory, W.K., (1910): The orders of mammals. *Bull. Amer. Museum Nat. History* 27, 1–524.

Halpin, K., Hyatt, A.D., Fogarty, R., Middleton, D., Bingham, J., Epstein, J.H., Rahman, S.A., Hughes, T., Smith, C., Field, H.E., Daszak, P., (2011): Pteropid Bats are Confirmed as the Reservoir Hosts of Henipaviruses: A Comprehensive Experimental Study of virus Transmission. *Am. J. Trop. Med. Hyg.* 85, 946–951.

Halpin, K., Hyatt, A.D., Plowright, R.K., Epstein, J.H., Daszak, P., Field, H., Wang, L., Daniels, P.W., (2008): Henipavirus Ecology Research Group 2007 Emerging viruses: coming in on a wrinkled wing and a prayer. *Clin. Infect. Dis.* 44, 711–717.

Halpin, K., Young, P.L., Field, H.E., Mackenzie, J.S., (2000): Isolation of Hendra Virus From Pteropid Bats: A Natural Reservoir of Hendra Virus. *J. Gen. Virol.* 81, 1927–1932.

Hatten, B.A., Allen R., Sulkin, S.E., (1968): Immune response in Chiroptera to bacteriophage X174. *J. Immunol.* 101, 141–150.

Hill, J.E., Smith, J.D., (1984): Bats: A natural history. Austin: Univ. Texas Press.

Jones, G., Jacobs, D.S., Kunz, T.H., Willig, M.R., Racey, P.A., (2009): Carpe noctem: The importance of bats as bioindicators. *Endangered Species Research.* 8, 93–115.

Kalka, M.B., Smith, A.R., Kalko, E.K.V., (2008): Bats limit arthropods and herbivory in a tropical forest. *Science* 320, 71.

Kumar, S., Tamura, K., Nei, M., (2004): MEGA3: integrated software for molecular evolutionary genetics analysis and sequence alignment. *Brief Bioinform* 5, 150–163.

Kunz, T.H., (ed.), (1982): Ecology of Bats. Plenum Press: New York.

Kunz, T.H., Lumsden, L.F., (2003): Ecology of cavity and foliage roosting bats. In: Kunz, T.H., Fenton, M.B., (eds.). Bat Ecology. Univ. Chicago Press. 3–89.

Kurta, A., Bell, G.P., Nagy, K.A., Kunz, T.H., (1989): Energetics of pregnancy and lactation in free-ranging little brown bats (*Myotis lucifugus*). *Physiol. Zool.* 62, 804–818.

Kurtz, C.C., Carey, H.V., (2007): Seasonal changes in the intestinal immune system of hibernating ground squirrels. *Dev. Com. Immunol.* 31, 415–428.

Lau, S.K.P., Woo, P.C., Li, K.C., Huang, Y., Tsoi, H.W., Wong, B.H., Wong, S.S., Leung, S.Y., ChanK, H., Yuen, K.Y., (2005): Severe acute respiratory syndrome coronavirus-like Virus in Chinese horseshoe bats. *Proc. Nat'l. Acad. Sci. USA* 102, 14040–14045.

Lefranc, M-P., LeFranc, G., (2001): The immunoglobulin Facts Book. Academic Press, NY; 457 pp.

Leroy, E.M., Kumulungui, B., Pourrut, X., Rouquet, P., Hassmanin, A., Yaba, P., Delicat, A., Paweska, J.T., Gonzales, J.P., Swanepoel, P., (2005): Fruit bats as reservoirs of Ebola Virus. *Nature* 438, 575–576.

Li, W., Shi, Z., Yu, M., Ren, W., Smith, C., Epstein, J.H., Wang, H., Eaton, G.B.T., Zhang, S., Wang, L.F., (2005): Bats are natural reservoirs of SARS-like coronaviruses. *Science* 310, 676–679.

Lochmilla, R.L., Deerenberg, C., (2000): Trade-offs in evolutionary immunology; just what is the cost of immunity. *Oikos* 88, 87–98.

Lorch, J.M., Meyer, C.U., Behr, M.J., Boyles, J.G., Cryan, P.M., et al., (2011): Experimental infection of bats with *Geomycs destructus* causes white-nosed syndrome. *Nature* 480, 376–378.

Luis, A.D., Hudson, P.J., (2006): Hibernation patterns in mammals: a role for bacterial growth? *Funct. Ecol.* 20, 471–477.

Mackenzie, J.S., Field, H., (2004): Emerging encephalitogenic viruses: lyssaviruses and henipa-viruses transmitted by frugivorous bats. *Arc. Virol. Suppl.* 18, 97–111.

McColl, K.A., Chamberlain, T., Lunt, R.A., Newberry, K.M., Middleton, D., Westbury, H.A., (2002): Pathogenesis studies with Australian bat lyssavirus in gray-headed flying foxes (*Pteropus poliocephalus*). *Australian Vet. J.* 80, 636–641.

McCormack, W.T., Tjoelker, L.W., Thompson, C.B., (1991): Avian B cell developmental generation of an immunoglobulin repertoire by gene conversion. *Annu. Rev. Immunol.* 9, 219–241.

McMurry, D.N., Stroud, J., Murphy, J.J.R., Carlomagno, MA., Greer, D.L., (1982): Role of immunoglobulin classes in experimental histoplasmosis in bats. *Dev. Comp. Immunol.* 6, 557–567.

Messenger, S.L., Rupprecht, C.E., Smith, J.S., (2003): Bats, emerging virus infections, and the rabies paradigm., In: Kunz, T.H., Fenton, M.B., (eds.). *Bat Ecology*. Chicago: Universiy of Chicago Press, 622–679.

Meteyer, C.U., Barber, D., Mandl, J.N., (2012): Pathology in euthermic bats with white nose syndrome suggests a natural manifestation of immune reconstitution inflammatory syndrome. *Virulence* 3, 583–588.

Mian, I.S., Bradwell, A.R., Olson, A.J. 1991. Structure, function and properties of antibody binding sites. *J. Mol. Biol.* 217, 133–151.

Middleton, D.J., Morrissy, C.J., Van der Heide, B.M., Russell, G.M., Braun, M.A., Westbury, H.A., et al., (2007): Experimental Nipah Virus Infection in Pteropid Bats (*Pteropus poliocephalus*). *J. Com. Path.* 136, 266–272.

Mindell, D.P., Dick, C.W., Baker, R.J., (1991): Phylogenetic relationships among megabats, microbats and primates. Proc. Nat'l. Acad. Sci. (USA) 88, 10322–10326.

Moore, M.S., Reichard, J.D., Murtha, T.D., Nabhan, M.L., Plan, R.E., Ferreira, J.S., et al. (2013): Hibernating little brown myotis (*Myotic lucifugus*) shows variable immunological responses to white-nosed syndrome. PloS ONE 8(3), e58976. doi:10.1371

Mueller, M.A., Paweska, J.T., Leman, P.A., Drosten, C., Grywna, K., Kemp, A., et al, (2007): Coronavirus antibodies in African bat species. *Emerg. Infect. Dis.* 13, 1367–1370.

Murphy, W.J., Pringle, T.H., Crider, T.A., Springer, M.S., Miller, W., (2007): Using genomic data to unravel the root of the placental mammal phylogeny. *Genome Res.* 174, 413–421.

Muscarella, R., Fleming, T.H., (2007): The Role of Frugivorous Bats in Tropical Forest Succession. *Biol. Rev. Camb. Philos. Soc.* 82, 573–590.

Ohta, Y., Flajnik, M., (2006): IgD like IgM is a primordial immunoglobulin class perpetuated in most jawed vertebrates. *Proc. Natl. Acad. Sci. USA* 103, 10723–19728.

Ota, T., Rast, J.P., Litman, G.W., Amemiya, C.T., (2003): Lineage restricted retention of a primitive immunoglobulin heavy chain isotype within the Dipnoi reveals an evolutionary paradox. *Proc. Nat'l Acad. Sci. USA* 100, 2501–2506.

Papenfuss, A.T., Baker, M.L., Feng, Z.-P., Tachedjian, M., Crameri, G., Cowled, C., et al., (2012): The immune gene repertoire of an important viral reservoir, the Australian black flying fox. *BMC Genomics*.

Pettigrew, J.D., (1986): Flying primates? Megabats have advanced pathway from eye to midbrain. *Science* 231, 1304–1306.

Puechmaillie, S.J., Frick, W.F., Kunz, T.H., Racey, P.A., Voigt, C.C., Wibbett, G., et al., (2011): White-nosed syndrome: is this emerging disease a threat to European bats? *Trends Ecol. Evol.* xx, 1–7.

Radic, M.Z., Mackle, J., Erikson, J., Mol, C., Anderson, W.F., Weigert, M., (1993): Residues that mediate DNA binding of autoimmune antibodies. *J. Immunol.* 150, 4966–4977

Radl, J., Schuit, H.R.E, Mestecky J, Hijmans W. (1974): The origin of monomeric and polymeric forms of IgA in man. *Adv. Med. Bio.* 45, 57–65.

Ratcliffe, M.J.H., (2006): Antibodies, immunoglobulin genes and the bursa of Fabricius in chicken B cell development. *Dev. Com. Immunol.* 30, 101–118.

Reynaud, C-A., Dahan, A., Anquez, V., Weill, J.C., (1989): Somatic hyperconversion diversifies the single VH gene of the chicken with a high incidence in the D region. *Cell* 59, 171–183.

Shaw, T.I., Srivastava, A., Chou, W.-C., Liu, L., Hawkinson, A., Glenn, T.C., et al. (2012): Transcriptome Sequencing and Annotation for the Jamaican Fruit Bat (*Artibeus jamaicensis*). *PLoS ONE* 7, e48472.

Sétien, A. A., Brochier, B., Tordo, N., De Paz, O., Desmettre, P., Péharpré, D., et al. (1998): Experimental rabies infection and oral Vaccination in Vampire bats (*Desmodus rotundus*). *Vaccine*, 16, 1122–1126.

Seymour, C., R., Dickerman, W., Martin, M. S., (1978): Venezuelan Encephalitis Virus Infection in Neotropical Bats. The American Journal of Tropical Medicine and Hygiene 27, 297–306.

Shi, Z., Hu, Z., (2008): A review of studies on animal reservoirs of the SARS coronavirus. *Virus Res.* 133, 74–87.

Shilton, L.A., Altringham, J.D., Compton, S.G., Whittaker, R.J., (1999): Old World fruit bats can be long-distance seed dispersers through extended retention of viable seeds in gut. *Proc. Royal Soc. Ser. B*; 266, 219–223.

Simmons, N.B., (2005): Order Chiroptera. In: Wilson, D.E., Reeder, D.M., (eds.). Mammal Species of the World: A taxonomic and Geographic Reference. 2nd Ed. Washington, D.C: Smithsonian Institution Press, 159–174.

Simmons, N.B., Seymour, K.L., Habersetzer, J., Gunnell, G.F., (2008): Primitive Early Eocene bat from Wyoming and the evolution of flight and echolocation. *Nature* 451, 818–821.

Simpson, G.G., (1945): The principles of classification and a classification of mammals. *Bull. Amer. Museum Nat. History* 85, 1–350.

Solem, S.T., Stenvik, J., (2006): Antibody repertoire development in teleost—a review with emphasis on salmonids and *Gadus morhua* L. *Dev. Com. Immunology* 30, 57–76.

Sulkin, S.E., Allen, R., Sims, R., Singh, K.V., (1966): Studies of Arthropod-Borne Virus Infections in Chiroptera. *Amer. J. Trop. Med. Hyg.* 15, 418–427.

Sun, X-Z, Wertz, N., Lager, K., Sinkora, M.. Stepankova, K., Tobin, G., et al. (2012): Antibody repertoire development in fetal and neonatal piglets XXII. l rearrangements precedes k rearrangement during B cell lymphogenesis in swine. *Immunology* 137, 149–159.

Swanepoel, R., Leman, P.A., Bart, F.J., Zachariades, N.A., Braack, L.E., Ksiazek, T.G., et al. (1996): Experimental inoculation of plants and animals with bola virus. *Emerg. Infect. Dis.* 2, 321–325.

Tamura, K., Peterson, D., Peterson, N., Stecher, G., Nei, M., Kumar, S., (2011): MEGA5: Molecular Evolutionary Genetics Analysis using Maximum Likelihood, Evolutionary Distance, and Maximum Parsimony Methods. *Mol. Biol. Evol.* 28, 2731–2739.

Teeling, E.C., Madsen, O., Van Den Busche, R.A., deJong, W.W., Stanhope, M.J., Springer, M.S., (2002): Microbat paraphyly and the convergent evolution of a key innovation in Old World rhinolophoid microbats. *Proc. Nat'l. Acad. Sci. USA* 99, 1431–1436.

Teeling, E.C., Springer, M.S., Madsen, O., Bates, P., O'Brien, J.J., Murphy, W.J., (2005): A molecular phylogeny for bats illuminates biogeography and the fossil record. *Science* 307, 580–584.

Tomlinson, I.M., Williams, S.C., Ignatovich, O., Corbett, S.J. and Winter, G. 1996. VBASE sequence directory. MRC Centre for Protein Engineering, Cambridge, UK.

Turmelle, A., Ellison, J., Mendonça, M., McCracken, G., (2010): Histological assessment of cellular immune response to the phytohemagglutinin skin test in Brazilian free-tailed bats (Tadarida brasiliensis). *Journal of Comparative Physiology B: Biochemical, Systemic, and Environmental Physiology*, 180, 1155–1164.

Veilleux, J.P. (2008): Current status of white-nosed syndrome in the North-eastern United States. *Bat Res. News.* 49, 15–17.

Wellehan, J.F.X., Green, L.G., Duke, D.G., Bootorabi, S., Heard, D.J., Klein, P.A., et al. (2009): Detection of specific antibody responses to vaccination in variable flying foxes (*Pteropus hypomelanus*). *Comp Immunol Microbiol* 32, 379–394

Warnecke, I., Turner, J.M., Bollinger, T.K., Lorch, J.M., Misra, V., et al., (2012): Inoculation of bats with European *Geomyces destructus* supports the novel pathogen hypothesis for the origin of white-nose syndrome. *Proc. Nat'l Acad. Sci* 109, 6999–7003.

Wibbelt, G., Speck, S., Field, H., (2009): Methods for assessing diseases in bats. In: Kunz, T.H., Parsons, S., (eds.). Ecological and Behavioral Methods for the Study of Bats. Baltimore: Johns Hopkins University Press 775–793.

Williams-Guillén, K., Perfecto, I., Vandermeer, J., (2008): Bats limit insects in a Neotropical agroforestry ecozystem. *Science* 320, 703.

Williamson, M.M., Hooper, P.T., Selleck, P.W., Gleeson, L.J., Daniels, P.W., Westbury, H.A., et al. (1998): Transmission studies of Hendra Virus (equine morbilli-virus) in fruit bats, horses and cats. *Aust. Vet. J.* 76, 813–818.

Williamson, M.M., Hooper, P.T., Selleck, P.W., Westbury, H.A., Slocombe, R.F., (2000): Experimental Hendra Virus Infectionin Pregnant Guinea-pigs and Fruit Bats (*Pteropus poliocephalus*). *J. Com. Path.* 122, 201–207.

Wimsatt, W.A., (1970): Biology of Bats. Academic Press, N.Y.

Wong, S., Lau, S., Woo, P., Yuen, K.Y., (2007): Bats as a continuing source of emerging infections in humans. *Res. Med. Virol.* 17, 67–91.

Wynne, J.W., Di Rubbo, A., Shiell, B.J., Beddome, G., Cowled, C., Peck, G.R., et al. (2013): Purification and Characterization of Immunoglobulins from the Australian Black Flying Fox (*Pteropus alecto*) Using Anti-Fab Affinity Chromatography Reveals the Low Abundance of IgA. *PLoS ONE* 8, e52930.

Zemlin, M., Klinger, M., Link, J., Zemlin, C., Bauer, K., Engler, A., et al. (2003): Expressed murine and human CDR-H3 intervals of equal lengths exhibit distinct repertoires that differ in their amino acid composition and predicted range of structures. *J. Mol. Biol.* 334, 733–749.

Zhang, G., Cowled, C., Shi, Z., Huang, Z., Bishop-Lilly, K.A., Fang, X., et al. (2013): Comparative Analysis of Bat Genomes Provides Insight into the Evolution of Flight and Immunity. *Science* 339, 456–460.

Zhao, Y., Ciu, H., Whittington, C.M., Wei, Z., Zhang, X., Zhang, Z., et al. (2009): *Ornithorhynchus anatinus* (Platypus) links the evolution of immunoglobulin genes in eutherian mammals and nonmammalian tetrapods. *J. Immunol.* 183, 3285–3293.

Zhao, Y., Pan-Hammarstrom, Q., Yu, S., Wertz, N., Zhang, X., Li, N., et al. (2006): Identification of IgF, a hinge-region containing Ig class and IgD in *Xenopus tropicalis*. *Proc. Natl. Acad. Sci. (USA)* 103, 12087–12092.

CHAPTER 4

MARSUPIAL AND MONOTREME IMMUNOGLOBULIN GENETICS

ROBERT D. MILLER and VICTORIA L. HANSEN

CONTENTS

ABSTRACT

Much of the history of mammalian immunology has focused on only one of the three living lineages of mammals: the eutherians, more commonly called the placentals. This is not surprising given that humans and nearly all economically important mammals are eutherian. This chapter reviews what is known about immunoglobulin genetics in the other two lineages, the marsupials and the monotremes. Marsupials appear to have a fairly minimal complement of heavy chain isotypes and limited variable region diversity. Instead they appear to rely more on light chain complexity for generating a diverse antibody repertoire. Monotremes, in contrast have a more diverse collection of heavy chain isotypes and have retained more heavy chain variable region gene complexity than have the marsupials. Monotremes, more than the other two mammalian lineages have also retained more of the characteristics shared with our reptile-like ancestors. This is true of their immunoglobulin genes in addition as evidenced by a novel heavy chain isotype in the platypus with characteristics of both IgG and IgY.

4.1   INTRODUCTION

In the late 1970s, R. B. Ashman lamented the lack of progress on the study of immune systems of noneutherian mammals but predicted, or perhaps hoped for, a brighter future for this field (Ashman, 1977). He would be pleased to know that advances in comparative genetics, genomics, and whole genome sequencing has significantly advanced the fields of marsupial and monotreme immunology in the 21st century. Notable progress has been made in two representative species, the South American gray short-tailed opossum, *Monodelphis domestica*, and the duckbill platypus, *Ornithorhynchus anatinus*. This chapter summarizes what is known about marsupial and monotreme immunoglobulin (Ig) genetics and the corresponding relationships to B cell ontogeny and antibody repertoire development.

4.1.1 MAMMALIAN RELATIONSHIPS AND LIFE HISTORY

To put this chapter into perspective it is important to remember that there are two living subclasses of extant mammals: Subclass Prototheria, containing Order Monotremata (hereafter referred to as the monotremes), and Subclass Theria (Fig. 1). The Therians include two infraclasses: the Marsupialia and the Placentalia, hereafter referred to as the marsupials and eutherians, respectively. These lineages last shared a common ancestor at least 185 million years (MY) and perhaps greater than 200 MY ago (O'Leary et al., 2013). Research on the immune systems of monotremes and marsupials is well established and has been driven by interest in both evolutionary and veterinary immunology. Of particular interest has been the interplay between the immune system, maternal immunology, and differences in reproductive strategies among the monotremes, marsupials, and eutherians.

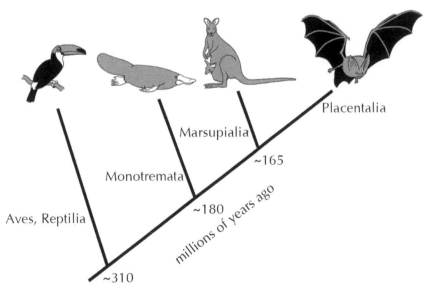

FIGURE 1 Phylogenetic relationships among the major amniote lineages. The numbers at each of the nodes represent time since the last common ancestor (based on Kumar and Hedges 1998; O'Leary et al., 2013).

Marsupials, like eutherians, are viviparous, however, they give birth to young that are in an extremely altricial state. Marsupials and eutherians last shared a common ancestor 145 to 165 MY ago. There is evidence that marsupials once inhabited a greater geographic range as fossils of mammals resembling metatherians have been found in North America and China (Luo et al., 2003). Today the greatest number and diversity of marsupial species is found in Australasia.

Monotreme biogeography is currently limited to Australia and Indonesia although, as with marsupials, the fossil record reveals a once larger geographic range as well (Pascual et al., 1992). In addition to the platypus there are four living recognized species of echidna (spiny anteaters) belonging to the genera *Tachyglossus* and *Zaglossus*. Monotremes have retained many characteristics shared with mammals' reptile-like ancestors, the most distinctive of which is the laying of eggs. Egg-laying mammals raise a number of questions regarding the evolution of transmission of maternal immunity to offspring, as well as providing models to investigate the origins of features of the immune system that are mammal specific: (e.g., the root origins of IgG and IgE) (Vernersson et al., 2002). Lamentably, information on the development and function of monotreme immune systems remains sparse. No monotreme species is currently bred in captivity for research purposes resulting in limited access to material for these species. However, probably due to their iconic place in the fauna of Australia, the platypus has played a more prominent role in monotreme research and immunology. The platypus is, so far, the only monotreme species for which there is currently a whole genome sequence available.

4.2 MARSUPIAL POSTNATAL IMMUNOLOGY

At birth most marsupial species are developmentally similar to fetal eutherians (Deane and Cooper, 1988). Upon leaving the birth canal neonatal marsupials crawl up their mother's abdomen to find a teat. Neonates latch on by their mouths and begin to suckle for several weeks, a period of time that varies between species. The teats are usually, but not always, inside a pouch structure referred to as a marsupium. The opossum *M. domestica*, for example, is a species that lacks a pouch and the young are exposed while attached to the teats. Marsupials essentially complete the equivalent of fetal development while continuously attached to the teats, after which they will begin to leave the teat but remain in the pouch or nest, suckling intermittently as necessary similar to a newborn eutherian.

The newborn marsupial thymus is primarily undifferentiated epithelium, and neonatal marsupials are generally unable to generate humoral or cellular adaptive immune responses until late in the first or second postnatal week (Kalmutz, 1962, La Via et al., 1963, Rowlands et al., 1972, Hubbard et al., 1991, Old and Deane, 2000, Wang et al., 2012a). Not surprisingly neonatal marsupials are dependent entirely on maternal factors for immune protection for a sustained period of time after birth. Milk plays an obvious important role in conferring protection.

Marsupial lactation is more complicated than that of eutherians (Adamski and Demmer 2000, Daly et al., 2007, Kuruppath et al., 2012). Following a colostrum phase, there are three distinct phases referred to as early, switch, and late. Some investigators refer to these phases as 2A, 2B, and 3; where phase 1 corresponds to prenatal changes in the mammaries during gestation. The early lactation phase (phase 2A) produces milk that is generally high in carbohydrates but low in fat content. This early phase corresponds to when the newborn is continuously attached to the teat. Late phase milk (phase 3) is lower in carbohydrates but increased fat content and its production correspond to when the neonates are not yet weaned but are independent of the teats. Some species of marsupials, members of the kangaroo family in particular can have more than one neonate (joeys) at different stages of development. Hence there can be two mammary glands side-by-side producing different phases of milk.

Although marsupials do have some form of placental structure, typically late in gestation, most marsupials do not obtain maternal Ig *in utero*. Only one species, the tammar wallaby *Macropus eugenii*, has been shown to transfer maternal IgG to the fetus via the yolk sac (Deane et al., 1990). All other marsupials studied depend entirely on milk for maternal IgG and IgA. Maternal IgG in the newborn opossum, for example, can be detected by the end of the first postnatal day (Samples et al., 1986). The transfer of maternal Ig through milk follows a pattern that mirrors the different phases of the milk. At the start of the early milk phase there is a spike of IgA that rapidly declines. There is a second peak of IgA transfer during the switch (phase 2B) when the neonate is transitioning to leaving the teat (Adamski and Demmer, 1999). Presumably the early transfer of IgA may play an important role in the early establishment of a gut microbiome. The second transfer may be preparing the neonate for greater exposure to ingested antigens and potential pathogens in solid food. There appears to be a peak of IgG detected in the early lacation phase, which declines, but is followed by a second increase in IgG in the late phase as well (Adamski and Demmer, 2000). Mammary expression of the poly Ig receptor (pIgR) and the neonatal IgG Fc receptor (FcRN) appears to mirror the expression of the different Ig isotypes. It is intriguing to speculate that, in addition to varying the nutrient content of milk to suit the stage of development of the suckling young, the mammary glands are also adjusting the class of antibody transferred to meet the needs for protection.

4.3   MARSUPIAL IMMUNOGLOBULIN GENETICS

4.3.1   CONSTANT REGION ISOTYPES

IgH chain constant region sequences have been reported for a variety of marsupial species. However, the exact genomic content and organization of the *IgH* locus has only been determined for one marsupial species, the opossum *M. domestica*. *M. domestica* may have the simplest, or most generic, of all mammalian *IgH* loci (Fig. 2). There are four functional IgH constant region genes, IgM, IgG, IgE and IgA. The IgG, IgE and IgA are single copy genes. There is a second pseudogene copy of $C\mu$ upstream of the functional $C\mu$. Both copies of $C\mu$ have three J_H gene segments just upstream, one of which is a pseudogene; an arrangement that appears to be the result of an $[\psi J_H - J_H - J_H - C\mu]$ duplication (Wang et al., 2009). The J_H gene segments upstream of the pseudogene copy of $C\mu$ are not used during V(D)J recombination (Wang et al., 2012a).

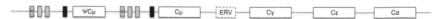

FIGURE 2   Diagram of the opossum *IgH* constant region (not to scale). The ψ symbol designates pseudogenes. Gray boxes represent J_H gene segments and solid black boxes designate identified switch regions. It should be noted that sequences resembling canonical mammalian switch regions were only identified upstream of the two $C\mu$ genes. The box labeled ERV indicates the expected location of $C\delta$ exons but they appear to have been replaced with ERV and LINE retroelements.

IgD is absent from the opossum genome and has not been reported in any marsupial species. The region of the IgH locus downstream from the Cμ exons where one would expect to find the Cδ genes contains a stretch of inserted retro-elements including endogenous retrovirus (ERV) and LINE elements, that appear to have deleted or replaced IgD from the opossum germline (Fig. 3) (Wang et al., 2009). Whether this is the case for other marsupial species is not yet known.

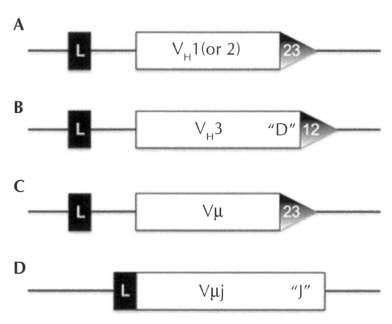

FIGURE 3   Diagram illustrating the basic structure of (A) a typical opossum germline V_H gene, (B) the partially germline joined opossum V_H3 gene, (C) a typical opossum germline Vμ gene, and (D) the germline joined opossum Vμj gene.

4.3.2   *GERMLINE VARIABLE REGION DIVERSITY*

What emerged from one of the first studies of expressed antibody diversity was the presence of limited heavy chain V gene (V_H) complexity (Miller et al., 1998). All amniote V_H genes group into one of three Clans (I, II, and III) based on nucleotide sequence identity. In analyzes of opossum Ig heavy chain cDNAs, only two V_H gene subgroups were found and both were Clan III members. As it turns out, all marsupial V_H genes described so far are Clan III members; furthermore, all marsupial V_H genes practically form a single major subclade within Clan III (Baker et al., 2005). During the evolution of the *IgH* locus in marsupials there appears to have been a major bottleneck in the diversity of V_H genes. It is not unusual to find limited germline V_H gene diversity in individual mammalian species (e.g., rabbits), however, in this case it is an entire class of diverse mammals. This suggests that the genetic bottleneck in V_H gene diversity occurred very early in marsupial evolution (Baker et al., 2005).

In the opossum, genomic analysis revealed three V_H gene subgroups. V_H1 is the only multimember family, makes up the majority of germline V_H genes, and contributes to the majority of expressed heavy chain V_H domains (Table 1, Wang et al., 2012a). The $V_H2.1$ subgroup, composed of a single member, is also expressed early in development at a frequency proportional to its representation in the germline genome (Baker et al., 2005, Wang et al., 2012a). The third subgroup, $V_H3.1$, also a singleton, is unusual in that it is partially germline joined and will be discussed in its own evolutionary context later in this chapter.

TABLE 1 Number and complexity of V, D, and J gene segments at the Ig heavy and light chain loci in the opossum, *Monodelphis domestica.*

IgH

V_H subgroups	Numbers of Gene Segments (Total/Functional[1])					
	Total V_H	V_H1	V_H2	V_H3	D	J_H
3	26/21	24/19	1/1	1/1	9	6/4

Igκ

Vκ subgroups	Numbers of Gene Segments (Total/Functional[1])									
	Total Vκ	Vκ1	Vκ2	Vκ3	Vκ4	Vκ5	Vk6	Vκ7	Jκ	Cκ
7	122/89	32/25	45/33	22/17	5/3	5/5	1/1	12/5	4	1

Igλ

Vλ subgroups	Numbers of Gene Segments (Total/Functional[1])						
	Total Vλ	Vλ1	Vλ2	Vλ3	Vλ4	Jλ	Cλ
4	64/58	54/48	7/7	2/2	1/1	8	8

[1]Functional includes gene or gene segments that have an open reading frame and appear to have all the necessary components to be expressed based on genomic sequence, independent of whether they have been found in a cDNA sequence or not.

There are nine recognized D_H gene segments in the opossum, and all are both functional and used for V(D)J recombination (Wang et al., 2012). They vary in length and repertoire analysis revealed that the shorter D_H gene segments are overrepresented in productive rearrangements. As stated earlier in the chapter, of the four functional J_H gene segments only two are used and these are the two immediately upstream of the functional Cμ exons (Wang et al., 2012a).

4.3.3   GERMLINE JOINED V GENES IN THE MARSUPIAL GENOMES

One of the more unusual features of the opossum *IgH* locus is the presence of a single, partially germline joined V_H gene (Wang et al., 2009). Called $V_H3.1$, it is so far the only such case reported in a mammal and is a V_H gene with a pre-joined D_H (Fig. 3). $V_H3.1$ was recognized as being a partially germline joined V_H due to its extended length and the presence of a recombination signal sequence (RSS) containing a 12 base pair spacer, typical of D_H gene segments, rather than a 23 bp RSS at the end of V_H genes (Wang et al., 2009). $V_H3.1$ was only discovered through the analysis of the whole genome sequence and had been absent from previous analyzes of expressed *IgH* cDNA sequences (Miller et al., 1998). However, its use and germline joined nature were confirmed recently when transcripts containing recombined $V_H3.1$ segments were detected in mature, young opossums (Wang and Miller, 2012). These transcripts contained evidence that when $V_H3.1$ undergoes V(D)J recombination it is joined directly to a J_H gene segment. The late detection of $V_H3.1$ recombinants most likely reflects its rare use in the IgH repertoire. This may be due to a direct V_H to J_H recombination being unusual and out of order for normal V(D)J recombination during B cell development. Alternatively, B cells rearranging $V_H3.1$ are at a functional disadvantage due to having a long complementarity-determining-region-3 (CDR3) resulting from the fixed D_H segment at the end of this V gene (Wang and Miller, 2012). $V_H3.1$ or its equivalent has not been reported for any other marsupial species and may be unique to *M. domestica*.

The presence of a germline joined V_H in the opossum raises a number of interesting questions regarding the origin of such genes. This has been studied in sharks where germline joined V_H are more common and it is clearly due to ectopic expression of the RAG recombination activating genes in germ cells (Lee et al., 2000). A similar explanation for the origin of $V_H3.1$ in the opossum is likely, although it resulted in only a partial rearrangement of a V_H and D_H. This is a more straightforward scenario than has been proposed for the only other known germline joined V genes found in mammals. Marsupials and monotremes are unique in having an extra T cell receptor (TCR) chain called TCRμ (Parra et al., 2007). In the marsupials TCRμ is unusual in that it uses a complete germline joined V gene called Vμj to encode one of the V domains (Fig. 3). Vμj is found in all marsupial species and apparently the germline joining event has a single ancient common origin for all species (Parra et al., 2007, 2012). Vμj is unique from other germline joined V genes in that it is missing the intron separating the leader exon from the V exon (Fig. 3). This has lead to speculation that the origin of Vμj also involved a retro-transposition event (Parra et al., 2007, 2012). It is noteworthy that monotremes have a homologue of TCRμ, however, the gene segments corresponding to Vμj are not germline joined and still require V(D)J recombination for expression (Wang et al., 2011). This indicates that the Vμj germline joining event was unique and early in the marsupial lineage.

Although Vμj and $V_H3.1$ appear to have followed different evolutionary origins, the presence of both in at least *M. domestica* indicates the role that ectopic RAG expression in germ cells has shaped the germline Ig and TCR repertoires in marsupials. The functional role or advantage to the presence of the partially germline joined $V_H3.1$ remains unclear. In sharks, germline joined V_H genes are expressed early in ontogeny and may play a functional role in young animals (Rumfelt et al., 2001). This does not seem to be the case for opossum $V_H3.1$ as it appears late and sparingly in the developing antibody repertoire (Wang et al., 2012a).

4.3.4 MARSUPIAL LIGHT CHAINS

Marsupials, like all mammals, have both the Igκ and Igλ light chains (Lucero et al., 1998; Miller et al., 1999; Belov et al., 2001, 2002). Like the *IgH* locus, the complete genomic composition and complexity of the light chain loci has only been established for a single marsupial species, the opossum *M. domestica* (Wang et al., 2009). One of the more noteworthy observations from this analysis was the greater germline V gene complexity for light chains as compared to that of heavy chains (Table 1, Baker et al., 2005; Wang et al., 2009). This appears to be a pattern common to all marsupial species studied so far (Baker et al., 2005). Indeed it has been proposed that light chains may make a greater contribution to marsupial antibody repertoire diversity than does the heavy chain (Baker et al., 2005). The limited IgH but complex Igκ and Igλ diversity found in early developing B cells in the opossum supports this hypothesis (Wang et al., 2012).

The overall organization of the *Igκ* and *Igλ* loci in the opossum are well conserved for a mammal. The *Igκ* locus contains a single *Cκ* gene located at the 3′ end of the locus. There are four *Jκ* genes and all are used in the expressed repertoire (Wang et al., 2009, 2012). The *Igκ* locus is the most complex with regards to V genes, containing seven different subgroups (Miller et al., 1999; Wang et al., 2009). The *Igλ* locus is also well conserved and contains eight Cλ genes, each with its own Jλ gene segment upstream (Lucero et al., 1998; Wang et al., 2012). The repeated Jλ-Cλ organization is conserved in *Igλ* loci in all therian mammals. Phylogenetic analyzes of Cλ from marsupials and other mammalian species implicate that these genes cluster by species (Lucero et al., 1998). Some investigators have explained this pattern of evolution as being the result of gene duplication, deletion, and replacement following speciation (Bengten et al., 2000). Concerted evolution may provide a preferable alternative explanation. Since the Cλ genes in each species function redundantly and must interact with the same heavy chains, there would be selection to homogenize the sequences through some gene conversion-like mechanism.

4.3.5 POSTNATAL B CELL ONTOGENY AND ANTIBODY REPERTOIRE DEVELOPMENT

As was stated earlier in this chapter, much of the immune system development in marsupials appears to take place postnatally. One of the more thorough analysis of B cell ontogeny in a marsupial was recently published for the opossum *M. domestica* (Wang et al., 2012a). Based on expression of early B cell markers such as CD79a and CD79b, initiation of B cell ontogeny could be detected in *M. domestica* embryos within the final 24 hours of gestation. Birth in the opossum takes place approximately 14.5 days post copulation and within the first 24 hours following birth there is evidence of V(D)J recombination. The diversity of V gene recombinants is relatively low, most likely due to the low number of pre-B cells at this stage. The majority of heavy chain V(D)J recombinants lack N region additions to their junctions in spite of concomitant Terminal deoxynucleotidyl transferase (Tdt) expression (Wang et al., 2012a). Indeed, for the first two postnatal weeks the endogenous Ig heavy chain repertoire is fairly limited.

The next developmental B cell stage detected is defined by the expression of the VpreB surrogate light chain. VpreB can be identified on postnatal day 6 in the opossum (Wang et al., 2012b). Unlike eutherian mammals, which can have up to three VpreB genes (VpreB1, 2, and 3), the opossum only has a VpreB3 homologue. The function of VpreB3 is not completely understood and evidence from the expression of this gene in chicken B cells suggests that it is not expressed on the cell surface. The opossum genome also appears to lack a gene for the $\lambda 5$ surrogate light chain. It is possible, therefore, that the marsupials do not have a cell surface pre-B cell receptor (BCR) similar to eutherians, but rather are more like nonmammalian vertebrates such as birds. How quality control of heavy chain V(D)J recombination and subsequent initiation of light chain rearrangement is regulated during marsupial B cell development, without the "conventional" pre-BCR as it is known from humans and mice, is not fully understood. However, likely VpreB3 expression does play a role on stimulating light chain gene rearrangement in the opossum due to the close timing of these two events (Wang et al., 2012a, b).

Light chain gene rearrangement, beginning with the *Igλ* locus can be first detected on postnatal day 7, followed one day later by *Igκ* rearrangements. Unlike the heavy chain repertoire the light chain repertoire is diverse from the start. An 8- to 9-day-old opossum has similar light chain diversity to what is found in the adult repertoire (Wang et al., 2012a). This observation is consistent with an earlier hypothesis based on germline V gene complexity that light chains may contribute more to the antibody diversity than do heavy chains (Baker et al., 2005).

One conclusion that can be drawn from B cell ontogeny studies in the opossum is that it is unlikely that this species is able to generate endogenous, antigen specific antibody responses until at least the second postnatal week of life. This conclusion is entirely consistent with previous studies of antibody responses in other newborn marsupial species. In most cases where it has been tested, neonatal marsupials are unable to generate antigen specific T-dependent antibody responses until the 7th postnatal day or later (Kalmutz 1962; La Via et al., 1963).

Analyzes of B cells in developing opossums also enabled investigation into the role of somatic mutation in diversifying the primary antibody repertoire. Species with limited germline V gene diversity, as in marsupials, often rely on somatic mutation to contribute additional diversity not achieved through V(D)J recombination alone (reviewed in Butler, 1997). This process typically involves a gut associated lymphoid organ like the appendix in rabbits or Peyer's patches in sheep. Reports of early detection of B cell markers in gut tissues of neonates lead to speculation that a similar process may be going on in marsupials (Old and Deane, 2003). However, there is little evidence in the opossum that their primary antibody repertoire is being diversified through additional somatic mutation (Wang et al., 2012a). Analyzes of large sequence databases of expressed Ig heavy and light chain V(D)J recombinants when compared with a reasonably high quality germline genomic sequence reveal no evidence of mutation. Indeed, the extent and importance of affinity maturation in marsupial memory B cell responses is not yet clear.

Lastly, when the analysis of B cell development in marsupials was extended to later developmental time-points, the timing of the appearance of isotype switch recombined B cells was assessed. One observation is that IgA production could not be detected in the gut or other organs until the animals were 8 weeks of age (Wang et al., 2012a). This is noteworthy as it corresponds with the time point when opossums are fully weaned. In other words, although they have been off the teats for nearly 4 weeks, with the possibility of ingesting antigens and have a well established gut microbiome, there has been little stimulation of IgA production in the gut associated lymphoid tissue. This observation suggests that maternal antibodies, likely IgA, in the milk are playing an important role on regulating gut microbes and pathogens throughout the lactation period.

4.4   MONOTREME IMMUNGLOBULIN GENETICS

Monotremes are a puzzling lineage of mammals because they have retained a number of characteristics usually associated with nonmammalian vertebrates. This was made evident when in 1884 Caldwell sent from Australia to the British Royal Society the four-word telegram "Monotremes oviparous, ovum meroblastic." His message was that they were egg laying and the egg is structured more like that of a bird, reptile or fish, rather than the holoblastic egg of a marsupial or eutherian (Caldwell, 1887). In addition to being egg-laying, they expel waste through a cloaca like a bird or reptile and the males have venom glands that are active during breeding season in the platypus, but may be vestigial in the echidnas. Monotreme genomics has also revealed a number of ancestral characteristics. Their sex chromosomes (which are unusual in there being 10 of them per diploid cell!) have conserved synteny with both the XY system found in marsupials and eutherians, as well as the WZ system found in birds (Grützner et al., 2004). Curiously the MHC region is located on the sex chromosomes in monotremes as well (Dohm et al., 2007).

Monotreme immunology has been greatly enhanced over the past decade with the development of molecular resources including a whole genome sequence of the duckbill platypus, *O. anatinus* (Warren et al., 2008). Fortunately this has included the study of monotreme immunoglobulins. Like the rest of monotreme anatomy and physiology, monotreme immune systems share characteristics with nonmammalian tetrapods. For example like marsupials, the monotremes have a clear homologue of the TCRμ T cell receptor chain, but the platypus TCRδ locus also contains V_H-related V genes similar to what has been found in birds and amphibians (Parra et al., 2010, 2011, 2012a, b, Wang et al., 2011).

4.4.1 MONOTREME IG HEAVY CHAIN GENETICS

4.4.1.1 MONOTREME CONSTANT REGIONS AND ISOTYPES

The discovery that platypus and echidna have both IgG and IgE pushed the origin of these uniquely mammalian heavy chain isotypes back as far as the earliest mammals (Vernersson et al., 2002, 2004). The most complete view of the antibody isotypes found in monotremes comes from genomic analyzes in the platypus. The platypus *IgH* locus contains exons for a single IgM and IgD, two IgG subclasses, two IgA subclasses, and a single IgE (Zhao et al., 2009). Nested between the IgD and IgG_2 exons are the genes encoding a novel isotype. Zhao and colleagues named this isotype IgO (for *Ornithorhyncus*), whereas Gambón-Deza and colleagues described these genes as being IgY (Gambón-Deza et al., 2009; Zhao et al., 2009). The reason for the different designations is understandable. This isotype had not been seen before in mammals and appeared unique to the platypus, hence the IgO. On the other hand, both groups recognized that IgO shared similarity to IgG, IgE and the IgY found in birds and reptiles. Platypus IgO/IgY appears to be an immunoglobulin missing link, although phylogenetic analyzes put it much closer to mammalian IgG than to avian IgY (Zhao et al., 2009). Platypus IgD is also unusual for a mammal. It shares more structural similarity to the IgD of reptiles and fish by having 10 C_H domains, rather than the typical three found in eutherian IgD (Gambón-Deza et al., 2009; Zhao et al., 2009).

4.4.1.2 VARIABLE REGION GENES AND ANTIBODY DIVERSITY

Earlier in this chapter it was noted that all marsupial V_H genes are similar, even across distantly related species (Baker et al., 2006). This is not true of monotremes. The platypus *IgH* locus contains only a single V_H subgroup that belongs to Clan III (Johansson et al., 2002). Genomic analysis estimated there to be 44 total V_H genes (Gambón-Deza et al., 2009). V(D)J recombination in the platypus produces among the longest and most diverse CDR3 found in any mammal, which is thought to compensate for limited germline V_H diversity (Johansson et al., 2002). In contrast to platypus, the short-beaked echidna *T. aculeatus* germline V_H repertoire is highly diverse (Belov and Hellman, 2003). The echidna uses at least seven different subgroups that are derived from all three V_H Clans (Wong et al., 2009).

4.4.1.3   MONOTREME IG LIGHT CHAIN GENETICS

Like all mammals, the monotremes have both Igκ and Igλ (Nowak et al., 2004, Johansson et al., 2005). Igλ V region diversity has been analyzed in the platypus, where there are only two Vλ subgroups. As in the platypus antibody heavy chain CDR diversity, both long and sequence, is thought to compensate for limited germline Vλ diversity (Johansson et al., 2005). The platypus Jλ–Cλ genes are organized in tandem pairs like in other mammals. The exact number of Jλ-Cλ pairs has not been determined for the platypus but based on sequence it appeared to be at least four.

The monotreme Igκ locus also has typical mammalian organization. There appears to be a single Cκ gene and, although the exact number is not known, there seems to be at least eight to ten Jκ gene segments (Nowak et al., 2004). The platypus and echidna Igκ loci appear to contain at least four and nine Vκ subgroups, respectively (Nowak et al., 2004). Therefore the monotreme Igκ diversity likely relies more on germline complexity for generating antibody diversity than does the Igλ locus.

4.5   CONCLUSIONS

In conclusion for the marsupial section of this chapter, much as been learned about antibody genetics and B cell ontogeny in marsupials, taking advantage of a limited number of model species for which resources have been developed. These resources include a high quality genome sequence for at least one species, the gray short-tailed opossum, and captive bred, pedigreed colonies for research (Samollow, 2006). However, most comparative analyzes of the immune systems within the marsupial lineage have found them to be remarkably homogeneous, particularly for immunoglobulins and T cell receptors (Baker et al., 2005, 2010; Parra et al., 2007,

2010). The opossum Ig loci are, with the possible exception of missing IgD, among the most generic and simplified of Ig genes among mammals. It is tempting to speculate that much of what has been discovered in the opossum may also be true for other marsupials, which is a bit surprising given the diversity of organization and complexity that exists within the eutherian mammals (Butler, 1997). In the end, the appearance of homogeneity may yet be an artifact due to the limited number of species examined.

Monotremes hold a special position in mammalian evolution and the results that emerge from their study never ceases to astound. Several important conclusions have emerged from the analysis of monotreme Ig genetics. The evolution of uniquely mammalian antibody classes such as IgG and IgE clearly occurred very early in mammalian evolution and the relationship these two antibody isotypes have to non-mammalian IgY is most evident from genes found in the platypus. Monotremes also continue to illustrate how closely related lineages are often on their own evolutionary paths towards generating antibody diversity. The platypus and the echidna have retained very different levels of germline diversity.

KEYWORDS

- B cells
- development
- diversity
- immunoglobulins
- marsupials
- monotremes

REFERENCES

Adamski, F.M., Demmer, J. (1999): Two stages of increased IgA transfer during lactation in the marsupial, *Trichosurus Vulpecula* (Brushtail possum). *J Immunol.*, 162, 6009–6015.

Adamski, F.M., Demmer, J. (2000): Immunological protection of the Vulnerable marsupial pouch young: two periods of immune transfer during lactation in Trichosurus Vulpecula (brushtail possum). *Dev Comp Immunol.*, 24, 491–502.

Ashman, R.B. (1977): Marsupial immunology: A brighter future? *Dev Comp Immunol.*, 1, 283–284.

Baker, M.L., Belov, K., Miller, R.D. (2005): Unusually similar patterns of antibody V segment diversity in distantly related marsupials. *J Immunol.*, 174, 5665–5671.

Baker, M.L., Wang, X., Miller, R.D. (2010): Marsupial immunoglobulin and T cell receptor biology and genomics. In: Deakin, J., Waters, P., Graves, J. (Eds.), *Marsupial Genetics and Genomics.* (pp. 357–380). Berlin: Springer-Verlag.

Baker, M.L., Wares, J.P., Harrison, G.A., Miller, R.D. (2004): The relationship of the marsupial families and the mammalian subclasses based on recombination activating gene-1. *J Mammal Evol.*, 11, 1–16.

Belov, K., Harrison, G.A., Miller, R.D., Cooper, D.W. (1999): Isolation and sequence of a cDNA coding for the heavy chain constant region of IgG from the Australian brushtail possum, *Trichosurus Vulpecula*. *Mol Immunol.*, 36, 535–541.

Belov, K., Harrison, G.A., Miller, R.D., Cooper, D.W. (1999): Molecular cloning of the brushtail possum (*Trichosurus Vulpecula*) immunglobulin E heavy chain constant region. *Mol Immunol.*, 36, 1255–1261.

Belov, K., Harrison, G.A., Miller, R.D., Cooper, D.W. (2001): Characterization of the kappa light chain of the brushtail possum (*Trichosurus Vulpecula*). V*et Immunol Immunopath.*, 78, 317–324.

Belov, K., Harrison, G.A., Miller, R.D., Cooper, D.W. (2002): Molecular cloning of four lambda light chain cDNAs from the Australian brushtail possum (*Trichosurus Vulpecula*). *Eur J Immunogenet.*, 29, 95–99.

Belov, K., Harrison, G.A., Rosenberg, G.H., Miller, R.D., Cooper, D.W. (1999): Isolation and comparison of the IgM heavy chain constant region from Australian (*Trichosurus Vulpecula*) and American (*Monodelphis domestica*) marsupials. *Dev Comp Immunol.*, 23, 649–656.

Belov, K., Hellman, L. (2003): Immunoglobulin genetics of Ornithorhynchus anatinus (platypus) and Tachyglossus aculeatus (short-beaked echidna). *Comp Biochem Phys A, 136*(4), 811–819.

Bengten, E., Wilson, M., Miller, N., Clem, L.W., Pilstrom, L., Warr, G.W. (2000): Immunoglobulin isotypes: Structure, function, and genetics. In: Origin and evolution of the Vertebrate immune system. *Curr Top Microbiol.*, 248, 189–219.

Butler, J.E. (1997): Immunoglobulin gene organization and the mechanism of repertoire development. *Scand J Immunol.*, 45, 455–462.

Caldwell, H. (1887): The embryology of Monotremata and Marsupialia. *Phil. Trans. R. Soc Lond B.*, 178, 463–486.

Daly, K.A., Digby, M., Lefe'vre, C., Mailer, S., Thomson, P., Nicholas, K., et al. (2007): Analysis of the expression of immunoglobulins throughout lactation suggests two periods of immune transfer in the tammar wallaby (*Macropus eugenii*). V*et Immunol Immunopathol.*, 120, 187–200.

Deane, E.M., Cooper, D.W. (1988): Immunological development in pouch young marsupials. In: Tyndale-Biscoe, C.H., Janssens, P.A. (Eds.) *The Developing Marsupial.* (pp. 190–199). Berlin: Springer-Verlag.

Deane, E.M., Cooper, D.W., Renfree, M.B. (1990): Immunoglobulin g levels in fetal and newborn tammar wallabies (*Macropus eugenii*). *Reprod Fertil Dev.*, 2, 369–375.

Deane, E.M., Miller, R.D. (2000): Marsupial immunology: out of the pouch (editorial), *Dev Comp Immunol.*, 24, 443–444.

Dohm, J.C., Tsend-Ayush, E., Reinhardt, R., Grützner, F., Himmelbauer, H. (2007): Disruption and pseudoautosomal localization of the major histocompatibility complex in monotremes. *Genome Biol.*, 8(8), R175.

Gambón-Deza, F., Sánchez-Espinel, C., Magadán-Mompó, S. (2009): The immunoglobulin heavy chain locus in the platypus (Ornithorhynchus anatinus). *Mol Immunol.*, 46(13), 2515–2523.

Grützner, F., Rens, W., Tsend-Ayush, E., El-Mogharbel, N., O'Brien, P.C.M., Jones, R.C., et al. (2004): In the platypus a meiotic chain of ten sex chromosomes shares genes with the bird Z and mammal X chromosomes. *Nature*, 432, 913–917.

Hubbard, G.B., Saphire, D.G., Hackleman, S.M., Silva, M.V., Vandeberg, J.L., Stone, W.H. (1991): Ontogeny of the thymus gland of a marsupial (*Monodelphis domestica*). *Lab Animal Sci.*, 41, 227–232.

Johansson, J., Aveskogh, M., Munday, B., Hellman, L. (2002): Heavy chain V region diversity in the duck-billed platypus (Ornithorhynchus anatinus): long and highly Variable complementarity-determining region 3 compensates for limited germline diversity. *J Immunol.*, 168(10), 5155–5162.

Johansson, J., Salazar, J.N., Aveskogh, M., Munday, B., Miller, R.D., Hellman, L. (2005): High Variability in complementarity-determining regions compensate for a low number of V gene families in the lambda light chain locus of the egg-laying mammals. *Eur J Immunol.*, 35, 3008–3019.

Kalmutz, S.E. (1962): Antibody production in the opossum embryo. *Nature*, 193, 851–853.

Kumar, S., Hedges, S.B. (1998): A molecular timescale for Vertebrate evolution. *Nature*, 392, 917–920.

Kuruppath, S., Bisana, S., Sharp, J.A., Lefèvre, C., Kumar, S., Nicholas, K.R. (2012): Monotremes and marsupials: Comparative models to better understand the function of milk. *J Biosciences*, 37, 581–588.

La Via, M.R., Rowlands Jr., D.T., Block, M. (1963): Antibody formation in embryos. *Science*, 140, 1219–1220.

Lee, S.S., Fitch, D., Flajnik, M.F., Hsu, E. (2000): Rearrangement of immunoglobulin genes in shark germ cells. *J Exp Med.*, 191, 1637–1648.

Lucero, J.E., Rosenberg, G.H., Miller, R.D. (1998): Marsupial light chains: Complexity and conservation of lambda in the opossum *Monodelphis domestica*. *J Immunol.*, 161, 6724–6732.

Luo, Z-X., Ji, Q., Wible, J.R., Yuan, C-X. (2003): An Early Cretaceous tribosphenic mammal and metatherian evolution. *Science*, 302, 1934–1940.

Mikkelsen, T.S., Wakefield, M.J., Aken, B., Amemiya, C.T., Chang, J.L., Duke, S., et al. (2007): Genome of the marsupial *Monodelphis domestica* reveals lineage-specific innovation in coding sequences. *Nature*, 447, 167–178.

Miller, R.D., Belov, K. (2000): Immunoglobulin genetics of marsupials (review). *Dev Comp Immunol.*, 24, 485–490.

Miller, R.D., Bergemann, E.R., Rosenberg, G.H. (1999): Marsupial light chains: Ig kappa with four V families in the opossum *Monodelphis domestica*. *Immunogenetics*, 50, 329–335.

Miller, R.D., Grabe, H., Rosenberg, G.H. (1998): The V_H Repertoire of a Marsupial: *Monodelphis domestica*. *J Immunol.*, 160, 259–265.

Nowak, M.A., Parra, Z.E., Hellman, L.H., Miller, R.D. (2004): The complexity of expressed kappa light chains in the egg-laying mammals. *Immunogenetics*, 56, 555–563.

O'Leary, M.A., Bloch, J.I., Flynn, J.J., Gaudin, T.J., Giallombardo, A., Giannini, N.P., et al. (2013): The placental mammal ancestor and the post-K-Pg radiation of placentals. *Science*, 339, 662–667.

Old, J.M., Deane, E.M. (2000): Development of the immune system and immunological protection in marsupial pouch young. *Dev Comp Immunol.*, 24, 445–454.

Old, J.M., Deane, E.M. (2003): The detection of mature T- and B-cells during development of the lymphoid tissues of the tammar wallaby (*Macropus eugenii*). *J Anat.*, 203, 123–131.

Parra, Z.E., Baker, M.L., Hathaway, J., Lopez, A.M., Trujillo, J., Sharp, A., et al. (2008): Comparative genomic analysis and evolution of the T cell receptor loci in the opossum *Monodelphis domestica*. *BMC Genomics*, 9, 111.

Parra, Z.E., Baker, M.L., Schwarz, R., Deakin, J.E., Lindblad-Toh K., Miller, R.D. (2007): Discovery of a new T cell receptor in marsupials. *Proc. Natl Acad Sci USA*, 104, 9776–9781.

Parra, Z.E., Lillie, M., Miller, R.D. (2012): A model for the evolution of the mammalian T cell receptor a/d and m loci based on evidence from the duckbill platypus. *Mol Biol Evol.*, 29, 3205–3214.

Parra, Z.E., Mitchell, K., Dalloul, R.A., Miller, R.D. (2012): A second TCRd locus in Galliformes uses antibody-like V domains: insight into the evolution of TCRd and TCRm genes in tetrapods. *J Immunol.*, 188, 3912–3919.

Parra, Z.E., Ohta, Y., Criscitiello, M.F., Flajnik, M.F., Miller R.D. (2010): The dynamic TCRδ: TCRδ chains in the amphibian *Xenopus tropicalis* use antibody-like V genes. *Eur J Immunol.*, 40, 2319–2329.

Pascual, R., Archer, M., Jaureguizar, E.O., Prado, J.L., Godthelp, H., Hand, S.J. (1992): First discovery of monotremes in South America. *Nature*, 356, 704–706.

Rowlands, D.T., Blakeslee, D., Lin, H.H. (1972): The early immune response and immunoglobulins of opossum embryos. *J Immunol.*, 108, 941–946.

Rumfelt, L.L., Avila, D., Diaz, M., Bartl, S., McKinney, E.C., Flajnik, M.F. (2001): A shark antibody heavy chain encoded by a nonsomatically rearranged VDJ is preferentially expressed in early development and is convergent with mammalian IgG. *Proc Natl Acad Sci USA*, 98, 1775–1780.

Samollow, P.B. (2006): Status and applications of genomic resources for the gray, short-tailed opossum, *Monodelphis domestica*, an American marsupial model for comparative biology. *Aust J Zool.*, 54, 173–196.

Samples, N.K., VandeBerg, J.L., Stone, W.H. (1986): Passively acquired immunity in the newborn of a marsupial (*Monodelphis domestica*). *Am J Reprod Immunol Microb.*, 11, 94–97.

Vernersson, M., Aveskogh, M., Hellman, L. (2004): Cloning of IgE from the echidna (*Tachyglossus aculeatus*) and a comparative analysis of epsilon chains from all three extant mammalian lineages. *Dev Comp Immunol.*, 28(1), 61–75.

Vernersson, M., Aveskogh, M., Munday, B., Hellman, L. (2002): Evidence for an early appearance of modern postswitch immunoglobulin isotypes in mammalian evolution (II); cloning of IgE, IgG1 and IgG2 from a monotreme, the duck-billed platypus, *Ornithorhynchus anatinus*. *Eur J Immunol.*, 32, 2145–2155.

Wang, X., Miller R.D. (2012): Recombination, transcription and diversity of a partially germline joined VH in a mammal. *Immunogenetics*, 64, 713–717.

Wang, X., Olp, J.J., Miller R.D. (2009): On the genomics of immunoglobulins in the gray, short-tailed opossum *Monodelphis domestica*. *Immunogenetics*, 61, 581–596.

Wang, X., Parra, Z.E., Miller R.D. (2011): Platypus TCRµ provides insight into the origins and evolution of a uniquely mammalian TCR locus. *J. Immunol.*, *187*(10), 5246–5254.

Wang, X., Parra, Z.E., Miller, R.D. (2012b). A V*preB3* homologue from a marsupial, the gray short-tailed opossum, *Monodelphis domestica*. *Immunogenetics*, 64, 647–652.

Wang, X., Sharp, A.R., Miller, R.D. (2012a) Early postnatal B cell ontogeny and antibody repertoire maturation in the opossum, *Monodelphis domestica*. *PLoS ONE*, 7, e45931.

Warren, W.C., Hillier, L.W., Marshall Graves, J.A., Birney, E., Ponting, C.P., Grutzner, F., Wilson, R.K. (2008): Genome analysis of the platypus reveals unique signatures of evolution. *Nature*, 453, 175–183.

Wong, E.S.W., Papenfuss, A.T., Miller, R.D., Belov, K. (2009): Hatching time for monotreme immunology. *Aust J Zool.*, 57, 185–198.

Zhao, Y., Cui, H., Whittington, C.M., Wei, Z., Zhang, X., Zhang, Z. (2009): *Ornithorhynchus anatinus* (platypus) links the evolution of immunoglobulin genes in eutherian mammals and nonmammalian tetrapods. *J Immunol.*, 183, 3285–3293.

CHAPTER 5

ORGANIZATION OF THE IMMUNOGLOBULIN HEAVY- AND LIGHT-CHAIN LOCI IN THE RAT

PETER M. DAMMERS, JACOBUS HENDRICKS, PETER TERPSTRA, NICOLAAS A. BOS, and FRANS G. M. KROESE

CONTENTS

ABSTRACT

Rats of the genus *Rattus norvegicus* are undoubtedly one of the most popular animals used for experimental biomedical research. Despite the fact that the initial publications on immunoglobulin (IG) genes and their organization in the rat were shortly behind those of mouse and human, our knowledge on the complexity and organization of the IG loci in this rodent species has been hampered for years, due to lack of (genomic) nucleotide sequence information. The tide turned as of the establishment of most of the genomic nucleotide sequence from the Brown Norway (BN) rat strain. This genomic sequence information allows researchers to more accurately map the IG genes in this so commonly used species. To date, the organization of the rat IGH locus has been described in detail, whereas effort is undertaken to resolve the organization of the IGK and IGL loci. This chapter summarizes the current knowledge on the complexity and organization of the IGH, IGK, and IGL loci in the rat and reveals that the IG loci in this animal bear much resemblance to mouse and human.

5.1   INTRODUCTION

Rats belong to the largest order of mammals, named *Rodentia* (rodents; family Muridae). This order comprises more than 2,000 species, including mice (family Muridae), guinea pigs (family Caviidae), squirrels (family Sciuridae), beavers (family Castoridae) and hamsters (family Cricetidae) (Carleton and Musser, 2005). The most well-known rat species belong to the genus *Rattus* ("true rats" or "Old World" rats) of which the roof rat (*Rattus rattus*) and the brown rat (*Rattus norvegicus*) are the most common members. The evolutionary history of genus *Rattus* goes back to Asia, where the oldest fossil specimens of *Rattus* sp. were excavated from sediments that extend to the late Pliocene (2.5 MYA) (Carleton and Musser, 2005). Nowadays, both *Rattus rattus* and *Rattus norvegicus* are established worldwide in the temperate climate areas and parts of tropical and subantarctic zones. Most laboratory rats used today trace their heritage to Wistar ancestors (*R. norvegicus*), originally held at the Wistar Institute of Anatomy and Biology, Philadelphia PA, in the beginning of the twentieth century (Clause, 1993).

At present, a large number of genetically well-defined inbred rat strains are established that serve as models for important human disease traits, including susceptibility to cancer, hypertension, ischemia, obesity, diabetes, and autoimmune diseases. So, the rat became "from evil harbinger of pestilence to hero of modern medicine", as described by Clause (Clause, 1993), and has undoubtedly become one of the most frequently used animals in experimental biology and medical research.

As in other mammalian species, diversity in the immunoglobulin (IG) antigen-recognition site in the rat is established during early B-cell development by rearrangement of Variable region genes (or gene segments) located at the IG heavy (H)-chain and light (L)-chain loci. The Variable domain of the IGH chain is encoded by three different genes: Variable (IGHV), diversity (IGHD), and joining (IGHJ), whereas the IGK and IGL chain Variable domains are encoded by a combination of IGKV–IGKJ and IGLV–IGLJ, respectively (Roth, 1996). Recombination at the IGH, IGK and IGL loci is mediated (among other enzymes) by two "recombinase activation genes"—RAG-1 and RAG-2—that recognize a recombination signal sequence (RSS), flanking each of the IG Variable region genes (Roth, 1996; Fugmann et al., 2000). During recombination, RAG-1 and RAG-2 produce double-strand breaks between the IG Variable region genes to be joined and the flanking RSS. The joining-ends are subsequently subjected to hairpin opening nicks (generating small palindrome sequences called P-nucleotides), exonuclease activity, and nucleotide additions (N-nucleotides) by terminal deoxy-nucleotidyl transferase (TdT) (Gilfillan et al., 1993; Komori et al., 1993). The end result is the generation of highly Variable nucleotide sequences at the junctions of the rearranged gene-segments. Rats are able to produce the following eight Ab isotypes: IgM, IgD, IgG1, IgG2a, IgG2b, IgG2c, IgA, and IgE (Bazin et al., 1974). The constant region exons (IGHC) necessary to encode these different isotypes are located at the 3'-end of the IGH locus.

5.2   GENOMIC ORGANIZATION OF THE RAT IGH LOCUS

5.2.1   IGHV LOCUS

The vast majority of the genomic nucleotide sequence of the Brown Norway (BN) rat has been elucidated and this confirmed the location of the

IGH locus on chromosome 6q32–33 (Gibbs et al., 2004), as determined before by Pear et al. (1996). The IGH locus in rats bears much resemblance to that of mice, both with respect to its genomic organization as well as the nucleotide sequence of the coding regions (Bruggemann et al., 1986; Dammers and Kroese, 2001; Dammers et al., 2000; Hendricks et al., 2010; Lang and Mocikat, 1991). The rat IGH locus consists of a typical translocon organization (Marchalonis et al., 1998), comprised of 363 individual IGHV genes (of which 136 are functional), 21 IGHD genes (14 functional), and five IGHJ genes (four functional) (Hendricks et al., 2010). A detailed map of the organization of the rat IGH Variable region locus has been published by Hendricks et al. (2010). The IGH locus in rat is orientated from telomere (distal) towards centromere (proximal). Similar to mouse and human, the vast majority of rat IGHV genes are orientated towards the IGHD and IGHJ genes, and deletional joining, instead of inversional joining, is therefore most preferably used as major recombination mechanism at the IGH locus.

The size of the rat IGHV locus spans about 4.8 Mb and is therefore two times larger than the IGHV region in mouse (2.5 Mb) (Johnston et al., 2006) and five times larger than in human (0.9 Mb) (Matsuda et al., 1998; Pallares et al., 1999). The rat IGHV region comprises two and three times as many IGHV genes in comparison to mouse (195 IGHV genes) and human (123–129 IGHV genes), respectively. This indicates that the overall density of IGHV genes in the IGHV region is very similar between rat and mouse (76 and 78 genes per Mb, respectively), but lower in comparison to humans (137–143 genes per Mb). The intergenic distance between the IGHV genes is rather large in comparison to the size of the IGHV genes (~500 bp). For mouse and rat, the density of IGHV genes is somewhat higher at 3′ end of the IGHV region than at the 5′ end. The total number of functional IGHV genes (i.e., germline IGHV genes with an open reading frame in the coding regions and no defects in splice sites, recombination signals and/or regulatory elements) is more or less the same between mouse and rat (110 vs. 136), and significantly more in comparison to human (39–46). Furthermore, the mouse IGHV locus contains relatively more functional IGHV genes (56%), compared to rat and human (37% and 36%, respectively). In Table 1, the total numbers of IGHV genes in the IGH locus of rat, mouse, and human are depicted, according to current

IGH chromosomal maps (Hendricks et al., 2010; Johnston et al., 2006; Matsuda et al., 1998). For this table, numbers of human IGHV genes were obtained from the study of Matsuda et al. (1998). However, due to allelic variation and structural variants (i.e., deletions, insertions, and duplications that result in changes in gene copy number), the numbers of IGHV genes in the human IGH locus differs among individuals (Pallares et al., 1999; Watson et al., 2013; Lefranc, 2001). The human IGH locus is estimated to contain between 123–129 IGHV genes of which 39–46 are considered functional (Pallares et al., 1999). The data of Matsuda et al. (1998) are therefore not applicable for every individual.

TABLE 1   Numbers of IGHV genes in the IGH locus of rat, mouse, and human grouped by IMGT subgroup.

IMGT Subgroup	Previous mouse nomenclature	Total number of IGHV genes[a]		Human[b]	
		BN Rat		C57BL/6 Mouse	
IGHV1	J558	67	(25)	89	(52)	14	(9)
IGHV2	Q52	105	(43)	13	(9)	4	(3)
IGHV3	36–60	8	(4)	8	(6)	65	(19)
IGHV4	X24	4	(2)	2	(1)	32	(6)
IGHV5	PC7183	83	(27)	21	(10)	2	(1)
IGHV6	J606	19	(8)	5	(5)	1	(1)
IGHV7	S107(T15)	15	(6)	4	(3)	5	(0)
IGHV8	3609	19	(9)	16	(8)	—	
IGHV9	VGAM3.8	8	(4)	4	(4)	—	
IGHV10	VH10	19	(2)	3	(2)	—	
IGHV11	VH11(CP3)	12	(5)	2	(2)	—	
IGHV12	VH12(CH27)	3	(1)	1	(1)	—	
IGHV13	3609N	—		2	(1)	—	

TABLE 1   *(Continued)*

IMGT Subgroup	Previous mouse nomenclature	Total number of IGHV genes[a]					
		BN Rat		C57BL/6 Mouse		Human[b]	
IGHV14	SM7	—		4	(4)	—	
IGHV15	VH15	1	(0)	1	(1)	—	
IGHV16	VH16	—		1	(1)	—	
Unclassified	—	—		19	(0)	—	
Total		363	(136)	195	(110)	123	(39)

[a]Total numbers of IGHV genes grouped by IMGT subgroup (functional + ORF + pseudogenes) (20, 50). Numbers of functional IGHV genes are shown in parentheses. A germline IGHV gene is regarded functional if the coding region has an open reading frame without stop codon and if there are no defects in splice sites, RSS and/or regulatory elements (20). Numbers of IGHV genes for the different species were obtained from (13, 16, 17). Please note that the human IGHV subgroup nomenclature is not fully compatible between rat and mouse, for instance human IGHV3 subgroup members share the highest identity with members of the rat/mouse IGHV5 subgroup and human IGHV4 with rat/mouse IGHV3.
[b]Number of IGHV genes in the human IGH locus can Vary among individuals due to copy-number Variation (18, 19, 70).

 Nearly all nonfunctional IGVH genes in rat are pseudogenes that lack an open reading frame (ORF). Some nonfunctional genes, however, have an ORF. In ORF genes, alterations in the splice, regulatory, and/or RSS signal sequence(s), and/or amino acid constitution, and/or chromosomal position (i.e., orphan) renders the gene or product nonfunctional (Lefranc, 2001). Das et al. (2008) showed that there is a positive correlation between the number of nonfunctional and functional IGVH genes (in general, the more IGHV genes, the higher the number of nonfunctional genes in the IGH locus). This observation is assumed to result from the evolution of the IGVH genes. As proposed by Ota and Nei (1994), the evolution of IGVH genes is the consequence of two evolutionary processes: the birth-and-death process and diversifying selection. Whereas, some duplicated IGVH genes diversify and acquire new functions by mutations and evolutionary selection ("birth"; diversifying selection), others become functionally eliminated after obtaining deleterious mutations ("death"; pseudogenes) (Ota and Nei, 1994; Nei et al., 1997; Tanaka and Nei, 1989). As a result of this evolutionary process, IGHV genes can be grouped into genes with highly homologous sequences, the IGHV gene-families or subgroups. As in mice (Brodeur and Riblet, 1984), IGHV subgroup members in rat share at least 80% identity over the coding exon nucleotide sequence, whereas the sequence identity between members of different IGHV subgroups is generally less than 70% (Dammers et al., 2000).

Rat, mouse and human IGHV genes can be grouped into 13, 16, and 7 IGHV families, respectively. The IGHV genes in the BN rat can be sub-divided into 13 IGHV subgroups based on nucleotide sequence identity: IGHV1, IGHV2, IGHV3, IGHV4, IGHV5, IGHV6, IGHV7, IGHV8, IGHV9, IGHV10, IGHV11, IGHV12, and IGHV15 (Hendricks et al., 2010). In rat, most IGHV families are composed of various members, ranging from 3 to 99 (total genes, i.e., functional and nonfunctional), except for the IGHV15 family, which consists of only one (nonfunctional) member. The largest IGHV families in rat are represented by IGHV1, IGHV2, and IGHV5, which contain a total of 67, 99, and 79 IGHV genes, respectively. In the IGHV locus of mouse and rat, the various IGHV family members are often found clustered together (Hendricks et al., 2010; Johnston et al., 2010). However, the IGHV families are not completely spatially separated from each other and members of different IGHV families are frequently found intermingled with one another. Similar to mouse, the IGVH1 and IGHV8 family members in rat are located at the 5′end of the IGHV locus, whereas members of the IGHV2 and IGHV5 families are located at the 3′ end of the IGHV locus, closely to the IGHD region (Hendricks et al., 2010; Johnston et al., 2010). In comparison to mouse and rat, the IGHV family members in human are more extensively intermingled with each other and therefore clustering of IGHV family members is hardly observed (Matsuda et al., 1998). The almost identical IGHV locus organization between mouse and rat strongly implies a close evolutionary relationship between the two species.

5.2.2   IGHD LOCUS

The rat IGHD gene-cluster spans about 70 kB and is similar in size in comparison to mouse (Hendricks et al., 2010; Lang and Mocikat, 1991). In addition to the size of the loci, rat IGHD genes (both coding as well as RSS regions) also show high sequence identity to those of the mouse (Fig. 1). The IGHD locus in BN rat is comprised of 14 functional IGHD genes (Table 2), which include nine IGHD1 (DFL16), four IGHD4 (DST4) genes, and one IGHD5 (DQ52) gene (previous mouse nomenclature is

Comparative Immunoglobulin Genetics

shown in parentheses). The number of functional IGHD genes in rat is very comparable to the situation in mouse, where the IGH locus contains about 10–13 functional IGHD genes, depending on the mouse strain (Ye, 2004; Kurosawa et al., 1982; Chang et al., 1992; Feeney, 1990; Feeney and Riblet, 1993; Gerondakis et al., 1988; Lawler et al., 1987).

Functional IGHD genes

```
R|IGHD1-7   GCTTTTTGTGAAGGGATTTATTACTGTGTTTAT---TACTATGATGGTAGTTATTACTAC---CACAGTGGTACGTCCAACAGCAAAAACC
R|IGHD1-1   .................AC.C.........GTA.....C.G-AT.-A...C...------.........TA.....G..........
R|IGHD1-9   .................C............----......---A.C-A--GC..TAT.TAC........A..TA....G..........
R|IGHD1-8   .............................---.......TA....C...------.........
R|IGHD1-6   .................C..C.......-..------...C.GA..GTA.AG.G.G-------......T..TA....GT.........
M|IGHD1-1   .................C..C.......---...C.G.A..-A--GC..------......C..TA...T..........
R|IGHD1-4   .A.........C..AC.C.......AC........--...A.A.C..------.......A.TA...G..........
R|IGHD1-2   .A.........C..AC.C.......C...-----......--...A.G.C..-----.......A.TA...G..A....C..
R|IGHD1-3   AT...............C.........T.---A...C---A..A--GC..------.......A.TA.T..G..A........
R|IGHD1-5   .............A..A..C...........---A..----------A---.C...------......C.A..TA.A.TG..........

R|IGHD4-1   GGATTTTGAACTAGTTAGTGTCACAGTGGGTATAAATTCGGGGTACCACTGTAGGAAAAGCTGCAACGAAAACT
R|IGHD4-2   A..............C............G..........TA.TA.....A.............C....A
R|IGHD4-3   ..........A.....C........................A................CTC...CTG
M|IGHD3-1   ..........A.....C........C.C.GC.....C..........A........CA...C.....
R|IGHD4-4   ..............G..C.....TG........-..T...C.T...T.........T....T..T.....

R|IGHD5-1   GGTTTTGACTAAGCAAAGCATCACAGTGCTAACTGGGAGCACAGTGACTTGTGGCTCAACAAAAACC
M|IGHD4-1   ...............GG....C.................C....G.....AC...............
```

IGHD ORF+pseudogenes

```
R|IGHD2-1   GGATTTTGTATGGGCCTCTCTCACTGTGGGATACTTACCATAGTAGTATAGTTCAGTCCCAAAAGC
R|IGHD2-3   .....CC......T.C.............C....A..GA.....A...........TT.
M|IGHD5-3   .....C......T........C....A.....C.....C.T.G...C..AG.....T....TT.
R|IGHD2-2   .....C..A........T...........C...T..C...GT....A.T.A...T...GCA

R|IGHD3-1   ACAACCCATGGTGGCTTCAGGCAGCAGGCCTCTGCAGTGCCCCCAACCCAACATGCCATCTGCTCTGGGACCAGAAAGT
R|IGHD3-4   ...........................................A.....................................T.
R|IGHD3-2   .GT...T...........................-..T..............T..........T......
R|IGHD3-3   .GT................A..T..........AT.....T........A.....T.........T....GT.
M|UNDEF     .GT.........AA.......TA............-.A......CA...A.T.G..AC..--T..A......G
```

FIGURE 1 Alignment of the IGHD sequences of the BN rat. Sequences are described in Hendricks et al. (2010) and obtained from the UCSC (http://genome.ucsc.edu) (Meyer et al., 2013) using Baylor 3.4/rn4 rat genome assembly (Nov. 2004) (Gibbs et al., 2004). All rat IGHD genes have the same orientation in the locus (5′ to 3′ on the minus strand). In each IGHD subgroup, a mouse IGHD gene from the most homologous subgroup is included for comparison (R: rat, M: mouse). Dots and dashes denote nucleotide identities and gaps, respectively. The RSS heptamer and nonamer sequences are underlined. The IGHD region is marked in bold. The coordinates of the IGHD genes in Baylor 3.4/rn4 assembly are as follows: IGHD1–1 chr6:138,521,262–138,521,344; IGHD1–2 chr6:138,511,394–138,511,471; IGHD1–3 chr6:138,505,008–138,505,083; IGHD1–4 chr6:138,503,455–138,503,532; IGHD1–5 chr6:138,496,518–138,496,587; IGHD1–6 chr6:138,490,407–138,490,485; IGHD1–7 chr6:138,483,608–138,483,692; IGHD1–8 chr6:138,471,761–138,471,842; IGHD1–9 chr6:138,743,870–138,743,951; IGHD4–1 chr6:138,509,072–138,509,144; IGHD4–2 chr6:138,501,150–138,501,222; IGHD4–3 chr6:138,494,453–138,494,525; IGHD4–4 chr6:138,486,905–138,486,976; IGHD5–1 chr6:138,453,776–138,453,842; IGHD2–1 chr6:138,518,929–138,518,994; IGHD2–2 chr6:138,510,119–138,510,184; IGHD2–3 chr6:138,495,637–138,495,702; IGHD3–1 chr6:138,518,691–138,518,769; IGHD3–2 chr6:138,509,882–138,509,959; IGHD3–3 chr6:138,488,933–138,489,011; IGHD3–4 chr6:138,495,398–138,495,476. The rat IGHD3–1 sequence matches with a previous undefined (UNDEF) region in the mouse IGH locus at chromosomal position chr12:113,469,160–113,469,235 of Genome Reference Consortium assembly Dec. 2011 (GRCm38/mm10) (Church et al., 2009).

TABLE 2 Numbers of IGHD genes in the IGH locus of rat, mouse, and human grouped by IMGT subgroup.

IMGT subgroup[a]			Number of genes[b]		
Rat	Mouse	Human	BN Rat	C57BL/6 Mouse	Human
IGHD1	IGHD1 (DFL16)	IGHD4	9 (9)	1 (1)	4 (2)
—	IGHD2 (DSP2)	—	—	6 (6)	—
—	—	IGHD5	—	—	4 (3)
IGHD2	IGHD5	—	3 (0)	8 (0)	—
IGHD3	UNDEF[c]	—	4 (0)	6 (0)	—
IGHD4	IGHD3 (DST4)	IGHD1	4 (4)	2 (2)	5 (4)
IGHD5	IGHD4 (DQ52)	IGHD7	1 (1)	1 (1)	1 (1)
—	IGHD6	IGHD2	—	2 (0)	4 (4)
—	—	IGHD3	—	—	5 (5)
—	—	IGHD6	—	—	4 (4)
Total			21 (14)	26 (10)	27 (23)

[a]IGHD genes are grouped by IMGT nomenclature and arranged in corresponding subgroups. Grouping of the mouse IGHD6 subgroup with human IGHD2 is tentative.
[b]Numbers of IGHD genes for the different species were obtained from (Hendricks et al. (2010), Watson et al. (2013), Lefranc (2001), Ye (2004) and IMGT (mouse IGHD5 genes) (Lefranc et al., 2009). Numbers of functional IGHD genes are shown in parentheses.
[c]Previously undefined murine IGHD subgroup, provisionally consisting of six nonfunctional IGHD genes (pseudo/ORF).

As indicated in Fig. 1, rat IGHD genes are flanked on both sides by a typical RSS, characterized by a 12-bp spacer and the rather conserved heptamer and nonamer sequences (Ramsden et al., 1994). This allows the proper rearrangement of IGHD genes with an IGHV and an IGHJ gene at the 5′ and 3′ side, respectively. In addition to the functional IGHD genes, there are seven nonfunctional ORF genes containing non-canonical/aberrant RSS sequences, which probably render them nonfunctional. All these nonfunctional IGHD genes either belong to the subgroups IGHD2 (3 genes) or IGHD3 (4 genes). Rat IGHD2 genes show high nucleotide identity to mouse IGHD5 genes (Fig. 1), which are also considered to be nonfunctional (Ye, 2004). Rat IGHD3 homologous, however, have not been described for mouse, but alignment of the rat IGHD3–1 sequence to the mouse genome using the BLAT genome search program (Kent, 2002), revealed the presence of a previously undefined IGHD gene in the mouse IGH locus equivalent to the rat IGHD3 subgroup (Fig. 1; M|UNDEF). This murine IGHD gene is most probably also nonfunctional, since it contains a 2-bp deletion in the 3′ RSS spacer and has heptamer and nonamer sequences that carry aberrant (non-canonical) bases. A preliminary BLAT search (assembly Dec. 2011, GRCm38/mm10) (Kent, 2002; Church et al., 2009), indicates that this new IGHD gene most likely belongs to a new murine IGHD subgroup consisting of six (presumably nonfunctional) members.

The distribution of IGHD genes in the IGH locus is not completely similar between rat and mouse (Fig. 2). Except for the single functional DQ52 gene (rat IGHD5–1 and mouse IGHD4–1), which is located in close proximity (approx. 0.6 kB) to the IGHJ locus, the relative position and numbers of IGHD subgroup members are less well preserved between these species. For instance, the IGH locus of C57BL/6 mice harbors one DFL16 (IGHD1) gene, six DSP2 (IGHD2) genes, two DST4 (IGHD3) genes, and one DQ52 (IGHD4) gene, revealing that the IGHD locus of the BN rat contains relatively more DFL16 (IGHD1) genes, whereas genes belonging to the DSP2 subgroup, which is the largest in mouse, seem to be absent from the rat IGH locus. Typically, five clusters of tandem IGHD genes can be found in the rat IGH locus, generally consisting of a functional IGHD1 and IGHD4 gene separated from each other by an approx. 6 kB region harboring most frequently two pseudo(p)/ORF(r) genes of the IGHD2 and IGHD3 subgroup, respectively ([IGHD1–IGHD2r–IGHD3p–IGHD4] gene-cluster). A similar phenomenon is observed in mouse, where five out of six IGHD2 genes are flanked at the 3′ side by a pseudogene of the IGHD5 subgroup. Most likely, such clusters of tandem IGHD genes evolved by duplication of a common ancestral IGHD gene-cluster and may well result in a rapid expansion of certain IGHD subgroups during species evolution.

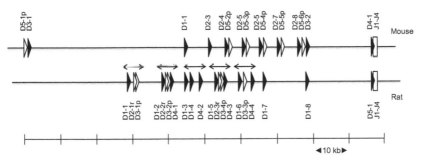

FIGURE 2 Comparison of the IGHD locus organization of BN rat vs. C57BL/6 mouse. Rat and mouse IGHD sequences are described by Hendricks et al. (2010) and Ye (2004), respectively, and retrieved from the IMGT (http://www.imgt.org) (2009). Relative positions were inferred using the BLAT genome search program (http://genome.ucsc. edu) (Kent, 2002; Meyer et al. (2013)) on the basis of genome assemblies Baylor 3.4/rn4 (Nov. 2004) and GRCm38/mm10 (Dec. 2011) (Gibbs et al., 2004; Church et al., 2009). IGHD genes are designated in abbreviated IMGT nomenclature. Solid and open triangles represent functional and pseudo(p)/ORF(r) genes, respectively. The IGHJ locus is marked by an open box and is approx. 0.6 kB downstream from gene DQ52 (rat D5–1 and mouse D4–1). For rat, the IGHD gene-clusters (see text) are indicated by bidirectional arrows. Rat IGHD1–9 is located 200 kB upstream of the IGHD gene-cluster and is not included in the figure.

The human IGHD gene locus, on the other hand, is about 40 kB and contains 27 IGHD genes (23 functional) subdivided into seven subgroups (Matsuda et al., 1998; Lefranc, 2001). The number of functional IGHD genes in the human IGH locus is therefore about twice the number of functional IGHD genes in rat and mouse. Figure 3 shows the evolutionary relationship between the functional IGHD genes of rat, mouse, and human, as inferred from the nucleotide sequences of the IGHD genes. This phylogenetic analysis shows that rat IGHD1 genes are closely related to mouse IGHD1 (DFL16), mouse IGHD2 (DSP2), and human IGHD4 genes. Also the rat IGHD5–1, mouse IGHD4–1 (DQ52), and human IGHD7–27 genes, seem to be relatively preserved among the three species. On the other hand, the human IGHD2, IGHD3, IGHD5, and IGHD6, form more isolated phylogenetic clusters. It seems likely that the human IGHD5 genes evolved from an ancestor shared with the human IGHD4 (rat/mouse IGHD1) subgroup, but the IGHD5 genes have substantially diverged from this group.

Comparative Immunoglobulin Genetics

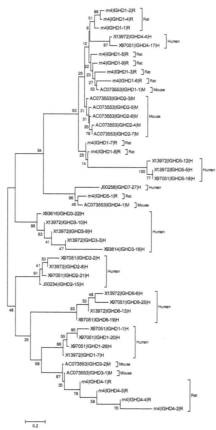

FIGURE 3 Evolutionary relationships of functional IGHD genes from rat, mouse and human. The evolutionary relationship was inferred using the Neighbor-Joining method (Nei and Kumar, 2000). The tree is drawn to scale, with branch lengths in the same units as those of the evolutionary distances used to infer the phylogenetic tree. Evolutionary distances were computed from IGHD 5' to 3' RSS nonamer sequences using the Kimura 2-parameter method (number of base substitutions per site), and modeled with a gamma distribution (shape parameter = 1). Bootstrap confidence Values of interior branches (500 replicates) are depicted near the branches. Values of 95% or higher are considered to represent the correct topology (Nei and Kumar, 2000). All ambiguous positions were removed for each sequence pair (partial deletion). There were a total of 95 positions in the final dataset. Evolutionary analyzes were conducted with MEGA5 software (Tamura et al., 2011). Sequence identifiers show GenBank accession number, IGHD gene number, and whether the sequence is derived from rat (R), mouse (M), or human (H), respectively. Mouse and human IGHD sequences were retrieved from the IMGT (http://www.imgt.org) (Lefranc et al., 2009). Rat IGHD sequences (rn4) were obtained from the UCSC (http://genome.ucsc.edu) (Meyer et al., 2013) using Baylor 3.4/rn4 rat genome assembly (Nov. 2004) (Gibbs et al., 2004).

5.2.3 IGHJ LOCUS

The rat IGHJ locus was initially partly described by Brüggemann et al. (1986) and further completed by Lang and Mocikat (1991). The IGHJ locus of rat is comprised of four functional IGHJ genes (IGHJ1 to IGHJ4), with intact 5' RSS and 3' splice signal sequences, and one IGHJ pseudogene (Jψ0; coding region is interrupted by a stop codon). The order of the IGHJ genes in the locus is Jψ0–IGHJ1–IGHJ2–IGHJ3–IGHJ4. Both IGHJ2 and IGHJ3 have a 23-bp RSS, whereas IGHJ1 and IGHJ4 (and the pseudogene Jψ0) carry a 22-bp RSS. Considering the preference of 23-bp over 22-bp RSS during recombination (Suzuki et al., 1992), this may result in a higher frequency of IGHJ2 and IGHJ3 gene usage in IGH transcripts. The rat IGHJ locus is about 2 kB in size and bears much resemblance to that of mouse and human, both in respect to organization as well as nucleotide and amino acid (coding region) sequence. In general, rat IGHJ coding regions share around 80% or more identity at both nucleotide and amino acid sequence level with the IGHJ genes of mouse (Lang and Mocikat, 1991). A similar degree of identity is also observed upon comparison with human IGHJ genes (Lang and Mocikat, 1991), although in human the IGHJ locus is comprised of six functional IGHJ genes and three IGHJ pseudogenes (Ravetch et al., 1981). The close evolutionary relationship among rat, mouse, and human IGHJ genes is illustrated by the phylogenetic tree depicted in Fig. 4. This phylogenetic analysis, based on the nucleotide sequences of the functional IGHJ genes, reveals that rat, mouse and, human IGHJ genes are related in the following way: rat/mouse IGHJ1 to human IGHJ2, rat/mouse IGHJ2 to human IGHJ1 and IGHJ4, rat/mouse IGHJ3 to human IGHJ5, and rat/ mouse IGHJ4 to human IGHJ6.

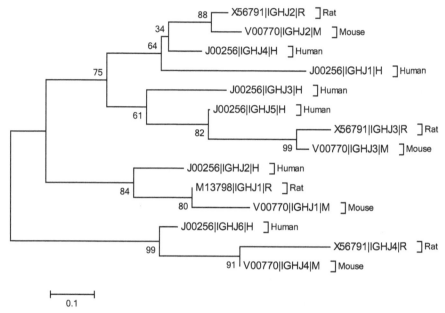

FIGURE 4 Phylogenetic tree of the functional IGHJ genes from rat, mouse and human (Neighbor-Joining method; (Nei and Kumar, 2000)). IGHJ sequences are described by (Gough and Bernard (1981)) and retrieved from the IMGT (http://www.imgt.org) (Lefranc et al., 2009). Evolutionary distances were computed from the IGHJ 5' RSS nonamer sequence up to the IGHJ 3' splice donor site (based on a total of 105 positions). See Fig. 3 legend for further details.

5.2.4 IGHC LOCUS

The eight serological-defined IGH isotypes in the rat (IgM, IgD, IgG1, Ig-G2a, IgG2b, IgG2c, IgE, and IgA) (7) are encoded by the IGHC genes: Cμ (IGHM), Cδ (IGHD), Cγ1 (IGHG1), Cγ2a (IGHG2A), Cγ2b (IGHG2B), Cγ2c (IGHG2C), Cε (IGHE), and Cα (IGHA), respectively. The coding and surrounding intron nucleotide sequences are described for many of the rat IGHC genes (Bruggemann et al., 1986). The chromosomal order of the IGHC genes in the rat was originally resolved by Brüggemann et al. (1986) and is: Cμ–Cδ– Cγ2c–Cγ2a–Cγ1–Cγ2b–Cε–Cα. To our knowledge, how-ever, an exact chromosomal map of the rat IGHC locus has never been pub-lished. On the basis of the rat IGHC exon nucleotide sequences that were retrieved for the IMGT/GENE-DB (Giudicelli et al., 2005; Lefranc et al.,

2005), we were able to establish a genomic map of the rat IGHC region using the Baylor 3.4/rn4 genome assembly (Nov. 2004) at the UCSC (http://
genome.ucsc.edu) (Meyer et al., 2013). As shown in Fig. 5, the size of rat
IGHC locus is about 220 kB and the IGHC genes are arranged in the following order: J_H–7.5 kB–Cμ–2 kB–Cδ–35 kB–Cγ2c–42 kB–Cγ2a–32 kB–
Cγ1–19 kB–Cγ2b–21 kB–Cϵ–8 kB–Cα. The number of IGHC genes in
the rat and the distance between them is rather similar to the IGHC gene
organization in mouse [J_H–6.5 kB–Cμ–4.5 kB–Cδ–55 kB–Cγ3–34 kB–
Cγ1–21 kB–Cγ2b–15 kB–Cγ2a–14 kB–Cϵ–12 kB–Cα] (Shimizu et al.,
1982), but is different from that observed in human, in which a tandem
gene-cluster [Cγ–Cγ–Cϵ–Cα] is found [J_H–8 kB–Cμ–8 kB–Cδ–±60 kB–
Cγ3–26 kB–Cγ1–19 kB–C$\psi\epsilon$2–13 kB–Cα1–±55 kB (incl. C$\psi\gamma$)–Cγ2–
18 kB–Cγ4–23 kB–Cϵ1–10 kB–Cα2] (Ravetch et al., 1981; Lefranc and
Lefranc, 1987). In contrast to human, the rat and mouse (52) IGHC locus
does not seem to contain any conserved IGHC pseudogenes. Except for
Cα, the IGHC genes in the rat are comprised of four exons encoding the
IGH chain constant domains and two exons coding for the membrane an-
chor (M1 and M2). The relative position of the most 5' (Cμ and Cδ) and 3'
(Cϵ and Cα) IGHC genes in the IGHC locus is similar between mouse and
rat. The Cμ, Cδ, and Cα loci are, however, not extensively described for
the rat. Genomic sequences of the exons Cμ2 and Cα3 were established
by Brüggemann et al. (1986), whereas the nucleotide sequence of the Cμ1
region was recovered from cDNA (Dammers et al., 2001). The rat Cμ
and Cα sequences bear high similarity to their counterpart in the mouse
and generally ≥90% sequence identity is revealed upon comparison (both
at nucleotide and amino acid level). A large proportion of the cDNA sequence of the rat Cδ gene was determined by Sire et al. (1982). The rat Cδ
locus spans nearly 20 kB and is therefore twice the size of the other IGHC
genes (Fig. 5). Comparison to the mouse reveals that the rat Cδ1 exon differs substantially from mouse Cδ1 (50–55% identity), whereas much more
identity is observed in the more C-terminal parts of the Cδ gene encoded
by the Cδ3 and CHS exons (85–90% identity) (Sire et al., 1982). The genomic organization of the rat Cϵ gene was described by Steen et al. (1984)
and is about 5 kB in size. Overall, the rat ϵ-chain yields ≥60% and ≥80%
nucleotide identity with the ϵ-chain in man and mouse, respectively. Of all rat
IGHC genes, Cγ genes have been described most extensively (Bruggemann

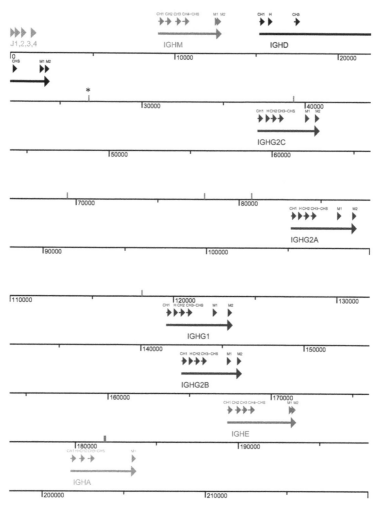

FIGURE 5 Genomic organization of the entire IGHC region of the BN rat. The 220 kB map was constructed on the basis of rat Baylor 3.4/rn4 genome assembly (Nov. 2004) at UCSC (http://genome.ucsc.edu) (Meyer et al., 2013) and Genvision software (DNASTAR, Madison, WI; http://www.dnastar.com). Direction is from telomere to centromere on chromosome 6q32 (minus strand in UCSC genome browser). The region corresponds to the assembly coordinates chr6:138450912–138230912. Nucleotide sequences of the IGHC exons were obtained using IMGT/GENE-DB (http://www.imgt.org) (Lefranc et al., 2009). The IGHJ locus is shown for map orientation. *Tick marks indicate positions of (small) assembly gaps in the Baylor 3.4/rn4 assembly (first 6 gaps approx. 10 bp; last gap approx. 130 bp). Long arrows represent the loci of individual IGHC genes, including the introns, but excluding the 5′ and 3′ untranslated regions (UTR). IGHC exons are indicated by short arrows and annotated with standard IMGT labels (Lefranc et al., 2009).

et al., 1986, 1988, 1989; Bruggemann, 1988). The rat Cγ1 and Cγ2a genes share 94% nucleotide identity with each other and best resemble the single mouse Cγ1 gene (87% and 86%, respectively). The rat Cγ2b gene, on the other hand, bears high nucleotide sequence identity to the mouse Cγ2a and Cγ2b genes (82% and 81%, respectively). Furthermore, the rat Cγ2c gene seems to be the equivalent of mouse Cγ3 gene (87% identity), as revealed by nucleotide sequence identity and effector function (Bruggemanne tal., 1988). Similar to other IGH genes, the IGHC genes in mammals most probably evolved from series of gene duplication(s) followed by mutation and selection of new genes. Some of these duplications occurred before species divergence, whereas others occurred in recent species evolution. In this regard, rat and mouse Cγ genes are most likely derived from a common set of three ancestral genes that evolved to Cγ2c, [Cγ2a–Cγ1], and Cγ2b in rat, and Cγ3, Cγ1, and [Cγ2b–Cγ2a] in mouse (39). The pairs of closely related Cγ2a/Cγ1 genes in rat and Cγ2b/Cγ2a genes in mouse are expected to result from a duplication event in recent evolution of either species. Also the presence of two Cγ gene-clusters [Cγ–Cγ–Cε–Cα] in the human IGHC locus can be explained by a segmental-duplication in recent human evolution.

5.3   GENOMIC ORGANIZATION OF THE RAT IGK AND IGL LOCI

The IGK and IGL chains in rats are transcribed from two loci of which only one copy of either locus is present in the rat haploid genome (Frank et al., 1987; Sheppard et al., 1981; Steen et al., 1987). The IGK and IGL loci are located on chromosome 4 and 11, respectively (Perlmann et al., 1985; Wahlstrom et al., 1988). In rodents, the IGK and IGL chains are not equally expressed among peripheral B cells and most (>90%) express IGK chains. In contrast to the rat IGH locus, limited information is available on the genomic organization of the rat IGK and IGL loci. Initial Southern blotting experiments by Breiner et al. (1982) using Vκ probes revealed the presence of dozens of Vκ genes in the rat genome and that they presumably could be subdivided into subgroups similar to mouse. The current IMGT/ GENE-DB (Giudicelli et al., 2005) lists 163 (135 functional) IGKV genes for the IGK locus of the BN rat that are subdivided over 21 IGKV subgroups. The largest IGKV subgroups in rat are IGKV1 (of which 22 are functional), IGKV4 (19 functional), and IGKV12 (21 functional). Together, members of these subgroups comprise almost half (46%) of the functional IGKV gene repertoire. In comparison, the mouse IGK locus on chromosome 6 consists of 169 IGKV genes (98 functional; current IMGT/GENE-DB) (Giudicelli et al., 2005), which belong to 20 subgroups. The total number of IGKV genes is therefore very similar between rat and mouse, but the rat IGK locus contains relatively more functional IGKV genes (83% vs. 68%).

In addition to the IGKV genes, the IGK locus harbors seven IGKJ genes (IGKJ1, IGKJ2–1, IGKJ2–2, IGKJ2–3, IGKJ3, IGKJ4, and IGKJ5) and only one IGKC (Cκ) gene (Frank et al., 1987; Breiner et al., 1982; Burstein et al., 1982; Sheppard and Gutman, 1981). As in mouse, IGKJ3 is probably not functional, because of a mutation in the splice-donor site, leaving six functional IGKJ genes available (Burstein et al., 1982; Sheppard and Gutman, 1982). The rat IGKJ genes bear much resemblance to their murine homologs (>90% nucleotide identity for the coding regions). The same degree of nucleotide sequence identity is observed for the IGKC genes of rat and mouse (88.5%) (Sheppard and Gutman, 1981). An interesting observation was made by Sheppard and Gutman (1981) and Frank et al. (1987), who demonstrated that on short-term evolutionary scale the mutation rate in the IGKC coding region is higher in comparison to the surrounding noncoding regions. This results in a rapid divergence of the IGKC region in the rat lineage and the creation of many allelic variants. A phenomenon which is also observed for the IGLC gene (Frank and Gutman, 1988).

The rat IGL and related loci (l5 and V_{preB}) have not been as extensively studied as those of mouse and an exact physical map of these loci has still to be established. In mouse, the IGL locus spans a region of about 180 kB on chromosome 16 and is arranged from a limited number of IGL genes. The IGL genes in this species are organized in two [V_nJCJC] gene-clusters, about 94 kB separated from each other, which have the following order: IGLV2–18.5 kB–IGLV3–40.4 kB–IGLJ2–1.3 kB–IGLC2–2.0 kB–IGLJ4–1.2 kB–IGLC4 and IGLV1–14.4 kB–IGLJ3–1.3 kB–IGLC3–2.1 kB–IGLJ1–1.1 kB–IGLC1 (Gerdes and Wabl, 2002). The IGLJ4 and

IGLC4 combination is considered nonfunctional due to a defective splice donor-site (Blomberg and Tonegawa, 1982). Only three IGLV genes are described for the mouse IGL locus. The number of combinations that can be generated during IGLV–IGLJ rearrangement is therefore very restricted. In case of the rat, only three IGLC genes and one IGLV gene are described (Steen et al., 1987; Frank and Gutman, 1988). Two of these IGLC genes (originally named Cλ2 and Cλ1) are located at approximately 3 kB from each other. Each of these IGLC genes seems to be preceded by two IGLJ genes, instead of one in case of the mouse. One of these IGLC genes (Cλ1) does not seem to be functionally expressed, as both Jλ1 genes upstream of Cλ1 have aberrant RSS and splice donor-sites. Also one of the Jλ2 genes is not functional, leaving only the Jλ2–Cλ2 combination apparently able to be functionally expressed. A third IGL gene (Cλ1.2) was also described by Frank and Gutman (Frank and Gutman 1988) and initially thought to represent another IGLC pseudogene. Cλ1.2, however, may well represent the rat homologue of the mouse λ5 gene (unpublished observations; accession number Z68145). Rat Cλ2 bears the highest resemblance to the murine IGLC3 gene (>90% sequence identity in coding and surrounding noncoding region), whereas the rat Cλ1 gene is most closely related to both IGLC1 and IGLC4 (Steen et al., 1987; Frank and Gutman, 1988). The rat Cλ2–Cλ1 cluster described before (Steen et al., 1987; Frank and Gutman, 1988) may therefore well be the homologue of the mouse IGLC3–IGLC1 cluster. In addition to the IGLJ and IGLC genes, Aquilar and Gutman (*66*) showed that the IGL locus in rats also comprises about 10–15 IGLV genes (including some pseudogenes), representing at least four distantly related IGLV subgroups.

At present, the rat IGL locus seems to have a rather low complexity, apparently consisting of only one [VnJJCJJC] cluster. According to the current IMGT/GENE-DB (Giudicelli et al., 2005), the rat IGL locus on chromosome 11 consists of seven functional IGLV (representing three subgroups: IGLV1, IGLV2, and IGLV3), four IGLJ (two functional), and four functional IGLC genes. Whether the two additional IGLC genes listed in the IMGT database represent the members of a second IGL cluster in the rat, as observed in mouse, is currently not known.

5.4 CONCLUSION

The rapid evolution of IG loci suggests that these loci are subjected to high diversifying-selection pressure, to establish a large repertoire of antigen-receptors on B cells. This evolutionary process results in variation of complexity and organization of IG loci among different mammalian species and provides optimal protection against threatening pathogens. Knowledge on the IG complexity and organization is prerequisite for the appropriate evaluation of the functional repertoire expressed by B cells. With the background information on the IG loci in the rat that is presented in this chapter, it will be feasible to maximize the usefulness of the rat as an experimental model for many important human disorders.

KEYWORDS

- **IGHC genes**
- **IGHD genes**
- **IGHJ genes**
- **IGHV genes**
- **immunoglobulin genes**
- **rat IGH locus**

REFERENCES

Aguilar, B.A., Gutman, G.A., Transcription and diversity of immunoglobulin lambda chain Variable genes in the rat. Immunogenetics. (1992): 37(1), 39–48.

Alcaraz, G., Bourgois, A., Moulin, A., Bazin, H., Fougereau, M. Partial structure of a rat IgD molecule with a deletion in the heavy chain. Ann Immunol (Paris). (1980): 131C(3), 363–388.

Bazin, H., Beckers, A., Querinjean, P. Three classes and four (sub)classes of rat immunoglobulins: IgM, IgA, IgE and IgG1, IgG2a, IgG2b, IgG2c. Eur J Immunol. (1974): 4(1), 44–48.

Blomberg, B., Tonegawa, S. DNA sequences of the joining regions of mouse lambda light chain immunoglobulin genes. Proc Natl Acad Sci USA. (1982): 79(2), 530–533.

Breiner, A.V., Brandt, C.R., Milcarek, C., Sweet, R.W., Ziv, E., Burstein, Y., et al., Somatic DNA rearrangement generates functional rat immunoglobulin kappa chain genes: the J kappa gene cluster is longer in rat than in mouse. Gene. (1982): 18(2), 165–174.

Brodeur, P.H., Riblet, R. The immunoglobulin heavy chain Variable region (Igh-V) locus in the mouse. I. One hundred Igh-V genes comprise seven families of homologous genes. Eur J Immunol. (1984): 14(10), 922–930.

Bruggemann, M. Evolution of the rat immunoglobulin gamma heavy-chain gene family. Gene. (1988): 74(2), 473–482.

Bruggemann, M., Delmastro-Galfre, P., Waldmann, H., Calabi, F. Sequence of a rat immunoglobulin gamma 2c heavy chain constant region cDNA: extensive homology to mouse gamma 3. Eur J Immunol. (1988): 18(2), 317–319.

Bruggemann, M., Free, J., Diamond, A., Howard, J., Cobbold, S., Waldmann, H. Immunoglobulin heavy chain locus of the rat: striking homology to mouse antibody genes. Proc Natl Acad Sci USA. (1986): 83(16), 6075–6079.

Bruggemann, M., Teale, C., Clark, M., Bindon, C., Waldmann, H. A matched set of rat/mouse chimeric antibodies. Identification and biological properties of rat H chain constant regions mu, gamma 1, gamma 2a, gamma 2b, gamma 2c, epsilon, and alpha. J Immunol. (1989): 142(9), 3145–3150.

Burstein, Y., Breiner, A.V., Brandt, C.R., Milcarek, C., Sweet, R.W., Warszawski, D., et al., Recent duplication and germline diversification of rat immunoglobulin kappa chain gene joining segments. Proc Natl Acad Sci USA. (1982): 79(19), 5993–5997.

Carleton, M.D., Musser, G.G., Order of Rodentia. In: Wilson, D.E., Reeder, D.M., editors. Mammal Species of the World: A Taxonomic and Geographic Reference. 3. Baltimore, MD: The Johns Hopkins University Press; 2005. pp. 745–1600.

Chang, Y., Paige, C.J., Wu, G.E., Enumeration and characterization of DJH structures in mouse fetal liver. The EMBO journal. (1992): 11(5), 1891–1899.

Church, D.M., Goodstadt, L., Hillier, L.W., Zody, M.C., Goldstein, S., She, X., et al., Lineage-specific biology revealed by a finished genome assembly of the mouse. PLoS Biol. (2009): 7(5), e1000112.

Clause, B.T., The Wistar Rat as a right choice: establishing mammalian standards and the ideal of a standardized mammal. J Hist Biol. (1993): 26(2), 329–349.

Dammers, P.M., Bun, J.C., Bellon, B., Kroese, F.G., Aten, J., Bos, N.A., Immunoglobulin VH-gene usage of autoantibodies in mercuric chloride-induced membranous glomerulopathy in the rat. Immunology. (2001): 103(2), 199–209.

Dammers, P.M., Kroese, F.G., Evolutionary relationship between rat and mouse immunoglobulin IGHV5 subgroup genes (PC7183) and human IGHV3 subgroup genes. Immunogenetics. (2001): 53(6), 511–517.

Dammers, P.M., Visser, A., Popa, E.R., Nieuwenhuis, P., Bos, N.A., Kroese, F.G., Immunoglobulin VH gene analysis in rat: most marginal zone B cells express germline encoded VH genes and are ligand selected. Curr Top Microbiol Immunol. (2000): 252: 107–117.

Das, S., Nozawa, M., Klein, J., Nei, M. Evolutionary dynamics of the immunoglobulin heavy chain Variable region genes in Vertebrates. Immunogenetics. (2008): 60(1), 47–55.

Feeney, A.J., Lack of N regions in fetal and neonatal mouse immunoglobulin V-D-J junctional sequences. J Exp Med. (1990): 172(5), 1377–1390.

Feeney, A.J., Riblet, R. DST4: a new, and probably the last, functional DH gene in the BALB/c mouse. Immunogenetics. (1993): 37(3), 217–221.

Frank, M.B., Besta, R.M., Baverstock, P.R., Gutman, G.A., The structure and evolution of immunoglobulin kappa chain constant region genes in the genus Rattus. Mol Immunol. (1987): 24(9), 953–961.

Frank, M.B., Gutman, G.A., Two pseudogenes among three rat immunoglobulin lambda chain genes. Mol Immunol. (1988): 25(10), 953–960.

Fugmann, S.D., Lee, A.I., Shockett, P.E., Villey, I.J., Schatz, D.G., The RAG proteins and V(D)J recombination: complexes, ends, and transposition. AnnuRevImmunol. (2000): 18: 495–527.

Gerdes, T., Wabl, M. Physical map of the mouse lambda light chain and related loci. Immunogenetics. (2002): 54(1), 62–65.

Gerondakis, S., Bernard, O., Cory, S., Adams, J.M., Immunoglobulin JH rearrangement in a T-cell line reflects fusion to the DH locus at a sequence lacking the nonamer recognition signal. Immunogenetics. (1988): 28(4), 255–259.

Gibbs, R.A., Weinstock, G.M., Metzker, M.L., Muzny, D.M., Sodergren, E.J., Scherer, S., et al., Genome sequence of the Brown Norway rat yields insights into mammalian evolution. Nature. (2004): 428(6982): 493–521.

Gilfillan, S., Dierich, A., Lemeur, M., Benoist, C., Mathis, D. Mice lacking TdT: mature animals with an immature lymphocyte repertoire. Science. (1993): 261(5125): 1175–1178.

Giudicelli, V., Chaume, D., Lefranc, M.P., IMGT/GENE-DB: a comprehensive database for human and mouse immunoglobulin and T cell receptor genes. Nucleic Acids Res. (2005): 33(Database issue): D256–261.

Gough, N.M., Bernard, O. Sequences of the joining region genes for immunoglobulin heavy chains and their role in generation of antibody diversity. Proc Natl Acad Sci USA. (1981): 78(1), 509–513.

Hellman, L., Pettersson, U., Bennich, H. Characterization and molecular cloning of the mRNA for the heavy (epsilon) chain of rat immunoglobulin, E. Proc Natl Acad Sci USA. (1982): 79(4), 1264–1268.

Hellman, L., Steen, M.L., Sundvall, M., Pettersson, U. A rapidly evolving region in the immunoglobulin heavy chain loci of rat and mouse: postulated role of (dC-dA)n.(dG-dT)n sequences. Gene. (1988): 68(1), 93–100.

Hendricks, J., Terpstra, P., Dammers, P.M., Somasundaram, R., Visser, A., Stoel, M., et al., Organization of the Variable region of the immunoglobulin heavy-chain gene locus of the rat. Immunogenetics. (2010): 62(7), 479–486.

Johnston, C.M., Wood, A.L., Bolland, D.J., Corcoran, A.E., Complete sequence assembly and characterization of the C57BL/6 mouse Ig heavy chain V region. J Immunol. (2006): 176(7), 4221–4234.

Kent, W.J., BLAT–the BLAST-like alignment tool. Genome Res. (2002): 12(4), 656–64.

Komori, T., Okada, A., Stewart, V., Alt, F.W., Lack of N regions in antigen receptor Variable region genes of TdT-deficient lymphocytes. Science. (1993): 261(5125): 1171–1175.

Kurosawa, Y., Tonegawa, S. Organization, structure, and assembly of immunoglobulin heavy chain diversity DNA segments. J Exp Med. (1982): 155(1), 201–218.

Lang, P., Mocikat, R. Immunoglobulin heavy-chain joining genes in the rat: comparison with mouse and human. Gene. (1991): 102(2), 261–264.

Lawler, A.M., Lin, P.S., Gearhart, P.J., Adult B-cell repertoire is biased toward two heavy-chain Variable-region genes that rearrange frequently in fetal pre-B cells. Proc Natl Acad Sci USA. (1987): 84(8), 2454–2458.

Lefranc, M.P., Giudicelli, V., Ginestoux, C., Jabado-Michaloud, J., Folch, G., Bellahcene, F., et al., IMGT, the international ImMunoGeneTics information system. Nucleic Acids Res. (2009): 37(Database issue): D1006–1012.

Lefranc, M.P., Lefranc, G. Human immunoglobulin heavy-chain multigene deletions in healthy individuals. FEBS Lett. (1987): 213(2), 231–237.

Lefranc, M.P., Nomenclature of the human immunoglobulin heavy (IGH) genes. Exp Clin Immunogenet. (2001): 18(2), 100–116.

Marchalonis, J.J., Schluter, S.F., Bernstein, R.M., Shen, S., Edmundson, A.B., Phylogenetic emergence and molecular evolution of the immunoglobulin family. Adv Immunol. (1998): 70: 417–506.

Matsuda, F., Ishii, K., Bourvagnet, P., Kuma, K., Hayashida, H., Miyata, T., et al., The complete nucleotide sequence of the human immunoglobulin heavy chain Variable region locus. J Exp Med. (1998): 188(11), 2151–2162.

Meyer, L.R., Zweig, A.S., Hinrichs, A.S., Karolchik, D., Kuhn, R.M., Wong, M., et al., The UCSC Genome Browser database: extensions and updates 2013. Nucleic Acids Res. (2013): 41(Database issue): D64–69.

Nei, M., Gu, X., Sitnikova, T. Evolution by the birth-and-death process in multigene families of the Vertebrate immune system. Proc Natl Acad Sci USA. (1997): 94(15), 7799–806.

Nei, M., Kumar, S. Molecular evolution and phylogenetics. New York: Oxford University Press; 2000.

Ota, T., Nei, M. Divergent evolution and evolution by the birth-and-death process in the immunoglobulin VH gene family. Mol Biol Evol. (1994): 11(3), 469–482.

Pallares, N., Lefebvre, S., Contet, V., Matsuda, F., Lefranc, M.P., The human immunoglobulin heavy Variable genes. Exp Clin Immunogenet. (1999): 16(1), 36–60.

Parker, K.E., Bugeon, L., Cuturi, M.C., Soulillou, J.P., Cloning of cDNA coding for the rat mu heavy chain constant region: differences between rat allotypes. Immunogenetics. (1994): 39(2), 159.

Pear, W.S., Wahlstrom, G., Szpirer, J., Levan, G., Klein, G., Sumegi, J. Localization of the rat immunoglobulin heavy chain locus to chromosome 6. Immunogenetics. (1986): 23(6), 393–395.

Perlmann, C., Sumegi, J., Szpirer, C., Levan, G., Klein, G. The rat immunoglobulin kappa light chain locus is on chromosome 4. Immunogenetics. (1985): 22(1), 97–100.

Ramsden, D.A., Baetz, K., Wu, G.E., Conservation of sequence in recombination signal sequence spacers. Nucleic Acids Res. (1994): 22(10), 1785–1796.

Ravetch, J.V., Siebenlist, U., Korsmeyer, S., Waldmann, T., Leder, P. Structure of the human immunoglobulin mu locus: characterization of embryonic and rearranged J and D genes. Cell. (1981): 27(3 Pt 2): 583–591.

Roth, D.B., V(D)J Recombination. In: Herzenberg, L.A., Weir, D.M., Blackwell, C., editors. Weir's Handbook of Experimental Immunology. 5 ed. Oxford: Blackwell Science; 1996. pp. 16–20.

Sakano, H., Maki, R., Kurosawa, Y., Roeder, W., Tonegawa, S. Two types of somatic recombination are necessary for the generation of complete immunoglobulin heavy-chain genes. Nature. (1980): 286(5774): 676–683.

Sheppard, H.W., Gutman, G.A., Allelic forms of rat kappa chain genes: evidence for strong selection at the level of nucleotide sequence. Proc Natl Acad Sci USA. (1981): 78(11), 7064–8.

Sheppard, H.W., Gutman, G.A., Complex allotypes of rat kappa chains are encoded by structural alleles. Nature. (1981): 293(5834): 669–671.

Sheppard, H.W., Gutman, G.A., Rat kappa-chain J-segment genes: two recent gene duplications separate rat and mouse. Cell. (1982): 29(1), 121–127.

Shimizu, A., Takahashi, N., Yaoita, Y., Honjo, T. Organization of the constant-region gene family of the mouse immunoglobulin heavy chain. Cell. (1982): 28(3), 499–506.

Sire, J., Auffray, C., Jordan, B.R., Rat immunoglobulin delta heavy chain gene: nucleotide sequence derived from cloned cDNA. Gene. (1982): 20(3), 377–386.

Steen, M.L., Hellman, L., Pettersson, U. Rat immunoglobulin E heavy chain locus. J Mol Biol. (1984): 177(1), 19–32.

Steen, M.L., Hellman, L., Pettersson, U. The immunoglobulin lambda locus in rat consists of two C lambda genes and a single V lambda gene. Gene. (1987): 55(1), 75–84.

Sudmant, P.H., Kitzman, J.O., Antonacci, F., Alkan, C., Malig, M., Tsalenko, A., et al., Diversity of human copy number Variation and multicopy genes. Science. (2010): 330(6004): 641–646.

Suzuki, H., Shiku, H. Preferential usage of JH2 in D-J joinings with DQ52 is determined by the primary DNA sequence and is largely dependent on recombination signal sequences. Eur J Immunol. (1992): 22(9), 2225–2230.

Tamura, K., Peterson, D., Peterson, N., Stecher, G., Nei, M., Kumar, S. MEGA5: molecular evolutionary genetics analysis using maximum likelihood, evolutionary distance, and maximum parsimony methods. Mol Biol Evol. (2011): 28(10), 2731–2719.

Tanaka, T., Nei, M. Positive darwinian selection observed at the Variable-region genes of immunoglobulins. Mol Biol Evol. (1989): 6(5), 447–459.

Wahlstrom, G., Pear, W.S., Steen, M.L., Szpirer, J., Levan, G., Klein, G., et al., Localization of the rat immunoglobulin lambda light chain locus to chromosome 11. Immunogenetics. (1988): 28(3), 182–183.

Watson, C.T., Steinberg, K.M., Huddleston, J., Warren, R.L., Malig, M., Schein, J., et al., Complete haplotype sequence of the human immunoglobulin heavy-chain Variable, diversity, and joining genes and characterization of allelic and copy-number Variation. Am J Hum Genet. (2013): 92(4), 530–546.

Ye, J. The immunoglobulin IGHD gene locus in C57BL/6 mice. Immunogenetics. (2004): 56(6), 399–404.

CHAPTER 6

GENERATION OF THE ANTIBODY REPERTOIRE IN RABBITS: ROLE OF GUT-ASSOCIATED LYMPHOID TISSUES

KARI M. SEVERSON and KATHERINE L. KNIGHT

CONTENTS

ABSTRACT

Animals use different strategies to generate a preimmune antibody repertoire. In rabbits, relatively little antibody diversity is generated by combinatorial joining of V(D)J genes at the immunoglobulin heavy chain (IgH) locus due to predominant rearrangement of a single V_H gene. Instead, progenitor cells produced in the bone marrow during B cell lymphopoiesis migrate to gut-associated lymphoid tissues (GALT) where they extensively proliferate and diversify their Ig genes by somatic hypermutation and gene conversion mechanisms in response to stimulation by the intestinal microbiota. Recent studies have identified bacterial molecules that contribute to, as well as endogenous molecules required for B cell proliferation and somatic diversification of Ig genes in GALT. In addition to generating a preimmune antibody repertoire in the presence of limited V_H gene usage during B cell development, rabbits are presented with an additional challenge of maintaining B cell populations throughout life, as B lymphopoiesis arrests in adult rabbits. Increasing evidence suggests that GALT also plays a key role in maintaining peripheral B cell populations in the absence of ongoing lymphopoiesis. In this chapter, we provide a detailed description of the key experiments and data demonstrating that antibody diversity in rabbits is generated by a two-step mechanism.

6.1   INTRODUCTION

The generation of antibody diversity was one of the most important questions in the history of immunology. Through the combined efforts of protein chemists, molecular biologists, and immunologists in the 1960s and 1970s, it was concluded that antibody diversity is generated by somatic recombination of germline-encoded immunoglobulin (Ig) V(D)J-C gene segments, also known as combinatorial joining. Since the original discoveries in mouse, studies of antibody diversity in other species have revealed that combinatorial diversity is just one mechanism, and perhaps a minor mechanism, by which some animals generate a preimmune antibody repertoire.

In humans and mice, a preimmune antibody repertoire is generated through the rearrangement and joining of V(D)J gene segments within progenitor B cells at the primary site of lymphopoiesis (bone marrow) throughout life. In other species, including chickens, sheep, and rabbits, a two-step mechanism occurs. In the first step, a limited number of V, D, and J-gene segments are used during V(D)J gene rearrangements at the primary site of lymphopoiesis, and second, diversification of the small number of used V(D)J genes occurs in the gut-associated lymphoid tissue (GALT) by varying mechanisms. In the following sections, we describe in detail, the two-step mechanism for the generation of antibody diversity in rabbits.

6.2 STEP 1: LIMITED V-GENE USAGE AND SUPPRESSION OF B LYMPHOPOIESIS IN THE BONE MARROW

Similar to humans and mice, the primary sites of B lymphopoiesis in rabbits are the fetal liver and bone marrow. Progenitor B cells expressing cytoplasmic IgM are first detected in the fetal liver at 23 days gestation where they peak 2 days after birth, and in the bone marrow where they peak 2–5 days after birth (Hayward et al., 1978). Unlike humans and mice, however, very little antibody diversity is generated in rabbits by the combinatorial joining of V, D, and J gene segments. Although the rabbit heavy chain locus contains at least 100 V_H gene segments (Currier et al., 1988; Gallarda et al., 1985; Ros et al., 2004), 11 D_H gene segments, and 6 J_H gene segments (Becker et al., 1989; Ros et al., 2004), a limited number of these genes are preferentially rearranged (Fig. 1). As a consequence, peripheral B cells have a limited variety of rearranged V, D, and J genes.

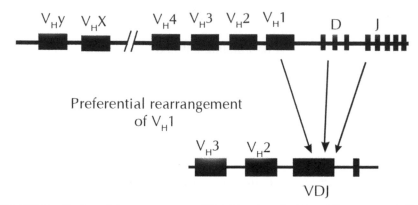

FIGURE 1 Preferential rearrangement of $V_H 1$. Most B cells (80 to 90%) use $V_H 1$ in VDJ gene rearrangements; the other 10 to 20% use gene segments at least 100 kB 5' of $V_H 1$ (e.g., $V_H x$ and $V_H y$) during VDJ gene rearrangements. No IgH gene rearrangement, including DJ, is usually found on the second IgH allele (Tunyaplin and Knight, 1997).

Rabbit Ig heavy chains contain allotypes, or genetic differences that induce an immune response in genetically distinct animals of the same species (Oudin, 1960; Perey and Good, 1968), and early studies of these V_H allotypes revealed interesting features of antibody diversity in rabbits. For example, 80% of serum antibodies display a1, a2, or a3 allotype specificities, also called $V_H a$ or a-positive allotypes, whereas 20% of serum antibodies lack a-positive allotypes but have x32 and y33, also called $V_H n$ or a-negative allotypes (Dray et al., 1963; Kim and Dray, 1972; Kim and Dray, 1973). The predominance of $V_H a$ allotype specificities in the periphery suggested that a limited number of V_H genes may be used during B lymphopoiesis. Experiments comparing cDNA sequences of peripheral VDJ genes to the genomic DNA sequence of the 3'-most/D-proximal V_H gene ($V_H 1$) provided further evidence for limited V_H gene usage in rabbits. Sequence analysis of eight VDJ genes cloned from leukemic rabbit B cells revealed that seven of the eight sequences were identical to $V_H 1$ (Becker et al., 1990). Additionally, when the genomic DNA sequence of $V_H 1$ from a^1/a^1, a^2/a^2, and a^3/a^3 homozygous rabbits was translated and compared to the partial amino acid sequence of pooled Ig from the same rabbits, the sequences were identical (Knight and Becker, 1990), directly demonstrating that the D-proximal V_H gene, $V_H 1$, is preferentially rearranged during VDJ-recombination.

6.2.1   ARREST OF B LYMPHOPOIESIS EARLY IN ONTOGENY

Another interesting feature of rabbit B cell development is that B lymphopoiesis is not continuous throughout life, as there is an arrest of B lymphopoiesis in adults. This B cell development differs from humans and mice, and also presents rabbits with a challenge for generating antibodies throughout life. Observations from early allotype suppression experiments first suggested that B lymphopoiesis may not be continuous. Administration of anti-allotype antibodies to neonatal rabbits to eliminate or suppress B cell production of a particular allotype, resulted in suppression that, surprisingly, was maintained for up to two years (Eskinazi et al., 1979; Harrison et al., 1973; Mage and Dray, 1965). One would expect that if B cells are continuously produced, then newly generated antibodies would outnumber those suppressed and the allotype suppression would not be maintained for such an extended period of time. Several years later, observations in rabbit bone marrow further supported the idea that B lymphopoiesis arrests after a few months of age. By performing VDJ sequence analysis and RNase protection assays using undiversified V-gene probes on bone marrow samples, Crane et al. (1996) found a lack of undiversified VDJ genes in adult bone marrow. Furthermore, the authors detected fewer B cell recombination excision circles (BRECs) in adult bone marrow as compared to young bone marrow samples by PCR analysis, providing direct evidence for an arrest of B lymphopoiesis in adult rabbits (Crane et al., 1996). Additionally, detailed flow cytometric analysis of pro-B and pre-B cell populations in the bone marrow of various aged rabbits (Fig. 2) demonstrated that progenitor B cell populations decline over time and are not detectable in the bone morrow by 16 weeks of age (Jasper et al., 2003).

Interestingly, a combination of in vitro and in vivo experiments suggested that the lack of newly made progenitor B cell populations in adult rabbits is not due to B cell-intrinsic factors, but instead, to changes in multiple B cell-extrinsic or bone marrow microenvironmental factors. To test if the arrest of B lymphopoiesis in adult rabbits is due to changes in the bone marrow microenvironment or to changes within progenitor cells themselves, Kalis et al. (2007) co-cultured adult bone marrow cells with mouse OP9 stromal cells, a cell line that supports B lymphopoiesis, and analyzed the co-cultures for pro-B and pre-B cell populations by flow cytometry. The authors reasoned that if the arrest of B lymphopoiesis in adult rabbits is

due to cell-intrinsic factors rather than to the bone marrow microenvironment, then pro-B and pre-B cell populations would not be produced during
co-culture with OP9 stromal cells. However, progenitor B cell populations
were detected following co-culture of adult bone marrow with OP9 stromal
cells, suggesting that adult progenitor cells are capable of differentiating in
vitro (Kalis et al., 2007). To test whether the same is true in vivo, the authors transferred adult bone marrow cells (lacking pre-B cells) from rabbits
containing a GFP transgene into normal, young irradiated recipients, and
found GFP[+] donor pre-B and B cells in the recipients, indicating that adult
progenitor cells are capable of differentiation when provided the correct
microenvironmental factors in vivo (Kalis et al., 2007). During this series

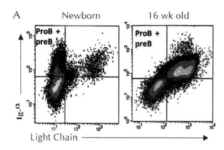

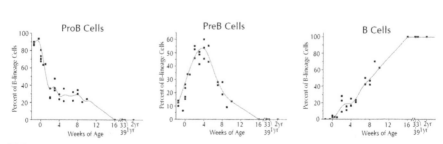

FIGURE 2   Decline of B lymphopoiesis after birth. A. Flow cytometric analysis of bone
marrow (BM) cells from newborn and 16-week-old rabbits, showing large numbers of
pro-B and pre-B cells (Ig-α^+L-chain$^-$) in BM from newborn rabbits and almost none from
16-week-old rabbits. B. Change in percentage of pro-B, pre-B, and B cells in BM over
time. ProB cell = Ig-α^+/cytoplasmic μ^- cells; pre-B cell = cytoplasmic μ^+/surface μ^-; B cell
= cytoplasmic μ^+/surface μ^+; Each point = data from a single rabbit (Jasper et al., 2003).

of in vivo experiments, Kalis et al. (2007) also irradiated adult rabbits, and discovered that progenitor B cell populations arise in the bone marrow of adults following irradiation, suggesting that the arrest of B lymphoiesis is not necessarily permanent, but more likely is suppressed. Taken together, these data demonstrate that the suppression of B lymphopoiesis in adult rabbits is due to changes in the bone marrow microenvironment.

6.2.2 MECHANISM OF ARREST OF B LYMPHOPOIESIS

To determine which factors are responsible for the suppression of B cell development in adult rabbits, a cDNA representational difference analysis (RDA) of young and adult bone marrow stromal cells was performed and revealed several factors that were differentially expressed in these two samples. One of these factors, encoding the extracellular matrix protein periostin, was decreased in adult bone marrow stromal cells. Further analysis by semi-quantitative RT-PCR on bone marrow from various aged rabbits confirmed this finding, as the decrease in periostin expression correlated with the decline of B lymphopoiesis (Siewe et al., 2011). To test if periostin is required for B lymphopoiesis, Siewe et al. (2011) co-cultured adult bone marrow cells with OP9 stromal cells in which periostin expression was knocked-down with siRNA, and the cultures were analyzed for progenitor B cells by flow cytometry. The number of progenitor B cells arising in these cultures was markedly reduced, indicating that periostin contributes to, but may not be essential for B cell development in the bone marrow (Siewe et al., 2011). Periostin knockout mice showed no deficit in either B or T cell development, suggesting that in vivo, other molecules (presumably extracellular matrix molecules) can compensate for the loss of periostin.

   In addition to looking for specific factors that may be required for suppression of B lymphopoiesis in adult rabbits, Bilwani and Knight (2012) took a different approach and assessed the number and differentiation status of cell populations comprising the bone marrow of various aged rabbits. Quite remarkably, the authors found that the number of mesenchymal stem cells (MSC) in the rabbit bone marrow decreased by 8 weeks of age, that these MSCs preferentially differentiate into adipocytes instead of osteoblasts, and that bone marrow essentially becomes filled with fat cells instead of with cells that are known to promote B cell development. The authors also determined that the adipocytes secrete a soluble factor that directly inhibits B lymphopoiesis in vitro (Bilwani and Knight, 2012). Studies are underway to identify this soluble factor and determine if it is required for B lymphopoiesis in vivo.

Years of work on rabbit B cell development in the bone marrow have revealed two interesting and unique features for the generation of antibody diversity in rabbits. First, very little diversity is generated by combinatorial joining of VDJ genes in progenitor B cells at the primary site of lymphopoiesis due to preferential rearrangement of $V_H 1$. Second, due to microenvironmental changes in the bone marrow, B lymphopoiesis arrests a few months after birth. These observations pose two major questions for the generation of antibody diversity and general humoral immunity in rabbits: How (and where) is a preimmune antibody repertoire generated in rabbits? How are B cells maintained so that humoral immune responses are initiated against a wide variety of foreign antigens throughout the lifespan of rabbits?

6.3   STEP 2: GALT AND THE GENERATION OF A PRE-IMMUNE ANTIBODY REPERTOIRE

Lack of Ig diversity generated from somatic recombination at the heavy chain locus led researchers to investigate other mechanisms by which a preimmune antibody repertoire is generated in rabbits. One possibility was that L-chains contribute significantly to diversity. Sequence analysis of two bacterial artificial chromosomes (BAC) containing 0.4 Mb of the V_κ locus leads to estimates of approximately 100 germline V_κ gene segments and 5 J elements that can recombine to generate light chains and contribute to light chain diversity (Ros et al., 2005). Unlike the IgH locus, there is currently no evidence for preferential rearrangement of particular V_κ gene segments. In fact, VJ sequence analysis of bone marrow cDNA from 1-day-old rabbits revealed that many different V_κ gene segments are expressed (Sehgal et al., 1999). Further, diversification of light chain genes occurs in the rabbit appendix by both somatic hypermutation and gene conversion mechansisms (Sehgal et al., 2002). Taken together, these data suggest that light chains contribute significantly to antibody diversity.

A second possibility for the generation of a large primary antibody repertoire was that Ig genes undergo extensive somatic diversification in the periphery. Several observations from VDJ sequence analysis in peripheral tissues indicated that IgH chain genes are diversified through both somatic gene conversion and somatic hypermutation mechanisms. For example, VDJ genes cloned from spleens and mesenteric lymph nodes of a^3/a^3 homozygous rabbits contained clusters of nucleotide changes present in V_H1 which resembled sequences of upstream V_H genes, suggesting that upstream V-genes may serve as donors for gene conversion (Fig. 3) (Becker and Knight, 1990). In separate studies, VDJ genes cloned from peripheral tissues displayed several base pair substitutions in the D- and J-regions, suggesting that somatic hypermutation also occurs (DiPietro et al., 1992; Short et al., 1991). Further characterization of the genomic DNA directly downstream of J_H gene segments, which does not contain an upstream donor for gene conversion, indicated that this region of genomic DNA contains point mutations characteristic of somatic hypermutation (Lanning and Knight, 1997). Taken together, these data indicate that Ig gene diversity is generated at least partially through combinatorial joining of light chain gene segments, but more predominantly through somatic diversification mechanisms. But, in which peripheral tissues does somatic diversification of Ig genes originate?

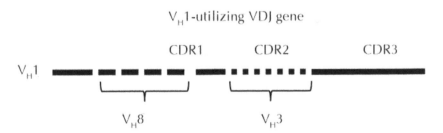

FIGURE 3 Somatic diversification of IgH genes by somatic gene conversion and somatic hypermutation. Schematic representation of somatically diversified V_H1-using VDJ gene in which upstream V_H8 and V_H3 gene segments were used as donors for somatic gene conversion. In addition, multiple single nucleotide changes, presumably due to somatic hypermutation are present, but not shown (example taken from Winstead et al., 1999).

6.3.1   GALT AS THE SITE OF DEVELOPMENT OF THE PRIMARY ANTIBODY REPERTOIRE

Early studies of rabbit organized GALT, which consists of the Peyer's patches, sacculus rotundus, and appendix, suggested that these tissues are important sites for B cell development and antibody responses. Histologic observations of the appendix provided the first clue that rabbit GALT may function similarly to the chicken bursa and be a site of B cell development because, similar to the bursa, the neonatal appendix is seeded by a few lymphocytes that subsequently develop into tightly packed B cell follicles (Archer et al., 1964). Additionally, rabbits lacking GALT due to surgical removal, have decreased antibody responses after immunization, suggesting that GALT is the site of antibody production (Archer et al., 1964; Cooper et al., 1968; Cooper et al., 1966). Later studies, following the discoveries of peripheral somatic gene conversion and somatic hypermutation, provided evidence that GALT is the site of Ig gene diversification in rabbits. For instance, Weinstein et al. (1994) analyzed DNA sequences of VDJ genes cloned from appendices of 6-week-old rabbits and found signs of somatic hypermutation and gene conversion. The authors also noticed that the sequences were clonally related, suggesting that the appendix is a site of ongoing diversification (Weinstein et al., 1994). Similarly, Lanning and Knight (1997) identified somatic hypermutation in VDJ genes cloned from appendices of rabbits between 4–6 weeks of age, and more recently, activation-induced cytidine deaminase (AID) transcripts were identified at the base of B cell follicles in appendices from 1-week-old rabbits (Zhai and Lanning, 2013). VDJ genes cloned from B cells isolated from the AID[+] regions of these follicles displayed evidence of somatic hypermutation and gene conversion, directly demonstrating that the appendix is a site of Ig gene diversification in very young rabbits (Zhai and Lanning, 2013). To directly test if GALT is required for somatic diversification of Ig genes, Vajdy et al. (1998) compared DNA sequences of VDJ genes cloned from the periphery of various aged normal and GALTless rabbits (where appendix, sacculus rotundus, and Peyer's patches were surgically removed shortly after birth). The authors predicted that if GALT is required for Ig gene diversification, then fewer mutations would be present in VDJ genes from rabbits lacking GALT than from normal rabbits. Indeed, fewer mutations were observed in peripheral VDJ genes from GALTless rabbits, indicating that GALT is required for the generation of antibody diversity during early B cell development (Fig. 4).

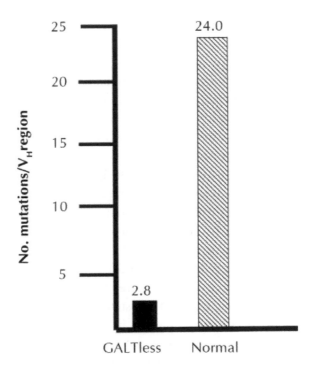

FIGURE 4   Requirement of GALT for somatic diversification of IgH genes. Comparison of the average number of nucleotide changes (mutations) in VDJ gene sequences from GALTless rabbits in which the sacculus rotundus, appendix, and Peyer's patches were removed shortly after birth. The mutations include those that arise from both somatic gene conversion and hypermutation. Data are from Vajdy et al. (1998).

6.3.2   REQUIREMENT OF MICROBIOTA FOR GALT DEVELOPMENT AND GENERATION OF THE PRIMARY ANTIBODY REPERTOIRE

GALT is colonized by a large number of commensal microorganisms, collectively referred to as the intestinal microbiota, which are required for immune system development and function in many species. A number of studies on germ-free (microbiologically sterile) rabbits or on rabbits with an altered microbiota demonstrated that commensal bacteria are required for B cell proliferation/B cell follicle formation in GALT and somatic diversification of Ig genes for generation of a preimmune antibody repertoire. Over 30 years ago, it was noted that germ-free rabbits contain small B cell follicles, have low titers of circulating antibodies, and display poor antibody responses following immunization (Stepánková et al., 1980; Tlaskalova-Hogenova and Stepánková, 1980); similar to observations in other species showing that commensal bacteria stimulate immune system development and function. In an even earlier surgical model, involving a reversible surgical ligation of the rabbit appendix at birth to prevent bacterial colonization, researchers observed a lack of B cell follicle formation in ligated appendices. Following removal of the ligation to allow bacterial colonization, B cell follicles appeared, demonstrating that intestinal bacteria are required for B cell follicle formation in the rabbit appendix (Perey and Good, 1968). Additionally, remote colony rabbits (which contain an altered microbiota due to separation from the rest of the rabbit colony and a diet of sterile food and milk from birth) displayed fewer somatic mutations in peripheral VDJ genes as compared to normal, conventionally raised rabbits. Upon administration of intestinal microbes from normal rabbits, the number of VDJ gene mutations in remote colony rabbits increased, suggesting that commensal bacteria are also required for somatic diversification of Ig genes (Lanning et al., 2000). Taken together, these observations provided evidence that intestinal bacteria stimulate both B cell follicle formation in GALT and somatic diversification of Ig genes to generate a preimmune antibody repertoire in rabbits, or what we collectively refer to as GALT development.

Not only do bacteria promote B cell proliferation and Ig gene diversification in GALT, but studies of B cell populations in *ali/ali* rabbits, which contain two mutant a^2 alleles, demonstrated that interactions between bacteria and GALT are also required for positive selection of B cells. As compared to normal rabbits where 80% of serum Ig display $V_H a$ (a-positive) allotype specificities and 20% of serum Ig display $V_H n$ (a-negative) allotype specificities, the opposite is true in *ali/ali* rabbits. At birth almost all B cells express $V_H n$; however, over time, $V_H n$ allotype specificities gradually decrease until, as adults, nearly all B cells express V_Ha (Chen et al., 1993; Kelus and Weiss, 1986). It is unlikely that the repertoire shift from V_Hn to V_Ha B cells in *ali/ali* rabbits is due to gene conversion, because the predominant V_Hn genes (V_Hx and V_Hy) are located upstream of the predominantly used V_Ha gene (V_H4), and during VDJ gene rearrangements in the bone marrow, the *V_H4* DNA would be excised and no longer be available as a donor for gene conversion (DiPietro et al., 1990). The repertoire shift is also not likely due to secondary VDJ gene rearrangements, as single cell PCR analysis of peripheral B cells from *ali/ali* rabbits using primers to distinguish VDJ gene rearrangements from unrearranged germline J_H genes revealed a single rearranged allele and a single germline allele in the majority of cells (Rhee et al., 2005). Instead, data suggest that the shift from V_Hn to V_Ha B cells is most likely due to a proliferative expansion of V_Ha, but not V_Hn B cells in the appendix.

Comparative propidium iodide analysis of V_Ha and V_Hn B cells isolated from appendices of *ali/ali* rabbits demonstrated that V_Ha B cells have higher DNA content than V_Hn B cells, suggesting that they may proliferate more than V_Hn B cells and may be selectively expanded in GALT (Pospisil et al., 1995). A kinetic flow cytometric analysis of V_Hn and V_Ha B cell populations isolated from the appendices and spleens of *ali/ali* rabbits demonstrated that the switch from V_Hn to V_Ha B cells occurs slightly earlier in the appendix than in the spleen, in accordance with the previously mentioned observation that positive selection of V_Ha B cells occurs in GALT. To directly test if GALT is the site of V_Ha B cell selection in *ali/ali* rabbits, Rhee et al. (2005) assessed peripheral B cell populations by flow cytometry in normal and GALTless ligated-appendix *ali/ali* rabbits (neonatal surgical removal of the sacculus rotundus and Peyer's patches and ligation of the lumen of the appendix to maintain sterility). Remarkably, the switch from V_Hn to V_Ha B cells did not occur in GALTless *ali/ali* rabbits (Fig. 5), demonstrating that GALT is the site of V_Ha B cell selection (Rhee et al., 2005). These data also suggested that an interaction between the intestinal microbiota and GALT promote positive selection of B cells in addition to stimulating GALT development. Taken together, the observations in normal and *ali/ali* rabbits sparked many additional questions, including: What bacterial species and bacterial molecules induce GALT development? Do bacteria directly stimulate B cells or do they up-regulate endogenous molecules that in-turn stimulate B cells?

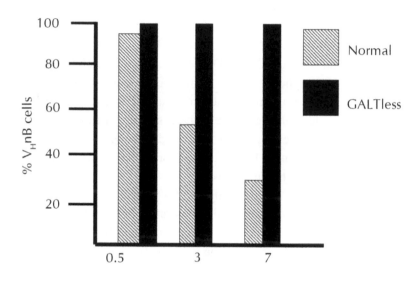

Months of Age

FIGURE 5   Selective expansion of $V_H a$ (loss of $V_H n$) B cells by gut microbiota. Whereas nearly all B cells in *ali/ali* rabbits (crosshatched box) are $V_H n^+$ soon after birth, the % of $V_H n$ B cells decreases over time until <30% are $V_H n$ (most are $V_H a$). In contrast, the number of $V_H n$ B cells does not decrease in the GALTless rabbits (solid bars) in which the sacculus rotundus and Peyer's patches were removed shortly after birth and the appendix was ligated to prevent bacterial colonization and GALT development; the $V_H a$ B cells did not expand in number, and continued to account for less than 10% of all B cells in the GALTless rabbits.

The correlation between underdeveloped GALT and fewer VDJ gene mutations in remote colony rabbits, which contain an altered microbiota, suggested that GALT development may be dependent on select bacterial species (Lanning et al., 2000). To directly test this hypothesis, Rhee et al. (2004) made use of the surgical appendix ligation model, and introduced individual or combinations of bacterial species into ligated appendices of young rabbits and three weeks later assessed the appendix for GALT development. They predicted that if select bacterial species promoted GALT development, then after introduction of certain bacteria, but not others, there would be large follicles of proliferating B cells and somatic diversification of VDJ genes. Indeed, by histology the authors reproducibly observed IgM⁺ Ki-67⁺ (proliferation marker) B cell follicles in appendices colonized by both *Bacillus subtilis* and *Bacteroides fragilis*, but not with *B. subtilis* or *B. fragilis* alone, nor with other individual bacterial species such as *E. coli* or *Clostridium subterminale*. Additionally, B cells isolated from both appendices and spleens of rabbits containing ligated appendices colonized by *B. subtilis* and *B. fragilis* contained somatic mutations in the VDJ genes, demonstrating that the combination of these two bacteria promote GALT development (Rhee et al., 2004).

6.3.3 BACTERIAL MOLECULES THAT CONTRIBUTE TO GALT DEVELOPMENT

To begin to address the mechanism by which bacteria stimulate B cell proliferation and VDJ gene diversification, various mutants of *B. subtilis* in combination with *B. fragilis* were injected into ligated appendices. Interestingly, *B. subtilis* strains deficient for sporulation did not promote GALT development, suggesting that either spores themselves or the act of sporulation is required for *B. subtilis* to stimulate B cells in the appendix (Rhee et al., 2004). Consistent with the idea that spores themselves are stimulatory, another related *Bacillus* species, the nonpathogenic Sterne strain of *B. anthracis*, when introduced alone into ligated appendices also induced numerous follicles of proliferating B cells. However, when a *B. anthracis* mutant lacking spore surface proteins (*cotO*) was injected into ligated appendices, significantly fewer IgM⁺Ki-67⁺ follicles were observed, suggesting that a molecule on the surface of spores stimulates B cell proliferation in the appendix (Severson et al., 2010). To test if *B. anthracis* spores stimulate B cells directly, B cells were incubated with spores in vitro, and B cell stimulation was accessed by a flow cytometry-based calcium flux assay. Interestingly, when incubated with spores, calcium flux was induced in B cells, indicating that spores themselves can directly stimulate B cells in vitro (Severson et al., 2010), leading the authors to further investigate which molecule on the surface of the B cells the spores may be binding.

IgM is a likely candidate for direct stimulation of B cells in the appendix, because all undiversified B cells in the appendix of young rabbits have a similar V_H region sequence and structure due to the preferential usage of V_H1 in V(D)J gene recombination in the bone marrow. B cell superantigens are molecules that bind to IgM outside of the traditional antigen binding-site, to a region that is common between all B cells (Fig. 6). Quite remarkably, introduction of a known B cell superantigen, protein A, together with *B. fragilis*, induced B cell follicle formation when introduced into ligated appendices, demonstrating that a known superantigen can promote GALT development (Rhee et al., 2004). Based on these observations, it was hypothesized that spores bind directly to IgM through a superantigen-like binding site. To test this hypothesis, spores were incubated with rabbit IgM and single-chain fragments of the variable region (scFv) containing different V_H and V_L domains, and binding was assessed by immunofluorescence microscopy. The expectation was that if spores bind to IgM through a superantigen-like binding site, then IgM will bind to spores independent of antigen specificity. Indeed, IgM and scFv molecules with varying or unknown antigen specificities bound strongly to spores, but surprisingly, IgM and scFv molecules containing V_κ light chains bound more strongly to spores than did molecules containing V_λ (Severson et al., 2010), suggesting that spores interact with IgM through an unconventional antigen binding-site largely involving the light chain region. Taken together these data suggest that one mechanism by which B cells are stimulated in GALT is through direct binding of bacterial spores to IgM on B cells. In addition, several in vivo experiments, in which receptor-ligand interactions were blocked by introduction of recombinant soluble receptors, demonstrate that, in addition to bacteria, GALT development also requires signaling through several endogenous molecules.

Superantigen-binding site(s)

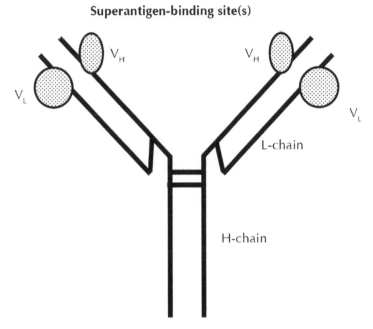

FIGURE 6   Location of proposed superantigen-binding sites on V_H and V_L regions of Ig molecules. Bacterial superantigens, such as protein A of *Staphylococcus aureus* or protein L of *Peptostreptococcus magnus*, may bind conserved regions of B cell surface IgM V_H (dotted ovals) and V_L (dotted circles) respectively, thereby providing a stimulatory signal to B cells.

6.3.4   ENDOGENOUS MOLECULES REQUIRED FOR GALT DEVELOPMENT

To identify endogenous molecules that may also be required for GALT development, Yeramilli and Knight (2010, 2011) generated a series of re-combinant adenoviruses encoding Ig fusion proteins of molecules known to be important for B cell activation in other species and/or tissues, including transmembrane activator calcium modulator and cyclophilin ligand interactor (TACI), complement receptor 2 (CR2/CD21), CD40, and CTLA4. They then injected each of the recombinant adenoviruses into newborn rabbits to deliver soluble receptors to developing tissues, and after approximately one week they assessed GALT development by im-munohistochemistry. Using this approach, the authors observed little to no B cell proliferation and follicle formation in appendices from rabbits injected with recombinant adenoviruses encoding TACI-Ig, CD21-Ig, or CD40-Ig. In contrast, appendices from rabbits injected with CTLA4-Ig adenovirus contained large follicles of proliferating B cells, whereas an-tibody responses to a T cell-dependent antigen were diminished in the periphery (Yeramilli and Knight, 2010, 2011). Taken together, these data demonstrated that signaling through TACI, CR2/CD21, and CD40, but not through B7-CD28 (receptors for CTLA-4), are all required for GALT de-velopment, and led the authors to further investigate how each of these molecules may function in GALT to support development of a preimmune antibody repertoire.

TACI serves as a receptor for two molecules, B cell-activating factor belonging to the TNF family (BAFF) and a proliferation-inducing ligand (APRIL), both of which are expressed in the rabbit appendix, where BAFF is expressed by B cells in the B cell follicles and APRIL is expressed in cells residing near the epithelium (Yeramilli and Knight, 2010). Notably, staining of tissue sections from conventional, ligated, or ligated appendi-ces colonized by *B. subtilis* and *B. fragilis* revealed that BAFF is only de-tected in B cell follicles from appendices colonized by bacteria, indicating that BAFF expression is bacterially induced (Yeramilli and Knight, 2010). These data suggest that appendix B cells up-regulate BAFF in response to bacterial stimulation where B cells are stimulated by BAFF to proliferate in an autocrine fashion.

Complement is a group of serum proteins that participates in a series of activation cascades, as part of the innate immune response, which ul-timately results in the coating and killing of bacteria. One such comple-ment protein, C3, is cleaved into multiple fragments, some of which bind to CR1/CD21 expressed on follicular dendritic cells (FDCs) and B cells; CR1/CD21 is part of the B cell co-receptor and is known to amplify B cell activation during humoral immune responses (Carroll, 2004). Com-parisons of C3 staining in tissue sections from conventional and ligated appendices demonstrated that C3 is up-regulated in B cell follicles in re-sponse to bacteria (Yeramilli and Knight, 2011). Additionally, in the lu-men of the rabbit appendix, C3 can be detected bound to the surface of bacteria, suggesting that commensal bacteria are coated with complement (Yeramilli and Knight, 2011). These data provide a scenario where complement-coated bacteria are delivered to FDCs or B cells within the B cell follicles of the appendix where they bind to CR1/CD21 and in-turn stimulate B cell proliferation (Fig. 7). Further experiments are needed to test this model and to determine which cells containing CR2/CD21 are required for B cell proliferation and the formation of B cell follicles in the appendix.

CD40-CD40L and B7-CD28 interactions are important for T cell-dependent B cell activation during an immune response. Based on the observations that B cell follicle formation proceeds regardless of T cell activation mediated by B7-CD28 interactions (Yeramilli and Knight, 2011), it is believed that GALT development (and thus development of a preimmune antibody repertoire) is a T cell-independent process. Although CD40-CD40L interactions are required for B cell proliferation and follicle formation, it is thought that the CD40L signal is coming from a cell type other than activated T cells, such as FDCs or macrophages. Further experiments are needed to determine which cell type(s) expressing CD40L promote GALT development.

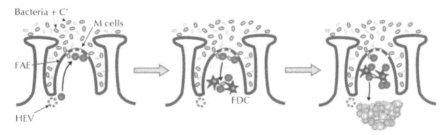

FIGURE 7 Model of intestinal microbiota-induced GALT development. B cells enter GALT through the HEVs and migrate toward the follicle-associated epithelium (FAE) where they interact with complement-coated (C') microbiota that cross the epithelial barrier through M cells (left). B cells then ferry bacteria to FDCs and become activated (center). Activated B cells migrate to the base of the follicle where AID is upregulated (Zhai and Lanning, 2013) and the Ig genes somatically diversify (right). The process of GALT development requires intestinal microbiota (Vajdy et al., 1998); complement activation (Yeramilli and Knight, 2010); CD40-CD40L interaction (Yeramilli and Knight, 2010); and BAFF (Yeramilli and Knight, 2010). Activated T cells, however, are not required for GALT development (Yeramilli and Knight, 2010). Bacteria are denoted as ovals; B cells are circular; a cluster of proliferating B cells is found at the base of follicle (right).

In-depth studies of rabbit GALT have revealed several key findings that are essential for fully understanding the mechanism by which antibody diversity is generated in rabbits. A combination of bacterial and endogenous molecules promotes B cell proliferation/follicle formation, somatic diversification of Ig genes, and/or positive selection of B cells, processes which are required for generation of a preimmune antibody repertoire. In the next section, we discuss recent findings supporting a mechanism by which the preimmune antibody repertoire generated in GALT is maintained in the absence of ongoing lymphopoiesis.

6.4   GALT AND THE MAINTENANCE OF B CELLS

In addition to generating a preimmune antibody repertoire, rabbits are faced with the additional challenge of maintaining B cell populations, since new B cells are not made in the bone marrow throughout life. Unlike in humans and mice, where a progenitor B cell population has been detected outside of the bone marrow (Golby et al., 2002), there is no evidence of B lymphopoiesis in locations other than the bone marrow of rabbits. Rather, due to the expression of the B1 cell marker, CD5, on rabbit B cells, it was hypothesized that rabbit B cells may be self-renewing in the periphery (Raman and Knight, 1992). In accordance with this finding, a new subset of immature transitional B cells was recently discovered in GALT, and this cell population, named transitional 1 diversified (T1d) B cells, displays an immature phenotype and declines with age in the bone marrow like other progenitor cell populations. In IgH-transgenic rabbits, which are B cell-deficient at birth but accumulate a few B cells in peripheral tissues over time (Jasper et al., 2007), and in conventional rabbits at 3–6 days after birth, T1d B cells were found in the dome and villus near the lumen of the appendix, demonstrating that this cell population seeds the appendix and is in a prime location for interaction with and stimulation by commensal bacteria (Yeramilli and Knight, 2011). In adult rabbits, T1d B cells are proliferating, somatically diversified, and still present long after the arrest of B lymphopoiesis, suggesting that this cell population is a long-lived and/or self-renewing B cell population (Yeramilli and Knight, 2011). Interestingly, T1d B cells bind BAFF and accumulate in rabbits injected with a TACI-Ig-expressing recombinant adenovirus, indicating that BAFF may be required for the maturation of T1d B cells into mature B cells in GALT and suggesting that T1d B cells may be required for the maintenance of peripheral B cell populations in the absence of ongoing lymphopoiesis (Yeramilli and Knight, 2011). Future experiments are needed to test whether T1d B cells are required for humoral immune responses throughout life.

In addition to T1d B cells, Yeramilli and Knight (2013) have also recently characterized splenic MZ B cells in rabbit. Quite interestingly, they observed an absence of MZ B cells in spleens from rabbits where GALT was removed at birth, suggesting that GALT is also required for the development of splenic MZ B cells (Yeramilli and Knight, 2013). This observation, in accordance with the identification of the T1d B cell population, demonstrates the importance of GALT for the generation and maintenance of peripheral B cell populations in adult rabbits no longer capable of generating new progenitor B cells.

6.5   MODEL FOR GENERATING A PRE-IMMUNE ANTIBODY REPERTOIRE

Using the data presented in the above sections of this chapter, we describe a model that summarizes the cumulative findings in the literature and the entire process by which we believe rabbits generate a preimmune antibody repertoire (Fig. 7). First, VDJ gene rearrangements occur in the bone marrow of young rabbits, where limited V-gene usage occurs. Immature T1 B cells generated by differentiation of progenitor B cell populations in the bone marrow migrate to GALT and seed the domes, where we hypothesize that they are stimulated by surface molecules of select intestinal bacteria or spores, as well as by BAFF to undergo proliferation and differentiation into mature B cells. The stimulated B cells then migrate to the base of the follicle where they proliferate to form organized follicles and diversify their Ig genes to become T1d B cells. The signals required for proliferation and diversification are T cell-independent and include CR2/CD21-complement and CD40-CD40L, both of which we predict originate from DCs that have captured Ig- and complement-coated bacteria,

FDCs, macrophages, NK cells, or epithelial cells which express CD40L, respectively. While in the appendix, B cells are positively selected before they seed the periphery, and the positive selection of B cells requires interactions between the commensal bacterial and GALT, but the bacterial molecules required for the positive selection remain unknown. Next, positively selected T1d B cells leave the appendix and seed peripheral tissues where they differentiate into mature B cells and provide the rabbit with a preimmune antibody repertoire that awaits contact with foreign antigens. During this entire process in GALT, B lymphopoiesis declines in the bone marrow, but the lack of newly generated B cells in the bone marrow is compensated by the self-renewing population of T1d B cells in GALT, as B cell proliferation continues throughout life. We additionally propose that the "self-renewing" properties of the T1d B cells require signals from commensal bacteria, but future experiments are needed to test this prediction directly.

6.6   TWO-STEP MECHANISM FOR GENERATING A PRE-IMMUNE ANTIBODY REPERTOIRE IN SPECIES OTHER THAN RABBITS

In addition to rabbits, generation of a preimmune repertoire in other species, including chicken, sheep, and cattle, occurs by a two-step process. Following B cell production at the primary site of lymphopoiesis, B cells migrate to GALT where Ig gene diversification takes place. In chickens, B cell development begins in the yolk sac at 5–6 days gestation and continues in the blood, spleen, and bone marrow shortly thereafter (Reynaud et al., 1994), where only a single functional V_H and V_λ gene exist and recombine with a limited number of D and J genes, producing little antibody diversity from combinatorial joining (Reynaud et al., 1987; Reynaud et al., 1994; Reynaud et al., 1989; Thompson and Neiman, 1987). Also similar to rabbits, B lymphopoiesis is not continuous throughout life in chickens, but only a few million-progenitor cells are produced (Weill and Reynaud, 1998). Progenitor B cells produced during gestation migrate to the Bursa of Fabricius where they proliferate and diversify their Ig genes solely by gene conversion (Reynaud et al., 1995; Reynaud et al., 1987;

Thompson and Neiman, 1987; Reynaud et al., 1989); but unlike rabbits, diversification of Ig genes in chicken is not dependent on stimulation by commensal bacteria, as it begins before hatch (Weill and Reynaud, 1998). In sheep, progenitor B cells are produced in the spleen between day 48–77 of gestation (Press, 1993), and similar to rabbits and chickens, B lympho-poiesis is not continuous throughout life (Press, 1996). Progenitor B cells migrate to the ileal Peyer's patch where they proliferate and diversify their Ig genes by somatic hypermutation, and similar to chicken but in contrast to rabbit, neither the proliferation nor diversification requires stimulation by the intestinal microbiota (Reynaud et al., 1995; Reynaud et al., 1991). Similar to that observed in chicken, B cells in cattle use a limited number of V_λ genes during B lymphopoiesis (Aitken et al., 1999; Parng, 1996), providing limited Ig diversity by combinatorial joining of light chain gene segments. Ig gene diversification occurs by both somatic hypermutation and gene conversion (Lucier et al., 1998; Parng et al., 1996), first in the spleen and then in the ileal Peyer's patch, independent of stimulation by commensal bacteria.

Although details of the mechanisms differ between rabbits, chicken, sheep, and cattle, the generation of a preimmune antibody repertoire in these species proceeds by a common two-step theme, unlike that which occurs in mice and humans where a preimmune antibody repertoire is generated by combinatorial joining of a variety of V, D, and J gene seg-ments. However, "nontraditional" B cell populations have been reported in both mice and humans, which display characteristics of rabbit B cells in GALT, suggesting that mice and humans may have a GALT counterpart. In mice, this unique B cell population was discovered in the colon of mice, and displays an activated phenotype based on the expression of various cell surface markers (Shimomura et al., 2008). Following recruitment into the colon, this B cell population is polyclonally expanded in response to bacterial products by a mechanism dependent on BAFF, but independent of stimulation through the BCR and TCR (Shimomura et al., 2008). In humans, Weller et al. (2008) identified a B cell population in the spleen and peripheral blood of children less than 2 years of age, in which the Ig genes were somatically diversified, but the B cells did not display signs of clonal selection, although the children received immunizations (Weller et al., 2008). Similar to rabbit B cells in GALT, this finding suggests that somatic diversification of this unique B cell population occurs outside of germinal centers and independent of an immune response. Future experiments are needed to determine if the intestinal microbiota is required for the development of these "nontraditional" B cell populations.

6.7 CONCLUSION

The generation of a preimmune antibody repertoire was originally discovered as a mechanism involving the combinatorial joining of V, D, and J gene segments at the Ig loci in mice and humans, but years of work in other species has demonstrated that alternative mechanisms exist. In chickens and rabbits, and likely also in sheep and cattle, generation of a preimmune antibody repertoire occurs by a two-step process where, following the generation of progenitor B cells at the primary site of lymphopoiesis, B cells migrate to GALT where they proliferate and diversify their Ig genes in response to various stimuli. In rabbits specifically, B cell proliferation and diversification require signals from both the intestinal microbiota, as well as from endogenous molecules. Recent studies have begun to address specific aspects of this complicated mechanism, but future studies are also needed to fully understand which bacterial molecules are required for stimulation of rabbit B cells in GALT and which cell types, in addition to B cells, are required for the generation of a preimmune antibody repertoire in rabbit.

KEYWORDS

- **B lymphopoiesis**
- **GALT**
- **gene conversion**
- **intestinal microbiota**
- **pre-immune antibody repertoire**
- **somatic hypermutation**

REFERENCES

Aitken, R., Hosseini, A., MacDuff, R. (1999): Structure and diversification of the bovine immunoglobulin repertoire. Veterinary Immunology and Immunopathology 72, 21–29.

Archer, O.K., Sutherland, D.E., Good, R.A. (1964): The Developmental Biology of Lymphoid Tissue in the Rabbit. Consideration of the Role of Thymus and Appendix. Lab Invest 13, 259–271.

Becker, R.S., Suter, M., Knight, K.L. (1990): Restricted utilization of V_H and D_H genes in leukemic rabbit B cells. Eur J Immunol 20, 397–402.

Becker, R.S., Zhai, S.K., Currier, S.J., Knight, K.L. (1989): Ig VH, DH and JH germline gene segments linked by overlapping cosmid clones of rabbit DNA. Journal of Immunology 142, 1351–1355.

Bilwani, F.A., Knight, K.L. (2012): Adipocyte-derived soluble factor(s) inhibits early stages of B lymphopoiesis. Journal of Immunology 189, 4379–4386.

Carroll, M.C. (2004): The complement system in B cell regulation. Molecular Immunology 41, 141–146.

Chen, H.T., Alexander, C.B., Young-Cooper, G.O., Mage, R.G. (1993): VH gene expression and regulation in the mutant Alicia rabbit. Rescue of VHa2 allotype expression. J Immunol 150, 2783–2793.

Cooper, M.D., Perey, D.Y., Gabrielsen, A.E., Sutherland, D.E. R., McKneally, M.F., Good, R.A. (1968): Production of an antibody deficiency syndrome in rabbits by neonatal removal of organized intestinal lymphoid tissues. Int Arch Allergy Appl Immunol 33, 65–88.

Cooper, M.D., Perey, D.Y., McKneally, M.F., Gabrielsen, A.E., Sutherland, D.E. R., Good, R.A. (1966): A mammalian equivalent of the avian bursa of Fabricius. The Lancet 1, 1388–1391.

Crane, M.A., Kingzette, M., Knight, K.L. (1996): Evidence for limited B-lymphopoiesis in adult rabbits. Journal of Experimental Medicine 183, 2119–2127.

Currier, S.J., Gallarda, J.L., Knight, K.L. (1988): Partial molecular genetic map of the rabbit V_H chromosomal region. J Immunol 140, 1651–1659.

DiPietro, L.A., Sethupathi, P., Kingzette, M., Zhai, S.K., Suter, M., Knight, K.L. (1992): Limited repertoire of used V_H gene segments in a V_Ha3-allotype-suppressed rabbit. International Immunol 4, 555–561.

DiPietro, L.A., Short, J.A., Zhai, S.K., Kelus, A.S., Meier, D., Knight, K.L. (1990): Limited number of immunoglobulin V_H regions expressed in the mutant rabbit "Alicia." Eur J Immunol 20, 1401–1404.

Dray, S., Young, G.O., Nisonoff, A. (1963): Distribution of allotypic specificities among rabbit g-globulin molecules genetically defined at two loci. Nature 199, 52–55.

Eskinazi, D.P., Knight, K.L., Dray, S. (1979): Kinetics of escape from suppression of Ig heavy chain allotypes in multiheterozygous rabbits. Eur J Immunol 9, 276–283.

Gallarda, J.L., Gleason, K.S., Knight, K.L. (1985): Organization of rabbit immunoglobulin genes.I. Structure and multiplicity of germline V_H genes. J Immunol 135, 4222–4228.

Golby, S., Hackett, M., Boursier, L., Dunn-Walters, D., Thiagamoorthy, S., Spencer, J. (2002): B cell development and proliferation of mature B cells in human fetal intestine. Journal of Leukocyte Biology 72, 279–284.

Harrison, M.R., Jones, P.P., Mage, R.G. (1973): Endogenous synthesis of membrane $b5$ by lymphocytes from rabbits recovering from $b5$ allotype suppression. Journal of Immunology *111*, 1595–1597.

Hayward, A.R., Simons, M.A., Lawton, A.R., Mage, R.G., Cooper, M.D. (1978): PreB and B cells in rabbits: Ontogeny and allelic exclusion of Kappa light chain genes. J Exp Med *148*, 1367–1377.

Jasper, P.J., Rhee, K.J., Kalis, S.L., Sethupathi, P., Yam, P.-C., Zhai, S.-K., Knight, K.L. (2007): B lymphocyte deficiency in IgH-transgenic rabbits. Eur J Immunol12:2290–2299.

Jasper, P.J., Zhai, S.K., Kalis, S.L., Kingzette, M., Knight, K.L. (2003): B lymphocyte development in rabbit: progenitor B cells and waning of B lymphopoiesis. J Immunol *171*, 6372–6380.

Kalis, S.L., Zhai, S.K., Yam, P.C., Witte, P.L., Knight, K.L. (2007): Suppression of B lymphopoiesis at a lymphoid progenitor stage in adult rabbits. International Immunology *19*, 801–811.

Kelus, A.S., Weiss, S. (1986): Mutation affecting the expression of immunoglobulin Variable regions in the rabbit. Proc Natl Acad Sci USA *83*, 4883–4886.

Kim, B.S., Dray, S. (1972): Identification and genetic control of allotypic specificities of two Variable region subgroups of rabbit immunoglobulin heavy chains. Eur J Immunol *2*, 509–514.

Kim, B.S., Dray, S. (1973): Expression of the a, *x*, and*y* Variable region genes of heavy chains among IgG, IgM, and IgA molecules of normal and a locus allotype-suppressed rabbits. J Immunol *111*, 750–760.

Knight, K.L., Becker, R.S. (1990): Molecular basis of the allelic inheritance of rabbit immunoglobulin VH allotypes:Implications for the generation of antibody diversity. Cell *60*, 963–970.

Lanning, D., Sethupathi, P., Rhee, K.J., Zhai, S.K., Knight, K.L. (2000): Intestinal microflora and diversification of the rabbit antibody repertoire. J Immunol *165*, 2012–2019.

Lanning, D.K., Knight, K.L. (1997): Somatic hypermutation: Mutations 3' of rabbit VDJ H-chain genes. J Immunol *159*, 4403–4407.

Lucier, M.R., Thompson, R.E., Waire, J., Lin, A.W., Osborne, B.A., Goldsby, R.A. (1998): Multiple sites of V lambda diversification in cattle. J Immunol *161*, 5438–5444.

Mage, R., Dray, S. (1965): Persistent altered phenotypic expression of allelic gG-immunoglobulin allotypes in heterozygous rabbits exposed to isoantibodies in fetal and neonatal life. J Immunol *95*, 525–535.

Oudin, J. (1960): Allotypy of rabbit serum proteins. I. Immuno-chemical analysis leading to the individualization of seven main allotypes. Journal of Experimental Medicine *112*, 107–124.

Parng, C.L., S. Hansal, R.A. Goldsby and B.A. Osborne (1996): Gene conversion contributes to Ig light chain diversity in cattle. J Immunol *157*, 5478–5486.

Perey, D.Y., Good, R.A. (1968): Experimental arrest and induction of lymphoid development in intestinal lymphoepithelial tissues of rabbits. Laboratory Investigation *18*, 15–26.

Pospisil, R., Young-Cooper, G.O., Mage, R.G. (1995): Preferential expansion and survival of B lymphocytes based on VH framework 1 and framework 3 expression: "Positive" selection in appendix of normal and VH-mutant rabbits. Proceedings National Academy of Sciences, USA *92*, 6961–6965.

Press, C., Mcl, Reynolds, J.D., McClure, S.J., Simpson-Morgan, M.W., Landsverk, T. (1996): Fetal lambs are delpleted of IgM+ cells following a single injection of an anti-IgM antibody early in gestation. Immunology *88*, 28–34.

Press, C.M., Hein, W.R., Landsverk, T. (1993): Ontogeny of leucocyte populations in the spleen of fetal lambs with emphasis on the early prominence of B cells. Immunology *80*, 598–604.

Raman, C., Knight, K.L. (1992): CD5+ B cells predominate in peripheral tissues of rabbit. JImmunology *149*, 3858–3864.

Reynaud, C.-A., Anquez, V., Grimal, H., Weill, J.-C. (1987): A hyperconversion mechanism generates the chicken light chain preimmune repertoire. Cell *48*, 379–388.

Reynaud, C.-A., Bertocci, B., Dahan, A., Weill, J.-C. (1994): Formation of the chicken B-cell repertoire: Ontogenesis, regulation of Ig gene rearrangement, and diversification by gene conversion. Advances in Immunology *57*, 353–378.

Reynaud, C.-A., Dahan, A., Anquez, V., Weill, J.-C. (1989): Somatic hyperconversion diversifies the single V_H gene of the chicken with a high incidence in the D region. Cell *59*, 171–183.

Reynaud, C.-A., Garcia, C., Hein, W.R., Weill, J.-C. (1995): Hypermutation generation the sheep immunoglobulin repertoire is an antigen-independent process. Cell *80*, 115–125.

Reynaud, C.-A., Mackay, C.R., Muller, R.G., Weill, J.-C. (1991): Somatic generation of diversity in a mammalian primary lymphoid organ: The sheep ileal Peyer's Patches. Cell *64*, 995–1005.

Rhee, K.J., Jasper, P.J., Sethupathi, P., Shanmugam, M., Lanning, D., Knight, K.L. (2005): Positive selection of the peripheral B cell repertoire in gut-associated lymphoid tissues. J Exp Med *201*, 55–62.

Rhee, K.J., Sethupathi, P., Driks, A., Lanning, D.K., Knight, K.L. (2004): Role of commensal bacteria in development of gut-associated lymphoid tissues and preimmune antibody repertoire. J Immunol *172*, 1118–1124.

Ros, F., Puels, J., Reichenberger, N., Van Schooten, W., Buelow, R., Platzer, J. (2004): Sequence analysis of 0.5 Mb of the rabbit germline immunoglobulin heavy chain locus. Gene *330*, 49–59.

Sehgal, D., Johnson, G., Wu, T.T., Mage, R.G. (1999): Generation of the primary antibody repertoire in rabbits: expression of a diverse set of Igk-V genes may compensate for limited combinatorial diversity at the heavy chain locus. Immunogenetics *50*, 31–42.

Sehgal, D., Obiakor, H., Mage, R.G. (2002): Distinct clonal Ig diversification patterns in young appendix compared to antigen-specific splenic clones. J Immunol *168*, 5424–5433.

Severson, K.M., Mallozzi, M., Driks, A., Knight, K.L. (2010): B cell development in GALT: role of bacterial superantigen-like molecules. Journal of Immunology *184*, 6782–6789.

Shimomura, Y., Ogawa, A., Kawada, M., Sugimoto, K., Mizoguchi, E., Shi, H.N., Pillai, S., Bhan, A.K., Mizoguchi, A. (2008): A unique B2 B cell subset in the intestine. Journal of Experimental Medicine *205*, 1343–1355.

Short, J.A., Sethupathi, P., Zhai, S.K., Knight, K.L. (1991): VDJ genes in V_Ha2 allotype-suppressed rabbits.Limited germline V_H gene usage and accumulation of somatic mutations in D regions. J Immunol *147*, 4014–4018.

Siewe, B.T., Kalis, S.L., Le, P.T., Witte, P.L., Choi, S., Conway, S.J., Druschitz, L., Knight, K.L. (2011): In Vitro requirement for periostin in B lymphopoiesis. Blood *117*, 3770–3779.

Stepánková, R., Kovaru, F., Krumal, J. (1980): Lymphatic tissue of the intestinal tract of germ-free and conventional rabbits. Folia Microbiol *25*, 491–495.

Thompson, C.B., Neiman, P.E. (1987): Somatic diversification of the chicken immunoglobulin light chain gene is limited to the rearranged Variable gene segment. Cell *48*, 369–378.

Tlaskalova-Hogenova, H., Stepánková, R. (1980): Development of antibody formation in germ-free and conventionally reared rabbits: the role of intestinal lymphoid tissue in antibody formation to E. coli antigens. Folia Biologica *26*, 81–93.

Tunyaplin, C., Knight, K.L. (1997): IgH gene rearrangements on the unexpressed allele in rabbit B cells. J Immunol *158*, 4805–4811.

Vajdy, M., Sethupathi, P., Knight, K.L. (1998): Dependence of antibody somatic diversification on gut-associated lymphoid tissue in rabbit. J Immunology *160*, 2725–2729.

Weill, J.C., Reynaud, C.A. (1998): Galt Versus bone marrow models of B cell ontogeny. Developmental and Comparative Immunology *22*, 379–385.

Weinstein, P.D., Anderson, A.O., Mage, R.G. (1994): Rabbit IgH sequences in appendix germinal centers: VH diversification by gene conversion-like and hypermutation mechanisms. Immunity *1*, 647–659.

Weller, S., Mamani-Matsuda, M., Picard, C., Cordier, C., Lecoeuche, D., Gauthier, F., Weill, J.C., Reynaud, C.A. (2008): Somatic diversification in the absence of antigen-driven responses is the hallmark of the IgM+ IgD+ CD27+ B cell repertoire in infants. Journal of Experimental Medicine *205*, 1331–1342.

Winstead, C.R., Zhai, S.K., Sethupathi, P., Knight, K.L. (1999): Antigen-induced somatic diversification of rabbit IgH genes: gene conversion and point mutation. Journal of Immunology *162*, 6602–6612.

Yeramilli, V.A., Knight, K.L. Somatically diversified and proliferating transitional B cells: implications for peripheral B cell homeostasis. Journal of Immunology *186*, 6437–6444.

Yeramilli, V.A., Knight, K.L. (2010): Requirement for BAFF and APRIL during B cell development in GALT. Journal of Immunology *184*, 5527–5536.

Yeramilli, V.A., Knight, K.L. (2011): Somatically diversified and proliferating transitional B cells: implications for peripheral B cell homeostasis. Journal of Immunology *186*, 6437–6444.

Zhai, S.K., Lanning, D. (2013): Diversification of the primary antibody repertoire begins during early follicle development in the rabbit appendix. Molecular Immun *54*, 140–147.

CHAPTER 7

THE IMMUNOGLOBULIN GENES OF DOMESTIC SWINE

J. E. BUTLER and NANCY WERTZ

CONTENTS

ABSTRACT

Developing the piglet as a model for developmental immunology required characterization of the porcine immunoglobulins (Igs) and the genes encoding them. Swine have genes encoding the same five classes of Igs as most other mammals including six IgG subclasses. Allelic variants for IgA and IgG subclasses are also recognized. The IGHC genes are arranged as in other mammals, preceded by switch regions including a short one for IgD. Whether IgD in swine is expressed as a B cell receptor (BCR) like IgM, is unknown. Sequences for ~30 IGHV genes have been reported but only the 15 most 3' IGHV genes in one haplotype have been mapped. Three of the IGHV genes account for ~60% of the preimmune heavy chain repertoire and this changes little after antigen exposure. Swine have only two functional DH (IGHD) segments and one IGHJ so disruption of the latter generates B cell knock-out pigs. There are nine functional IGLV genes and nine functional IGLK genes yet two IGLK and three IGLV genes comprise 70–80 of the preimmune light chain repertoire. Unlike mice, lambda rearranges >30 days before kappa and the question of whether there is a pre-BCR is unresolved.

7.1   INTRODUCTION

Swine provide the highest proportion (37%) of the world's meat supply by weight (www.worldwatch.org). Therefore, the health of domesticated pigs is important to agriculture worldwide. Swine are also: (1) vectors of epizootic disease, (2) used as a model for cystic fibrosis (Rodgers et al., 2008), (3) a potential source of humanized antibodies (Mendicino et al., 2011; Ramsoondar et al., 2011) and (4) a model for developmental immunology (Butler and Sinkora 2007; Butler et al., 2009a).

The domestic pig belongs to the family Suidae which is one of three Suiform artiodactyls, the other two families include the hippo and the peccaries, respectively. Some regard the Suiformes as the most primitive artiodactyls, although their lack of specialization may contribute to their value as animal models. At least seven species of Suidae are recognized, *Sus scrofa* being the ancestor of the domestic pig of which there are many subspecies (Ruvinsky and Rothschild, 1998). Domestic swine were derived from the Eurasian wild boar and may have been domesticated for ~5,000 years by the Chinese. There are many recognized breeds of pigs, two of the most familiar being the Yorkshire (called Large White in Europe) that was recognized as a breed in the 19th century and the Landrace ("old Celtic pig") recognized at least as early. The Large White has been a favorite among geneticists since it was inbred for many generations in Babrahm, England. Very little is known about the genetic variation among domestic breeds as regards the genes encoding their immunoglobulins (Igs) and even less about those in other families of Suidae. The data reviewed is this chapter have been derived from: (1) a mixture of American farm pigs, many with a Yorkshire/Landrace background, (2) a Duroc BAC library, (3) a Large White BAC library, and (4) a limited numbers of samples from mini-pigs and Chinese Meishan pigs. The familiar and IMGT nomenclature is used interchangeably throughout the text.

7.2 THE PIGLET MODEL FOR DEVELOPMENTAL IMMUNOLOGY

Characterization of Igs and Ig genes of swine was initiated because of their potential value to developmental immunology and therefore research has been largely funded by the National Science Foundation. The idea of using piglets as models was conceived in the 60s by various investigators. Reasons for their popularity include their mode of passive immunity and the precosial nature of their offspring. Like all artiodactyls, swine are classified as Group III mammals based on their means of transferring immunity from mother to offspring (Butler 1974; Fig. 1). The mode of passive immunity in Group III mammals is dependent on the structure of the placenta and the role of the mammary gland. There is no transport of maternal antibodies to the fetus *in utero* as is the case with humans, rodents, rabbits or carnivores so their precosial offspring depend entirely on suckling for live-saving passive immunity. The precosial nature of piglets allows them to be derived by Caesarian surgery and then reared in germfree isolators or SPF "autosows" where they can be reared on cow's milk/colostrum or special milk replacers (Butler et al., 2009a). Given that Eurasian-derived farm pigs have litters of 10–20 offspring, one gilt can supply animals for an entire experiment.

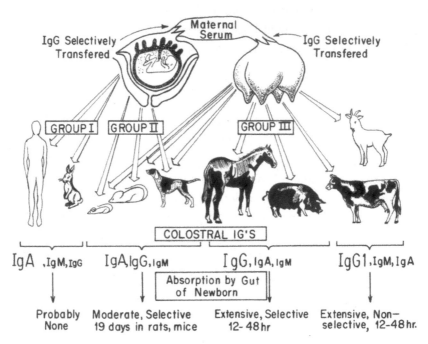

FIGURE 1 Transmission of passive immunity from mother to young among common mammals. Species are classified into groups based on whether Igs are transferred *in utero* or after birth via colostrum and milk. The size of the font for Igs depicts their relative concentrations (From Butler 1974).

Fetal piglets are of a size that allows for macroscopic identification of organs. Because B cell development begins at 20 days of gestation (DG) it allows investigators a 90-day window in which to study fetal B cell and antibody development without influence from maternal antibodies or other maternally derived regulatory proteins (Butler and Sinkora 2007). After birth, investigators can continue to study immune system development in piglets reared in isolators units or autosows for 5–8 weeks (Butler et al., 2009a). In this setting, the absorption and effect of colostrum-derived maternal antibodies, the role of normal gut flora and the direct effect of pathogens on immune system development can be accessed. Passive antibodies of defined quality and microorganisms of all types can be administered at any time within this window. Thus, the piglet model is particularly suited to study events in the "critical window of immune system development"

(Fig. 2). In our studies we have used the model to show that colonization of the gut is required for the development of adaptive immunity (Butler et al., 2002), which depends on recognition of Microbial-Associated Molecular Patterns (MAMPs) by pattern recognition receptors of the innate immune system (Butler et al., 2005).

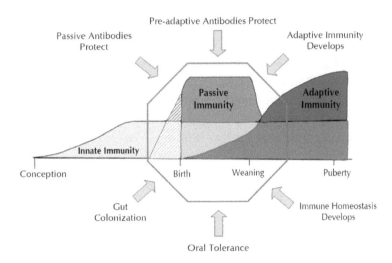

FIGURE 2   The critical window of immunological development. Arrows surrounding the window indicate the critical events that occur at or near birth. The "lined" triangle applies only to those mammals in which passive Igs are also transferred *in utero*. From Butler et al 2006b.

One of the earliest attempts to use piglets as a model for developmental immunology grew out of the desire to find an animal model for dietary allergy in infants to cow's milk. Thus, piglets recovered by Caesarian or directly from the birth canal are reared in autosows and fed milk/colostrum that is dispensed at regular intervals in response to Pavlovian signals. This allowed consumption of Igs and their absorption by the neonatal gut to be recorded together with data on the immune response to dietary proteins (Leece 1969; Klobasa et al., 1981; Butler et al., 2009a).

7.3   B CELL LYMPHOGENESIS AND IMMUNOGLOBULIN LEVELS

7.3.1   B CELL LYMPHOGENESIS AND PREIMMUNE REPERTOIRE DEVELOPMENT

The description of the Ig genome of swine is more meaningful if B cell development, antibody repertoire development and the levels and distribution of Igs are first reviewed. VDJ rearrangement first occurs in the yolk sac at 20 days of gestation (DG) a process that involves rearrangement of a half-dozen VH genes, two functional DH genes and the single functional JH (Butler et al., 1996; Eguchi-Ogawa et al., 2010; Mendicino et al., 2011; Sinkora et al., 2003). At the same time rearrangement occurs in the lambda locus but kappa rearrangements are delayed for at least 30 days and are first encountered in the bone marrow (Sun et al., 2012; Fig. 3). B cell lymphogenesis proceeds from yolk sac to the fetal liver, and after 60 days DG, to the bone marrow where it continues for at least five weeks after birth.

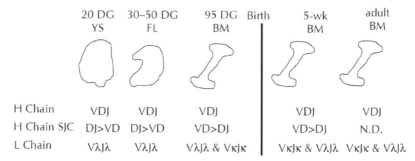

FIGURE 3   B cell lymphogenesis in swine. DG-days of gestation; YS = yolk sac; FL = fetal liver; BM = bone marrow; SJC = signal joint circles; N.D. = Not detectable.

The preimmune heavy and light chain repertoire in swine is generated from a few genes relative to the functional genomic potential (Table 1). Four VH genes comprise ~80% of the repertoire (Sun et al., 1998) three alone account for ~60% and seven account for up to 95% (Butler et al., 2006a, 2011a). At the same time two V-kappa (IGKV) genes and three V-lambda (IGLV) genes account for >70% of the repertoire (Table 1). Thus combinatorial diversity plays a small role in repertoire development in this species. Therefore, CDR3 diversity contributes >90% of the diversity in heavy chain rearrangements (Butler et al., 2000). CDR3 diversity in light chain rearrangements is very restricted (Table 2). Changes to the pre-immune repertoire after exposure to environmental antigens will be discussed in a subsequent section.

TABLE 1   A. Relationship between the genomic constitution of the heavy and light chain loci in swine and the potential combinatorial variants. Numbers in parentheses indicates the number of functional genes. B. Actual combinatorial variants when 70% of the pre-immune repertoire is considered. C. Theoretical combinatorial diversity in humans."

A

Genomic Constitution				
Ig Locus	V-genes	D-genes	J-genes	Combinational Potential
Heavy Chain	~30 (~20)	5 (2)	5 (1)	40
Lambda	22 (9)	NA	4 (2)	18
Kappa	14 (9)	NA	5 (1)	9

B

70% of Pre-immune Repertoire				
Ig Locus	V-genes	D-genes	J-genes	Combinational Potential
Heavy Chain	4	2	1	8
Lambda	3	NA	2	6
Kappa	2	NA	1	2

C

Heavy Chain	9,000
Lambda	200
Kappa	200

TABLE 2   CDR3 diversity and SHM in the preimmune repertoire of swine.

Transcript	Nr.	Mean Length ±S.D.	Range	C.V.	CDR3 diversity index	SHM
VDJ	175	41.2±9.8[a]	9 - 81	23.7[a]	383.4[a]	9.7±29.1[b]
VλJl	158	30.2±2.6	21 - 36	10.0	46.1	5.9±17.2
VκJk	89	26.3±1.6	18 - 30	6.1	9.0	2.3±8.6

Nr. = Number of rearrangements; CV = Coefficiant of variation.
[a]Significantly greater than for light chains.
[b]Not significantly higher than in light chains.

All major isotypes of swine Igs are transcribed *in utero* (McAleer et al., 2005) and IgM containing cells are present as early as 45 DG. IgG is present in serum as early as 60DG (Butler et al., 2001; Table 3) and the majority of IgG transcripts in the fetus are encoded by Cγ3 (IGHG3; Butler and Wertz 2006; Kloep et al., 2012).

TABLE 3   Concentration of Major Swine Immunoglobulins.

Sample	Serum			Colostrum/Milk			Bronchial-alveolar Lavage		
	IgM	IgG	IgA	IgM	IgG	IgA	IgM	IgG	IgA
Fetus, 60 DG	—	(0.29)[a]	—	NA	NA	NA	ND	ND	ND
Fetus, 90 DG	(0.57)	(3.65)	(0.27)	NA	NA	NA	ND	ND	ND
Newborn	(0.83)	(33.9)	(2.1)	NA	NA	NA	ND	ND	ND
5 Wks, Germfree[b]	(6.4)	(45)	(6.7)	NA	NA	NA	(0.14)	(0.41)	(1.7)
5 Wks, SIV infected[b]	(29.7)	(115)	(6.4)	NA	NA	NA	(0.5)	(0.92)	(1.1)
5 Wks, colonized[b]	(260)	(700)	(540)	NA	NA	NA	ND	ND	ND
5 Wks, PRRSV infected	(700)	30	(450)	NA	NA	NA	(184)	(72.9)	(53.6)
Sow, 60 DG	6.5	35	1.3	NA	NA	NA	ND	ND	ND
Sow, Parturition	5.0	26	1.8	9.1	95	21.2			
Sow, 3 Wks Postpartum	3.5	32	2.2	1.4	0.9	5.3	[IgA:IgG=0.7± 0.2[e]]		
Conv. Piglet, 1Wk	2.9	36	9.1	NA	NA	NA	ND	ND	ND
Conv. Piglet, 5 Wks	2.2	7.5	0.6	NA	NA	NA	ND	ND	ND
Autosow, CDCD, 5 Wks[c]	3.8	19	3	NA	NA	NA	ND	ND	ND
Autosow, CDCD +3.5gm IgG	1.1	6.5	0.7	NA	NA	NA	ND	ND	ND

[a]Concentrations in parenthesis are in ug/mL; all others are in mg/mL. Adapted from Butler et al. (2010).
[b]Piglets recovered by Caesarian and reared in isolator units.
[c]CDCD = Caesarian-derived colostrum-deprived.
ND = Not done; NA = Not applicable.

7.3.2   *IMMUNOGLOBULIN CONCENTRATIONS IN SERA AND SECRETIONS*

Transcription studies can determine if certain genes are used but immunochemistry is needed to show these are actually synthesized and in what amounts. Table 3 and Fig. 4 show that IgG is the major antibody isotype in serum and lacteal secretions. As the function of the mammary gland changes, the relative concentrations in lacteal secretion change as well as in the serum of the mother during the reproductive cycle (Fig. 4). IgA is the predominant Ig in the gut lumen, especially in blind loops, nasal

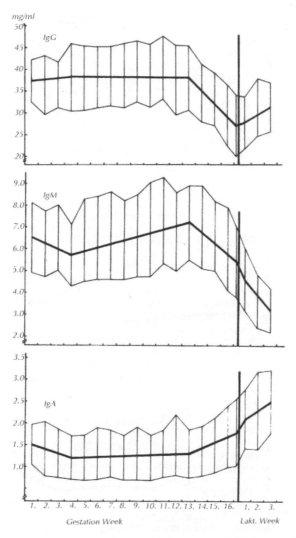

FIGURE 4 Levels of the major swine Igs in the serum of 1000 sows throughout the reproductive cycle. From Klobasa et al 1985.

secretions, parotid saliva and in bronchial-alveolar lavages of newborn and germfree piglets. Methods for the collection, handling and measurement of Igs for studies on mucosal immunity in swine and other large animals of veterinary importance have been reviewed (Butler, 2005, 2014). The same five isotypes of Ig common to human, mice and most other mammals occur in swine, although there are currently no reagents for quantifying the levels of IgE, IgD and the subclasses of IgG. Efforts to resolve this dilemma have been through Toolkit initiatives in the US (www.vetimm.org) and the UK (www.immunologicaltoolbox.com).

7.4   THE CONSTITUENCY AND ORGANIZATION OF THE PORCINE IG LOCI

7.4.1   THE PORCINE VARIABLE HEAVY CHAIN LOCUS

Porcine V_H genes were originally named VHA, VHB, etc. until their position in the locus was known after which they were given an IMGT designation with IGHV1 (a pseudogene in swine) being the most 3' V_H gene (Figures 5A, and 5B). Figure 5B provides a short list (16 of 32) of VH genes that have been reported. A more complete list can be found in Butler et al. (2006a) or on the CIgW website www.medicine.uiopwa. edu/ CIgW. Presently only the 15 most 3' V_H genes have been mapped (Eguchi-Ogawa et al., 2010; Fig. 5A). A number are pseudogenes and two functional genes (IGHV4 and IGHV10) and (IGHV6 and IGHV12) have been duplicated. V_H genes that have not yet been mapped may be alleles or lie upstream of IGHV15 (Fig. 5A). Alternatively, they may be V_H genes not present in the BAC library of the Large White breed on which Fig. 5A is based. The V_H genes of swine differ mainly in CDR1 and CDR2 and many genes share the same CDR1 or CDR2 regions (Fig. 5B). The variable heavy chain region also contains four D_H and five J_H segments although only two D_H and a single J_H are functional (Butler et al., 1996; Fig. 5A). The last observation was used to create B cell knockout pigs (Mendicino et al., 2011).

7.4.2   THE PORCINE CONSTANT HEAVY CHAIN LOCUS AND IGG SUBCLASS HETEROGENEITY

The CH portion of the heavy chain locus contains genes for the same five Ig isotypes found in most mammals including a segment encoding numerous IgG subclass genes (Fig. 5C). Figure 6 is an original dendrogram comparing the six Cγ genes and their putative allelic variants recovered from mixed breed farm pigs. The putative alleles proposed for five of the subclasses were confirmed using hemizygous pigs (Kloep et al., 2012). However, breed and individual variations occur (see Section 7.5). A slightly different dendogram is presented by Eguchi-Ogawa et al. (2012) in which IgG2-IgG4-IgG6 form a cluster (Group 3) which, from unpublished data on mAb, might be more correct.

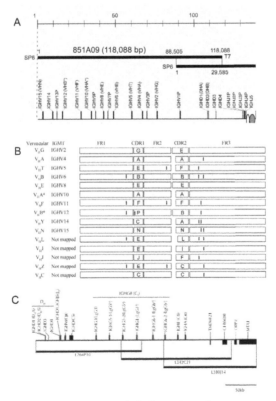

FIGURE 5   Organization of the heavy chain locus in swine.

FIGURE 5   *(Caption continued)*

A. Genomic map of the 3' portion of the variable region of the heavy chain locus. Both vernacular and IMGT nomenclature are given. VHA* and VHA are duplicated genes as are VHB* and VHB. P = pseudogenes. Refer to Eguchi-Ogawa et al 2010 for more detail. B. Diagram comparing the various segments of porcine V_H genes. V_H genes that are mapped (Fig. 5A) have been assigned an IMGT nomenclature. The capital Arabic letters in the CDR regions indicate the sequence is identical to that in the corresponding CDR region of other VH genes with the same arabic letter. Vertical lines indicate the location of sequence differences found in FR regions. C. Constant region of the heavy chain locus reconstructed from three BAC clones derived from a single haplotype from a Large White pig. It should be noted that IgG5[a] and IgG5[b] considered alleles when mixed breeds were studied (see Fig. 6), appear as separate genes in this haplotype, Also genes encoding IgG2 and IgG4 are absent. From Eguchi-Ogawa et al 2012.

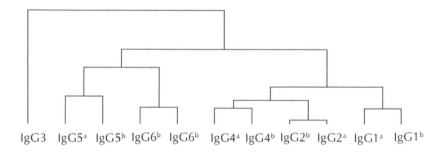

IgG3   IgG5[a] IgG5[b] IgG6[b] IgG6[b]   IgG4[a] IgG4[b] IgG2[b] IgG2[a]   IgG1[a]   IgG1[b]

FIGURE 6   Dendrogram comparing six porcine IgG subclass genes and their alleles obtained from transcripts (Butler et al., 2009b). Sequence alleles are designated and were later confirmed by Kloep et al. (2012), using hemizygous animals. This dendrogram differs somewhat from the one published by Eguchi-Ogawa et al. (2012) in which genes and alleles of IgG2, IgG4 and IgG6 form a cluster known as Group 3.

The heterogeneity of porcine IgG dates to the studies of Kaltreider and Johnson (1972) who used immunoelectrophoresis to identify four antigenically distinct IgGs. Other investigators have also presented data supporting IgG subclass and allotypic diversity (Metzger and Fougereau, 1967; Curtis and Bourne, 1971; Rejnek et al., 1966; Rapacz and Rapacz-Hasler, 1982; Van Zaane and Hulst, 1987). Despite these observations, physical chemical preparation of the various subclass proteins using ion-exchange chromatography and protein A affinity have been unsuccessful because of their overlapping charge properties (Dillender, 1989). Correspondingly "tight" subclasses also occur in mice, humans and horse. Fortunately the occurrence of natural or induced plasmacyto-mas has allowed IgG subclass proteins to be purified from the serum of patients with multiple myeloma or from the ascites of mice with induced plasmocytomas. Only recently has porcine IgG subclass preparation and purification been possible through genetic engineering and in vitro ex-pression (Butler et al., 2012).

The heavy chain constant region also contains a heavy chain enhanc-er and switch regions for all isotypes although the one for IgD is quite short (Fig. 5A). $S\mu$ and $S\varepsilon$ are the longest, $S\alpha$ moderate and the various $S\gamma$ regions one-third the length of $S\mu$ (Sun and Butler, 1997; Eguchi-Ogawa et al., 2012). Whether the short $S\delta$ is actually used to affect class switch or whether expression is by RNA splicing, has not been convinc-ingly demonstrated (Zhao et al., 2003). Switch regions for porcine CH genes also differ in their density of pentameric repeats; this is very high for $S\mu$, $S\varepsilon$ and $S\alpha$ whereas $S\gamma$s have only ~70 pentameric repeats (Egu-chi-Ogawa et al., 2012). In humans $S\gamma$ structure and pentameric density is correlated with usage (Pan et al., 1997, 1998).

$C\delta$ is least homologous among mammals (Butler et al., 2010) but re-tains the features of having multiple hinge exons as reported for human (Lefranc and LeFranc, 2001). Especially interesting is the near identical nature of the $C\mu 1$ and $C\delta 1$ domains and IgD can be expressed with the Cm1 domain (Zhao et al., 2003).

7.4.3   THE PORCINE LIGHT CHAIN LOCI

In swine nearly equal numbers of kappa and lambda light chains are used whereas ~95% of those in cattle are lambda (Butler 1997; Hood et al., 1967). A kappa deleting element (κDE) is located 23.22 kB downstream from porcine C kappa (IGKC) and is identical between cattle and swine (Schwartz et al., 2012a). The κDE in humans is involved in a rearrange-ment event that results in deletion of much of the kappa locus in lamb-da-expressing B cells (Siminovitch et al., 1985; Klobeck and Zachau, 1986). While the κDE may influence the kappa/lambda ratio, the fact that the element is identical in cattle and swine does not fit this model.

At least in mice, the predominant expression of kappa appears to be due to a more active Igκ 3' enhancer (Gorman et al., 1996).

Figure 7A is a map of the porcine kappa locus. The locus contains 14 IGKV genes spanning 89KB of which nine are potentially functional. Five are pseudogenes resulting from stop codons, lost exons or the loss of critical residues such as those for CYS 23 (IGKV5-4*02; Schwartz et al., 2012a). Non-canonical recombination signal sequences (RSSs) and octamers were also associated with some pseudogenes. There are five families (IGKV1, IGKV2, IGKV3, IGKV4 and IGKV7) of which IGKV2 has diversified into five genes and IGKV1 into four. IGKV3, IGKV4 and IGKV7 are clustered at the 3' end of the locus but are not expressed. Two orphan IGKV genes have also been identified on a separate BAC clone that may not be linked.

As in other mammals the porcine kappa locus contains a single gene although there are allelic differences (see next section). Also similar to many other mammals, there are five IGKJ segments (Butler et al., 2004; Schwartz et al., 2012a). The porcine V-kappa locus is one-fourth the size of that of the human and mouse (Zachau, 1995) and more similar in size to that of cattle in which eight bovine IGKV genes are believed functional (Ekman et al., 2009)

The lambda locus of swine is also similar in organization to that in many other mammals with multiple families of IGLV families upstream from tandem IGLJ-IGLC cassettes (Fig. 7B). Unlike mouse, IGLV genes are not found in these cassettes. The locus spans ~229 KB on chromosome 14. Twenty-two IGLV genes have been mapped; nine predicted to be functional (Schwartz et al., 2012b). This is similar to cattle but half the size of the human V-lambda genome. The IGLV genes are organized in two distinct clusters; the cluster dominated by the IGLV8 family is most 5' and the somewhat smaller IGLV3 family is located downstream. In addition to IGLV8 and IGLV3, IGLV1, IGLV2, IGLV5 and IGLV7 also occur (Fig. 7B) but these are not expressed (Wertz et al., 2013). These families do not form separate clusters but are interspersed. Five IGLV genes are predicted to be nonfunctional because they suffer from mutated start sites, frameshifts, premature stop codons, exon loss and loss of critical residues.

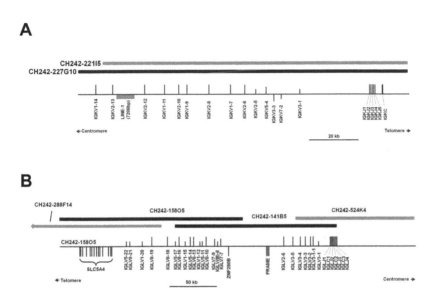

FIGURE 7 The organization of the porcine light chain loci. A. Organization of the kappa locus. For additional details see Schwartz et al 2012a. B. Organization of the lambda locus. For additional details see Schwartz et al 2012b. Both maps are used with permission of the authors.

In addition to the three tandem IGLJ-IGLC cassettes, there is a fourth downstream IGLJ, which lacks a companion IGLC. All three IGLC genes on one allele are sequence identical so their differential usage cannot be distinguished. However, the noncanonical heptamer associated the IGLJ1 and other mutated motifs predict that only IGLJ2 and IGLJ3 are used; this has been confirmed by expression studies (Wertz et al., 2013).

7.5 GENETIC VARIATION AMONG PORCINE IG GENES

The initial studies on the Ig gene repertoire of swine best resembles those for humans in that an outbred population is sampled; in both species polymorphisms and polygeny occur. Analyzing samples from mixed breeds castes a wide net, which increase the probability of identifying many genetic variants. However, the outcome is not representative of any one individual and it is therefore difficult to distinguish between genes and alleles of genes.

Variations among the Cγ (IGHC) genes of swine are a good example of the outcome of these different approaches. When studies are based on samples obtained from different animals and breeds, six expressed Cγ subclass genes could be identified of which five have two sequence alleles (Fig. 6; Butler et al., 2009b). This allelic designation was supported by analyzing expression in outbred hemizygous pigs (Kloep et al., 2012). On the other hand, when a single haplotype from a Large White Library was mapped, six Cγ genes were found but they were not the same as those predicted from the work of Kloep et al. (Fig. 5C). Rather IgG5[a] and IgG5[b] were located in the same haplotype and IgG2 and IgG4 were both absent (Eguchi-Ogawa et al., 2012). The absence of IgG2 and IgG4 in some animals was previously noted (Butler et al., 2009b). Also present in the same haplotype were two genes for IgG6. One was IgG6[a] and the other a hybrid gene that was named as IgG6[c]. With the exception of IgG5[b], all the Cγ genes were of the "a" allotype as was that for IgA (see below) which is consistent with the hemizygous pigs studied by Kloep et al. (2012). The IgG5[b] in the Large White haplotype (Fig. 5C) might not be expressed and would therefore have been overlooked in expression studies. Thus, the Cγ genes appear to be located in a flexible sub locus so IGHC genes may vary among haplotypes. Cγ polygeny and polymorphisms have also been reported from studies in humans (Lefranc et al., 1982; Keyeux et al., 1989; Wiebe et al., 1984).

There are two allelic variants of IgA (IGHA) in swine, which result from a splice acceptor site mutation in the CH2 domain of one haplotype. This results in a four amino acid deletion in the hinge of IgA[b] (Brown et al., 1995). At this point, no biological consequences for piglets homozygous for IgA[b] are known and distribution of the allotypes appears to be founder-based (Navarro et al., 2000). Both allelic variants are susceptible to proteases from *Haemophilus influenzae* (Mullens et al., 2011). The work of Kloep et al., and Eguchi-Ogawa et al., confirmed that the IgA[a] allotype is linked to the IgG[a] subclass genes (with exception of IgG5[b] in the Large White haplotype; Fig 5C). There are no known variants of IgM or IgE but those for the latter are quite prevalent in horses (Wagner et al., 2006).

Prior to the recent molecular genetics studies on porcine Cγ (IGHG) genes, the first evidence for polymorphism came from the work of Rapacz and Hasler-Rapacz (1982) who reported nine serologically distinct IgG heavy chain variants which they believed resided in four closely linked loci with at least two alleles at each autosomal locus. This early observation seems to partially fit with: (1) two allelic variants for each subclass (Fig. 6; Butler et al., 2009b; Rapacz and Hasler-Rapacz 1982) (2) the recent work of Eguchi-Ogawa et al. (2012) in which genes for IgG2 and IgG4 were absent in the Large White haplotype, (Fig. 5c) as well as in other swine (Butler et al., 2009b) and (3) the immunoelectrophoretic data of Kaltreider and Johnson (1972).

Although these polymorphisms have been recognized at the genetic level, efforts to prepare allotype-specific mAb to swine IgG and IgA allotypes have been only partially successful. Mabs recognizing IgA[a] and IgA[b] have been prepared but these are allotype-biased, rather than allotype-specific (Navarro, Nielsen, Butler, unpublished). Allotype bias in immunochemical reagents is well-known from studies in cattle in which most mAbs and polyclonal antibodies to bovine IgG2 are biased to an immunodominant epitope in the CH3 domain of IgG2a (Butler and Heyermann 1986; Butler et al., 1992). Similar bias has been seen with some mAbs to swine IgG1 (Butler et al., 2012).

Little is known about the allelic variants of porcine VH genes. In our earliest studies we speculated that the V_H genes sharing one CDR might be alleles (Fig. 5b). However, this was not supported by mapping of the 3' most V_H genes since IGHV5 (V_HT) shares CDR1 with IGHV8 (V_HF) and they are not alleles (Fig. 5b). The same applies to the sharing of CDR2 by IGHV5 (V_HT) and IGHV11 (V_HF). Whether any of the 17 V_H genes that have not been mapped are alleles of other mapped genes or are separate V_H genes remains to be seen.

More is known about allelic variation in the porcine kappa locus since several overlapping BAC clones from the same Duroc sow were available. This allowed 11 allelic variants of the 14 IGKV genes to be identified (Schwartz et al., 2012a). Allelic polymorphism was seen in all IGKV families, especially in IGKV2. The allelic variation among IGKV genes contrasts with those for J-kappa (IGKC) in which genes on both alleles for all five are identical (Fig. 7A; Schwartz et al., 2012a). Between the two Duroc alleles, one IGKC difference was seen but both were different from the IGKC sequence reported by Lammers et al. (1991). In addition to polymorphisms, polygeny also exists in the kappa locus. Using samples from mixed breeds, we identified three IGKV genes not present in the Duroc V-kappa genome (Butler et al., 2013).

Recent studies by Schwartz et al. (2012b) who mapped the porcine lambda locus using overlapping BAC clones from the same Duroc library as they used for kappa, provided information on polymorphism and gene order (Fig. 7B). Within the region of overlap all eight IGKV genes differed by at least one nucleotide and some like IGLV8–21, differed by eight amino acids in the deduced sequence. Another interesting feature was a change in the gene order in the most 5' cluster of IGKV genes. One sequence allele for IGLC-2 was also identified, but none for the other two IGLV.

Few mAb to porcine light chains are available, but Sinkora and colleagues (2001) identified three mAb to porcine lambda, one which appears to recognize an allelic variant. These same studied identified lambda-specific (27.7.1) and kappa-specific (27.2.1) mAbs.

7.6 THE EXPRESSED PRE-IMMUNE ANTIBODY REPERTOIRE

7.6.1 THE PREIMMUNE REPERTOIRE

Phenotypic differences among individuals in a species are often due to regulation of gene expression rather than genomic constituency. Dogs with very nearly identical genomes have given rise through selection to an amazingly diverse array of dog breeds. The Arctic wolf and Alaskan Malamute share an almost identical genome yet from birth the wolf cannot be trusted around humans. Therefore, factors controlling gene expression rather than genome difference may also determine the antibody repertoires.

Our research has focused on the expressed antibody repertoire and mostly on the preimmune repertoire and on the critical window in immune development (Fig. 2). Emphasis on the preimmune repertoire is based on the premise that fetal and germfree isolator piglets should be least affected by environmental and maternal influences (see Section 7.2). Thus, their preimmune repertoire should best reflect the germline repertoire, not the adaptive immune repertoire. As described in Section B, the developing preimmune repertoire can be followed during ~90 days of fetal life and thereafter for 5–8 weeks in germfree isolator piglets.

In all three loci, usage of variable Ig genes differs sharply from their genomic potential (Table 1). Although the VH genome is not completely mapped, it has been known for some time that a few VH genes comprised the expressed repertoire (Sun et al., 1998; Butler et al., 2006a; 2011a). Three genes (one a duplicate) account for ~60% of the repertoire. All but one member of the seven V_H genes that form >95% of the preimmune repertoire are among the 15 mapped genes at the 3' end of the locus (Fig. 5A).

The same selective pattern is seen in both the kappa and lambda loci. Genes of the IGKV2 family account for >90% of the repertoire (Butler et al., 2004) and among these, IGKV2–1 and IGKV2–10 account for 80% (Butler et al., 2013; Table 1). While there are nine potentially functional IGLV, those from the IGLV3 and IGLV8 families comprise the entire expressed repertoire. Furthermore, IGLV8–10 alone comprises 27% (Table 1).

Although lambda rearrangement occur at the first site of B cell lymphogenesis and >30 days before kappa (Fig. 3), no unique IGLV gene or surrogate-like light chain has been identified. However, only IGLV8 genes are used in yolk sac and fetal liver, but this includes four different IGLV8 genes that continue to be used throughout fetal life in all lymphoid tissues (Sun et al., 2012; Wertz et al., 2013). In addition to the restricted use of IGHV, IGLV and IGKV genes, swine use only two DH (IGHD) genes, one IGHJ gene, two IGLJ genes and primarily one IGKJ.

Antibody repertoire diversification in mammals depends on combinatorial diversity, junctional diversity in CDR3 and SHM. The limited combinatorial diversity in both heavy and light chain rearrangements shifts the focus to junctional diversity and SHM (Table 1). Junctional diversity in the light chain rearrangements is extremely limited (Butler et al., 2013) but extremely diverse in the heavy chain rearrangements (Butler et al., 2000; Table 2). Junctional diversity in CDR3 is dependent on certain exonucleases and the vigorous activity of terminal deoxynucleotide transferase (Tdt). The heavy chain CDR3 lengths tend to be Gaussian in the preimmune repertoire and range from 9–81 nucleotides long. This diversity is easily realized by spectratyping (Butler et al., 2007). CDR3 in lambda and kappa rearrangements are 27 ± 3 and 30 ± 1.2 respectively and spectratypic analysis yields only a diffuse single polynucleotide band. The frequency of SHM in heavy chain and lambda rearrangements is highest in the CDR1 and CDR2 regions (Butler et al., 2013). Thus the newborn piglets enter life with a diverse heavy chain repertoire of which >90% can be attributed to junctional diversity in CDR3 and to a lesser degree to SHM. Diversification in light chain rearrangements appears restricted to SHM.

7.6.2 DIVERSIFICATION OF THE PREIMMUNE REPERTOIRE AFTER ENVIRONMENTAL EXPOSURE

The development of adaptive immunity in piglets postpartum depends on bacterial colonization or viral infection and is associated with a significant increase in the antibody repertoire diversification index (RDI) which includes a 4–6 fold increase in SHM (Fig. 8). However, this occurs with minimal change in combinatorial diversity. Figure 9 illustrated that throughout fetal life more than 80% of IGHV genes are non-mutated. After birth, there is some increase in SHM in GF piglets but in piglets exposed to colonization, viral infection (C/V group) or those infected with helminth parasites (PIC), less than 10% of IGHV genes remain non-mutated. The number in the bars is the proportion comprised by the same IGHV genes that comprise the preimmune repertoire. In other words, swine diversify their adaptive antibody by SHM of the same small number of IGHV genes that comprise the preimmune repertoire. Whether a similar phenomenon takes places in the light chain repertoire after antigen exposure, has not been tested.

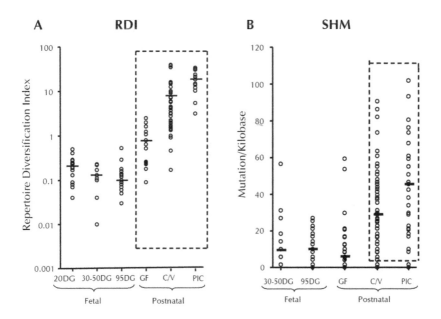

FIGURE 8   Diversification of the heavy chain repertoire in fetal piglets and piglets exposed postpartum to various antigenic stimulation. A. Diversification is measured using a diversification index (RDI). Horizontal bars indicate mean values. The RDI postpartum is significantly greater in C/V and PIC animals than in fetal piglets. C/V = Isolator piglets colonized with an exclusion flora or infected with swine influenza. PIC = conventional piglets infected with helminth parasites. GF = 5-week old germfree isolator piglets. B. Diversification measured in terms of the frequency of SHM. SHM is significantly greater in C/V and PIC piglets than in fetal piglets, but not greater in germfree (GF) isolator piglets. From Butler and Wertz 2012.

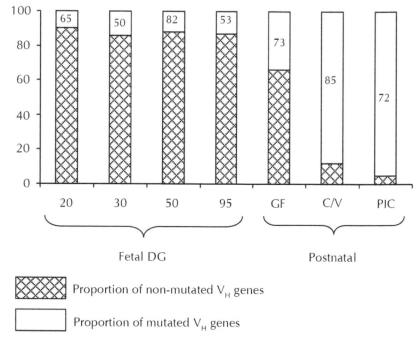

FIGURE 9   Environmental antigen results in an increase in SHM but not V_H gene usage. Designation of neonatal piglet groups is the same as in Fig. 8. The number in the open bar indicates the proportion of mutated V_H genes that is comprised of the same V_H genes used during fetal life. From Butler et al. 2012.

7.7   CONCLUSION

The most obvious feature of the porcine antibody repertoire is the disparity between the size of the functional kappa, lambda and heavy chain genomes and the size of the repertoire used for preimmune repertoire formation. Just 4 of 30 IGHV genes; 2 of 9 functional IGKV genes and 3 of 9 functional IGLV genes account for 70–80% of the repertoire (Table 1). The use of only two functional D_H genes, one functional J_H, one IGKJ segment and the 2 IGLJ genes further support the view that combinatorial diversity in all three swine loci contribute little to the preimmune repertoire (Table 1). Assuming the pattern seen for heavy chain rearrangements after antigen exposure (Fig. 9) also applies to light chain rearrangements, suggests that the majority of IGHV, IGKV and IGLV genes are never used. This suggests that variable region gene usage did not evolve in parallel with their diversification in the genome. The reason why gene duplication and genomic gene conversion especially target variable region genes remains speculative but this region is the site of relatively intense somatic DNA rearrangements and SHM, which may render it particularly susceptible to the processes that are responsible for gene duplication and genomic gene conversion (Butler et al., 2011b).

Extensive gene duplication and genomic gene conversion may at one time have been required for survival. Many sharks have > 200 fused VDJ so diversification by combinatorial and junctional diversity is not an option. SHM in sharks, bony fishes and amphibians is limited or absent and there are no germinal centers. Thus, the germline repertoire may be the same as the adaptive repertoire. Teleost have the largest number of V_H genes among all vertebrates, and although AID and Tdt are present in the genome, their role in repertoire diversification is unknown (Bengten et al., 2006; Solem and Stenvik, 2006). At this juncture there is little evidence for affinity maturation in Teleost (Solem and Stenvik, 2006). By contrast, the situation in birds and mammals is quite different because SHM (templated mutation in birds and non-templates in eutherian mammals) became a part of the arsenal of B cells. Thus, these higher vertebrates are less dependent on a vast array of variable region genes. As shown in the studies of Xu and David (2000) a transgenic mouse with single a V_H gene can make antibodies to most all antigens. Combined with the dominance of the heavy chain CDR3 in antibody specificity (Padlan, 1994; Amit et al., 1986) and in the generation of repertoire diversity (Table 2), the functional value of combinatorial diversity is diminished. This raises a question about the polygeny in variable heavy and light chain loci of mammals. Twenty years ago investigators were estimating there were 1000 V_H genes in mice, hundreds in human and ~200 in rabbits. We now realize these estimates were inflated as much as 10-fold above those currently recognized after genomes have been mapped. Even with the currently accepted numbers, their actual usage may be but a fraction of what is available in their genomes. For example, rabbits use their 3' most V_H genes in ~90% of their preimmune rearrangements (Knight, 1992). Our studies in swine follow a similar trend;

few variable region gene segments contribute to the expressed repertoire (Table 1). Unfortunately, there are no ontogenic studies that have quantified variable region gene usage in human or mic. Based on studies in rabbit and swine, we propose that the extreme polygeny in the variable portion of the heavy and light chain loci of mammals is an evolutionary vestige dating to a time before diversification by SHM and CDR3 junctional diversity in heavy chains developed.

ACKNOWLEDGEMENT

The authors are grateful to John Schwartz, Veterinary and Biomedical Science Deptartment, University of Minnesota for providing genome maps for porcine lambda and kappa loci.

KEYWORDS

- **B Cell Lymphogenesis**
- **immunoglobulin concentrations**
- **light/heavy chain repertoire**
- **Piglet model**
- **Porcine**

REFERENCES

Amit., A.G., Mariuzza, R.A., Phillips, S.E., Pliak, R.J., (1986): Three-dimensional structure of an antigen-antibody complex at 2.8 A resolution. Science 233, 747–753.

Bengten, E., Chen, L.W., Miller, N.W., Warr, G.W., Wilson, M., (2006): Channel cat fish immunoglobulins: Repertoire and expression. Dev. Com. Immunol. 30, 77–92.

Brown, W.R., Kacskovics, I., Amendt, B., Shinde, R., Blackmore, N., Rothschild, M., et al. (1995): The hinge deletion variant of porcine IgA results from a mutation at the splice acceptor site in the first Ca intron. J. Immunol. 154, 3836–3842.

Butler, J.E., Lemke, C.D., Weber, P., Sinkora, M., Lager, K.D., (2007): Antibody repertoire development in fetal and neonatal piglets. XIX. Undiversified B cells with hydrophobic HCDR3 σ preferentially proliferate in PRRS. J. Immunol. 178, 6320–6331.

Butler, J.E., (2005): Collection, handling and analysis of specimens for studies of mucosal immunity in large animals, in: Mucosal Immunity, Mestecky, J., Lamm, M.E., Strober, W., McGhee, J.R., Mayer, L., Bienenstock, J. (Eds.), 3rd Edition, Academic Press, NY. Pp. 1853–1868.

Butler, J.E., (1974): Immunoglobulins of the mammary secretions, in: Larson, B.L., Smith, V., (Eds.), Lactation, a Comprehensive Treatise. Academic Press, New York. Vol. III, pp. 217–255.

Butler, J.E., (1997): Immunoglobulin gene organization and the mechanism of repertoire development. Scand. J. Immunol. 45, 455–462.

Butler, J.E., (2013): Collection, handling and analysis of specimens for studies of mucosal immunity in animals of veterinary importance, in: Russell, M., Mestechy, J. (Eds.). Mucosal Immunology Fourth Edition, Elsevier. Appendix III. (in press).

Butler, J.E., Francis, D., Freeling, J., Weber, P., Sun, J., Krieg, M.A., (2005): Antibody repertoire development in fetal and neonatal piglets. IX. Three PAMPs act synergistically to allow germ-free piglets to respond to TI-2 and TD antigens. J. Immunol. 175, 6772–6785.

Butler, J.E., Heyermann, H., (1986): The heterogeneity of bovine IgG2. I. The A1 allotype is a major determinant recognized by rabbit antibodies to bovine IgG2. Mol. Immunol. 23, 291–296.

Butler, J.E., Lager, K.M., Splichal, I., Francis, D., Kacskovics, I., Sinkora, M., et al. (2009a): The Piglet as a Model for B cell and Immune System Development. Vet. Immunol. Immunopath. 128, 147–170.

Butler, J.E., Navarro, P., Heyermann, H., (1994): The heterogeneity of bovine IgG2. VI. The comparative specificity of monoclonal and polyclonal capture antibodies for IgG2a (A1) and IgG2a (A2). Vet. Immunol. Immunopath. 40, 119–133.

Butler, J.E., Sinkora, M., (2007): The isolator piglet: A model for studying the development of adaptive immunity. Immunol. Res. 39:33–51.

Butler, J.E., Sinkora, M., Wertz, N., Holtmeier, W., Lemke, C., (2006b): Development of the neonatal B- and T-cell repertoire in swine: Implications for comparative and veterinary immunology. Vet. Res. 37, 417–441.

Butler, J.E., Sinkora, M., Wertz, N., Kacskovics, I., (2010): Immunoglobulins, B cells and repertoire development, in: The porcine Immune System, Summerfield, A. (Ed). Develop. Comparative Immunology 33, 321–333.

Butler, J.E., Sun, J., Navarro, P., (1996): The swine immunoglobulin heavy chain locus has a single J_H and no identifiable IgD. International Immunology 8, 1897–1904.

Butler, J.E., Sun, J., Weber, P., Ford, S.P., Rehakova, Z., Sinkora, J., Lager, K., (2001): Antibody repertoire development in fetal and neonatal piglets. IV. Switch recombination primarily in fetal thymus occurs independent of environmental antigen and is only weakly associated with repertoire diversification. J. Immunol. 167, 3239–3249.

Butler, J.E., Sun, X-Z., Wertz, N., (2011b): Immunoglobulin polygeny: An evolutionary perspective, in: Friedberg, F., (Ed), Gene duplication. InTech, Rijeka, Croatia. pp.113–140.

Butler, J.E., Sun, X-Z., Wertz, N., Lager, K.M., Chaloner, K., Urban Jr., J., et al. (2011a): Antibody repertoire development in fetal and neonatal piglets. XXI. VH usage remains constant during development in fetal piglets and postnatally in pigs exposed to environmental antigen. Molec. Immunol. 49, 483–494.

Butler, J.E., Weber, P., Sinkora, M., Sun, J., Ford, S.J., Christenson, R., (2000): Antibody repertoire development in fetal and neonatal piglets. II. Characterization of heavy chain CDR3 diversity in the developing fetus. J. Immunol. 165, 6999–7011.

Butler, J.E., Weber, P., Sinkora, M., Baker, D., Schoenherr, A., Mayer, B., Francis, D., (2002): Antibody repertoire development in fetal and neonatal piglets. VIII. Colonization is required for newborn piglets to make serum antibodies to T-dependent and type 2 T-independent antigens. J. Immunol. 169, 6822–6830.

Butler, J.E., Weber, P., Wertz, N., (2006a): Antibody repertoire development in fetal and neonatal pigs. XIII. "Hybrid VH genes" and the preimmune repertoire revisited. J. Immunol. 177, 5459–5470.

Butler, J.E., Wertz, N., (2006): Antibody repertoire development in fetal and neonatal piglets. XVII. IgG subclass transcription revisited with emphasis on new IgG3. J. Immunol. 177, 5480–5489.

Butler, J.E., Wertz, N., (2012): The porcine antibody repertoire: Variations on the textbook theme. Frontiers in Immunology 3, 1–14.

Butler, J.E., Wertz, N., Deschacht, N., Kacskovics, I., (2009b): Porcine IgG: Structure, genetics and evolution. Immunogenetics 61, 209–230.

Butler, J.E., Wertz, N., Sun, X-Z., (2013): Antibody repertoire development in fetal and neonatal piglets. XIV. Two IGKV genes account for ~80% of the preimmune kappa repertoire. Mol. Immunol (pending).

Butler, J.E., Wertz, N., Sun, X-Z., Lunney, J.K., Muyldermanns, S., (2012): Resolution of an immunodiagnostic dilemma: Heavy chain chimeric antibodies for species in which plasmacytomas are unknown. Mol. Immunol. 53, 140–148.

Butler, J.E., Wertz, N., Wang, H., Sun, J., Chardon, P., Piumi, F., Wells, K., (2004): Antibody repertoire in fetal and neonatal pigs. VII. Characterization of the preimmune kappa light chain repertoire. J. Immunol. 173, 6794–6805.

Curtis, J., Bourne, F.J., (1971): Immunoglobulin quantitation in sow serum, colostrum and milk and the serum of young pigs. Biochim. Biophys. Acta. 236, 319–332.

Dillender M., (1990): The immune response of swine to phosphorylcholine. PhD thesis. University of Iowa.

Eguchi-Ogawa, T, Sun, X-Z., Wertz, N., Uenishi, H., Puimi, F., Chardon, P., et al. (2010): Antibody repertoire development in fetal and neonatal piglets. XI. The relationship of VDJ usage and the genomic organization of the variable heavy chain locus. J. Immunol. 184, 3734–3742.

Eguchi-Ogawa, T., Toki, D., Wertz, N., Butler, J.E., Uenishi, H., (2012): Structure of the genomic sequence comprizing the immunoglobulin heavy constant (IGHC) genes in *Sus scrofa*. Mol. Immunol. 52, 97–107.

Ekman, A., Niku, M., Liljavirta, J., Iivanainen, A., (2009): *Bos taurus* genome sequence reveals the assortment of immunoglobulin and surrogate light chain genes in domestic cattle. BMC Immunol. 10, 22.

Gorman, J.R., van der Stoep, N., Monroe, R., Cogne, M., Davidon, L., Alt, F.W., (1996): The Igk 3' enhancer influences the ratio of Igk versus Igl lymphocytes. Immunity 5, 242–252.

Hood, L., Gray, W.R., Saunders, B.G., Dreyer, W.J., (1967): Light chain evolution. Cold Spring Harbor Symp. Quant. Bio. 32, 133–146.

Kaltreider, H.B., Johnson, J.S., (1972): Porcine immunoglobulins. I. Identification of subclasses and preparation of specific antisera. J. Immunol. 109, 992–998.

Keyeux, G., Lefranc, G., Lefranc, M.P., (1989): A multigene deletion in the human IGH constant region locus involves highly homologous hot spots of recombination. Genomics 5, 432–441.

Klobasa, F., Werhahn, E., Butler, J.E., (1981): Regulation of humoral immunity in the piglet by immunoglobulins of maternal origin. Res. Vet. Sci. 31,195–206.

Klobasa, F., Habe, F., Werhahn, E., Butler, J.E., (1985): Changes in the concentration of serum IgG, IgA, and IgM of sows throughout the reproductive cycle. Vet. Immunol. Immunopath. 10, 341–353.

Klobeck, H.G., Bornkamm, G.W., Combriato, G., Mocikat, R., Pohlenz, H.D., Zachau, H.G., (1985): Subgroup IV of human immunoglobulin K light chains is encoded by a single germ-line gene. Nucleic Acids Res. 13, 6515–6529.

Kloep, A., Wertz, N., Mendicino, M., Butler, J.E., (2012): Linkage haplotype for IgG and IgA subclass genes. Immunogenetics 64; 469–473.

Knight, K.L., (1992): Restricted V_H gene usage and generation of antibody diversity in rabbit. Ann. Rev. Immunol. 10, 593–616.

Lammers, B.M., Bearman, K.D., Kim, Y.B., (1991): Sequence analysis of porcine immuno-globulin chain cDNAs. Mol. Immunol. 28, 877–880.

Leece, J.G., (1969): Rearing colostrum-deprived pigs in an automatic feeding device. J. Animal. Sci. 2, 27–33.

Lefranc, G., Chaabani, H., Van Loghem, E., Lefranc, M.P., De Lange, G., Helal, A.N., (1983): Simultaneous absence of the human IgG1, IgG2, IgG4 and IgA1 subclasses: immunological and immunogenetical considerations. Eur. J. Immunol. 13, 240–244.

Lefranc, M.P., Hammarstrom, L., Smith, C.L., Lefranc, G., (1991): Gene deletion in the human immunoglobulin heavy chain constant region locus: molecular and immunological analysis. Immunodef. Rev. 2, 265–281.

Lefranc, M.P., Lefranc, G., De Lange, G., Out, T.A., Van den Broek, P.J., Van Nieuwkoop, J., et al. (1983): Instability of the human immunoglobulin heavy chain constant region locus indi-cated by different inherited chromosomal deletions. Mol. Biol Med, 1, 207–217.

McAleer, J., Weber, P., Sun, J., Butler, J.E., (2005): Antibody repertoire development in fetal and neonatal piglets. XI. The thymic B cell repertoire develops independently from that in blood and mesenteric lymph nodes. Immunology (British) 114, 171–183.

Mendicino, M., Ramsoondar, J., Phelps, C., Vaught, T., Ball, S., Dai, Y., et al. (2011): Target-ed disruption of the porcine immunoglobulin heavy chain locus produces a null phenotype. Transgenic Research 20, 625–641.

Metzger, J.J., Fougereau, M., (1967): Characterization of two subclasses of γG immunoglobulin in swine. C.R. Hebd. Seances Acad. Sci. Ser. P. Sci. Nat., 265, 724–727.

Mullens, M.A., Register, K.B., Bayles, D.O., Butler, J.E., (2011): *Haemophilus parasuis* ex-hibits IgA protease activity but lacks homologs of the IgA protease genes of *Haemophilus influenzae*. Vet. Microbio. 153, 407–412.

Navarro, P., Christenson, R., Ekhardt, G., Lunney, J.K., Rothschild, M., Bosworth, B., Lemke, J., Butler, J.E., (2000): Genetic differences in the frequency of the hinge variants of porcine IgA is breed dependent. Vet. Immunol. Immunopath. 73, 287–295.

Padlan, E.A., (1994): Anatomy of the antibody molecule. Mol. Immunol. 31,169–217.

Ramsoondar, J., Mendicino, M., Phelps, C., Vaught, T., Ball, S., Monahan, J., et al. (2011): Tar-geted disruption of the porcine immunoglobulin kappa light chain locus. Transgenic Research 20, 643–653.

Rapacz, J., Hasler-Rapacz, J., (1982): Immunogenetic studies on polymorphism, postnatal pas-sive acquisition and development of immunoglobulin gamma [IgG] in swine. Proceedings of the second international congress genetics and applied livestock production, vol. III, Editorial Garsi, Madrid.

Rejnek, J., Kostka, J., Travenicek, J., (1966): Studies on the immunoglobulin spectrum of porcine serum and colostrum. Folia. Microbiol. 11, 173–178.

Rodgers, C.S., Stoltz, D.A., Meyerholz, D.K., Ostedgaards, L.S, Rohhlima, T., Taft, P.J., et al. (2008): Disruption of the CFTR gene produces a model of cystic fibrosis in newborn pigs. Science 321, 1837–1841.

Schwartz, J.C., Lefranc, M., Murtaugh, M.P., (2012a): Evolution of the porcine kappa locus through germline gene conversion. Immunogenetics 64, 303–311.

Schwartz, J.C., Lefranc, M., Murtaugh, M.P., (2012b): Organization, complexity and allelic diversity of the porcine immunoglobulin lambda locus. Immunogenetics 64, 399–407.

Siminovitch, K.A., Bakhshi, A., Goldman, P., Korsmeyer, S.J., (1985): A uniform deleting element mediates the loss of kappa genes in human B cells. Nature 316, 260–262.

Sinkora, J., Rehakova, Z., Samankova, L., Haverson, K., Butler, J. E., Zwart, R. (2001): Characterization of monoclonal antibodies recognizing immunoglobulin k and l chains in pigs by flow cytometry. Vet. Immunol. Immunopath. 80, 79–91.

Solem, S.T., Stenvik, J., (2006): Antibody repertoire development in teletost—a review with emphasis on salmanoids of *Gadus morhua L.* Dev. Com. Immunol. 30, 57–76.

Sun, J., Butler, J.E., (1997): Sequence analysis of swine switch m, Cm and Cµm. Immunogenetics 46, 452–460.

Sun, J., Hayward, C., Shinde, R., Christenson, R., Ford, S.P., Butler, J.E., (1998): Antibody repertoire development in fetal and neonatal piglets. I. Four V_H genes account for 80% of V_H usage during 84 days of fetal life. J. Immunol. 161, 5070–5078.

Sun, X-Z., Wertz, N., Sinkora, M., Tobin, G., Lager, K., Nara, P., et al. (2012): Antibody repertoire development in fetal and neonatal piglets. XXII. Rearrangement occurs in the lambda locus before kappa during B cell lymphogenesis. Immunology 137, 149–159.

Van Zaane, D., Hulst, M.M., (1987): Monoclonal antibodies against porcine immunoglobulin isotypes. Vet. Immunol. Immunopathol. 16, 23–26.

Wagner, B., (2006): Immunoglobulins and immunoglobulin gene of the horse. Devel. Comp. Immunol. 30, 155–164.

Wertz, N., Vazquez, J., Sun, J., Wells, K., Butler, J.E. Antibody repertoire development in fetal and neonatal piglets. XII. Three IGLV genes comprise 70% of the preimmune repertoire and there is little junctional diversity. Mol. Immunol.

Xu, J.L., Davis, M.M., (2000): Diversity in the CDR3 region of V_H is sufficient for most antibody specificities. Immunity. 13, 37–45.

Zachau, H.G., (1995): The human immunoglobulin k genes, in: Immunoglobulin genes, Honjo, T., Alt, F.W., (Eds), Academic Press, pp. 173–191.

Zhao, Y., Pan-Hammarstrom, Q., Kacskovics, I., Hammarstrom, L. (2003): The porcine Ig d gene: Unique chimeric splicing of the first constant region domain in its heavy chain transcripts. J. Immunol. 171, 1312–1318.

CHAPTER 8

BOVINE IMMUNOGLOBULIN GENETICS: NOVEL PHYLOGENETIC PERSPECTIVE

YFKE PASMAN and AZAD K. KAUSHIK

CONTENTS

ABSTRACT

Limited germline sequence divergence and combinatorial diversity in cattle, unlike rodents and humans, has resulted in unconventional antibody diversification strategies that involve: (a) generation of exceptionally long CDR3H (>50 codons) by using single long *IGHD2* gene (potentially capable of coding for 49 codons) and insertion of conserved short nucleotide sequence (CSNS) specifically at *IGHV-IGHD* junction; (b) somatic hypermutations without exposure to external antigen during B cell ontogeny. The presence of atypical CDR3H (up to 66 amino acids) in cattle antibodies is yet to be seen in any other species. The antibodies with exceptionally long CDR3H show restricted $V\lambda+V_H$ pairings where λ light chain provides only structural support. The λ-light chain is predominantly expressed in bovine antibody repertoire mostly encoded by restricted *IGLV1-IGLJ3-IGLC3* recombinations. Despite significant complexity at IGK locus, κ-light chains are expressed al low levels in the antibody repertoire predominantly coded by *IGVK2-IGKJ1-IGKC* recombination. Three IgM allotypes are defined where some allelic variants may arise via alternate splicing. Of four IgG1 allotypes described, unique presence of Pro-Ala-Ser-Ser in Cγ1 domain of IgG1c allotype may have a role in cell adhesion and migration function. Overall, generation of exceptionally long CDR3H, with or without CSNS insertions, and somatic hypermutations without prior antigen exposure compensate for limited germline divergence and contribute to antibody diversification in cattle. Such an atypical CDR3H with multiple cystienes generates minidomains by intra-CDR3H disulfide bridges creating novel configurational diversity in the antigen-binding site.

8.1　THE ADAPTIVE IMMUNE SYSTEM

The adaptive immune system in jawed vertebrates involves somatically selected and randomly expanded clonally diverse antigen receptors of the immunoglobulin (Ig) superfamily (Cannon et al., 2010) that originated more than 500 million years ago. Such an evolution of multiple gene recombination based diversity of Ig superfamily receptors of lymphocytes is due to acquisition of recombinases, RAG1 and RAG2, via horizontal transmission approximately 400–450 million years back (Agrawal et al., 1998; Litman et al., 2010). Despite increasing complexity of the adaptive immune system during vertebrate evolution, basic elements are relatively conserved as these evolved under continuous pathogen challenge. Essentially, B- and T-lymphocytes expressing Ig and T cell antigen receptor (TcR), respectively, that are encoded by RAG-based recombination of variable (*V*), diversity (*D*) and/or joining (*J*) and constant (*C*) region genes form the core of adaptive immunity. An absence of RAG1 and RAG2 in jawless vertebrates has resulted in fundamentally different parallel mechanisms of lymphocyte receptor diversity (Butler, 1998; Flajnik et al., 2004; Cooper et al., 2006; Bailey et al., 2013) reflective of convergent evolution. For example, lamprey and hagfish assemble variable lymphocyte receptors (VLRs) from leucine rich repeat modules by gene conversion. Further, no evidence of major histocompatibility complex (MHC) class I and II antigens, TcR and Ig exists in invertebrates together with the jawless vertebrates. The members of Ig superfamily are, however, found throughout species, including those involved in the innate protein responses in insects, fibrinogen related proteins in snails and V-region chitin–binding protein in amphioxus (Flajnik et al., 2004; Pancer and Cooper, 2006).

A species-specific evolutionary path of RAG-based Ig and TcR recombinations is evident from lower (cartilaginous) fish to higher order jawed vertebrates where clan I, II and III Ig heavy variable-region genes are selected and retained differently across species, with clan I genes being few or absent in many species (Das et al., 2008). Four vertebrate light-chains isotypes (σ, σ-cart, κ and λ) originated 450 million years ago before the appearance of cartilaginous fishes (Criscitiello and Flajnik, 2007), but only two isotypes (κ and λ) are found in reptiles and most higher order mammals (Das et al., 2008). Given varying germline sequence divergence and complexity across species, different post-recombination antibody (Ab) diversification strategies have evolved across species to sustain host defense (Table 1).

An Ig, composed of two identical heavy- (H) and light (L) chains, is the B cell antigen receptor (BCR) as well as the main effector of B-lymphocyte mediated humoral natural and adaptive immunity. In general, Ig heavy chain variable-region is encoded by programed recombination of germline V (*IGHV*), D (*IGHD*) and J (*IGHJ*) genes, whereas the light-chain

TABLE 1 Antibody diversification mechanisms across species.

Species	Germline diversity	Ig Transfer		Primary Lymphoid Organ	Mechansim of Ab Diversification
		Placental	Colostrum Ig		
Man	Extensive	+	+	Fetal Liver, Bone marrow	Combinatorial diversity
Rodent		+	+	Fetal Liver, Bone marrow	Combinatorial diversity
Rabbit		+	+	Appendix, GALT	Gene Conversion, Somatic hypermutations via gut microflora stimulation
Pig				Fetal Liver/Bone marrow, Ileal Payer's Patch, Thymus	Extensive junctional diversity
Sheep	Limited			Ileal Payer's Patch	Antigen independent somatic hypermutations
Cattle		-	+	Ileal Payer's Patch, Fetal Bone marrow and Lymph Node	Exceptionally long CDR3H generation via CSNS insertion, Antigen independent somatic hypermutations
Came				Not known	Gene conversion/replacement. Repertoire expansion via VHH diversity without light chain.
Horse				Not known	Somatic hypermutations (!), Gene conersion
Chicken			Yolk sac?	Bursa of Fabricius	Gene Conversion

variable region, both for kappa (κ) and lambda (λ), originates via recombination of V (*IGKV* or *IGLV*) and J (*IGKJ* or *IGLJ*) genes (Tonegawa, 1983; Jones and Simkus, 2009; Kaushik and Lim, 1996). IMGT nomenclature for immunoglobulin heavy and light chain genes has been used that takes into consideration the historical gene designations widely cited in the literature. The designation *IGHD* as per IGMT nomenclature must be viewed in proper context as it might refer to a heavy chain (*Cδ*) or diversity (*D*) mini-gene involved in encoding the variable-region of the heavy chain. The VDJ and VJ recombination generated combinatorial diversity is further enhanced via junctional flexibility (nucleotide deletions, non-templated or templated nucleotide additions) and somatic hypermutations (SHM) effected by activation-induced deaminase (AID) enzyme (Neuberger and Scott, 2000; Hackney et al., 2009). In rodents and humans where both placental and colostral Ig transfer occurs, extensive germline sequence divergence and combinatorial diversity is seen in developing B-cells in fetal liver and bone marrow (Kabat and Wu, 1991). By contrast, in species without placental Ig transfer and limited germline sequence divergence, B-cells develop in other lymphoid organs, (e.g., ileal Peyer's patches (IPP), Bursa of Fabricius) (Pink et al., 1985; Reynaud et al., 1985; Butler et al., 2000; Dufour et al., 1996) and employ alternative Ab diversification strategies (Table 1). An exception is rabbit where despite placental and colostral Ig transfer both gene conversion and SHM, induced by intestinal microflora stimulation, diversify Ab repertoire (Knight, 1992; Weinstein et al., 1994) as described in Chapter 6. Upon antigen (Ag) exposure in the periphery, however, the *VDJ* and *VJ* recombinations undergo SHM, a mechanism common to Ab diversification and affinity maturation in vertebrate species.

8.2 THE BOVINE IMMUNE SYSTEM

Development of humoral immunity differs across species because of selective influences of speciation events and evolutionary forces (Cohn and Langman, 1990). For example, bovine B cells bear characteristics common to B-1 and B-2 cells Naessens, 1997, considered to be different lineages or these develop via distinct B cell differentiation pathways. This chapter focuses on some unique comparative characteristics of the bovine immune system relevant to immunoglobulin genetics.

8.2.1 PASSIVE IMMUNITY VIA MATERNAL IG TO NEWBORN

Maternal Ig transfer to fetus during gestation is mostly prevented by syn-desmochorial placentation in cattle (Brandon et al., 1971; Schultz et al., 1971) although some IgG transfer may occur (Kuroiwa et al., 2009). Maternal Igs are predominantly transferred via colostrum to the newborn to provide passive protection (reviewed in (Butler et al., 2009; Butler and Kerli, 2004). Non-selective predominant colostrum IgG1 uptake occurs in the intestine of newborn via neonatal Fc receptor (FcRn) within 12–48 hours post-birth (Kacskovics et al., 2006), though some IgM and IgA transfer may occur. The neonatal FcRn is known to transport IgG across the placental barrier (Leach et al., 1996) in some mammals. While neonatal FcRn is capable of transporting Ig across mucosal surfaces, but it is unable to do so through syndesmochorial placentation in ruminants (Kacskovics, 2004). Binding of IgG to FcRn prolongs its serum half-life by influencing its metabolism (Kacskovics et al., 2006; Brambell et al., 1964; Cervenak and Kacskovics, 2009). FcRn is also suggested to protect albumin from intracellular catabolic degradation (Anderson et al., 2006). The FcRn receptors are confined to crypt epithelial cells of the large and small intestine of cattle (Cervenak and Kacskovics, 2009). Various bovine FcRn haplotypes correlate with serum IgG concentrations in the newborn consistent with their role in colostral IgG1 transport and enhanced IgG half-life (Laegreid et al., 2002). The FcRn distribution in bovine mammary epithelial cells varies before and after parturition in correlation with IgG1 transport during colostrum formation (Cervenak and Kacskovics, 2009). Since FcRn expression is seen in mammary gland, intestine and lung of ruminants (Mayer et al., 2002, 2004), IgG1 secretion may be FcRn-dependent in cattle. By contrast, FcRn receptors are not found in duodenal enterocytes of lambs (Mayer et al., 2004), another ruminant species. But

FcRn is identified in the ovine mammary gland (Kacskovics, 2004) and, also, the human placenta (Story et al., 1994). Given such constitutive biological differences across species, obviously different mechanisms operate for Ig transport in the mammary gland and placenta.

In general, IgG predominates in the colostrum of carnivores and ungulates whereas IgA is the principal colostral Ig in rodents and primates. Bovine colostrum is rich in IgG1 (>100 mg/mL), a predominant Ig class in the serum (Butler and Kerli, 2004; Hurley, 2003; Farrell et al., 2004). Unlike other species where IgA provides mucosal protection, ruminant IgG1, being relatively resistant to proteolysis, protects mucosal lining (Newby and Bourne, 1976). In cattle, IgG1 exceeds IgA by, at least, 10-fold in colostrum even though IgA levels are also high as compared to serum (Hurley, 2003; Farrell et al., 2004; Gapper et al., 2007. Thus, both IgG and IgA are transported to mammary gland of cattle where IgG1 transfers passive immunity to neonate while IgA provides the mucosal protection (Butler, 2006).

8.2.2 B LYMPHOCYTE DEVELOPMENT

In rodents and humans, B-cell development continues throughout life given persistent VDJ and VJ recombinations occurring in the bone marrow. In cattle, similar to sheep, chicken, rabbit and swine, Ig diversification occurs only during perinatal life in the ileal Peyer's patches (IPP), considered to be the primary lymphoid organ in ruminants (Yasuda et al., 2004, 2006). Such a contention was supported by the observation that removal of IPP in sheep affected Ig$^+$ cell population in the peripheral lymphoid organs including circulating blood (Yasuda et al., 2004). However, Vλ recombination associated diversification has been noted in the bovine fetal spleen before the establishment of B cell repertoire in the IPP (Lucier et al., 1998). In addition, evidence for B lymphopoesis, that is, pre-B like cells positive for intracellular Igμ, have been found in bovine fetal bone marrow and lymph node in parallel to IPP (Ekman et al., 2012). These observations suggest that IPP may not be the only primary lymphoid organ in cattle. Such differences in B cell development can be an outcome of divergent evolution across species (Yasuda et al., 2006; Alitheen et al., 2010).

Nevertheless, *de novo* synthesis of IgA in bovine thymic tissue culture (Butler et al., 1972) suggests that alternative B cell development pathways may coexist.

IgM$^+$ B cells are detectable in cattle fetus as early as 59 days of gestation (Schultz et al., 1973) when pro/pre-B (CD79α^+ IgM$^-$, CD21$^-$) cells (Ekman et al., 2010) appear in IPP and liver (Table 2). The jejunal Peyer's patch (JPP), rich in IgM$^+$ B cells, appears before IPP at mid gestation and persists throughout life. The JPP, however, develop into secondary lymphoid tissue with characteristic germinal centers around one month of age (Yasuda et al., 2004). The IPP involutes at sexual maturity similar to thymus and mostly comprises oligoclonally expanded IgM$^+$ B cells (David et al., 2003). Few IgG$^+$ B cells are noted in both IPP and JPP, however. A high rate of B cell proliferation occurs in IPP around birth that provides a stable B lymphocyte population (Lucier et al., 1998) apart from diversifying the Ab repertoire. Both productive and nonproductive V*DJ* and V*J* recombinations are known to occur in B-splenocytes of 125-days-old bovine fetus (Saini and Kaushik, 2002). The antibody diversity increases in peripheral lymphoid organs 1–2 weeks post birth (Yasuda et al., 2006), which may be modulated by bovine colostrum IgG1 uptake. Colostral Igs are known to suppress immune responsiveness of the neonate, probably via down-regulation of IgG expression on B-cell surface, but this phenomenon is not fully understood (Zhao et al., 2006). In neonates (<1 week), circulating B cells are ~5% of the total leukocytes and reach adult levels (~19%) at about 20 weeks of age (Senogles et al., 1978). A lack of expression of surrogate light chain (*Vpreb1*; *IGLL1*), *RAG1* and *RAG2* genes in adult tissues (Ekman et al., 2012) suggests decline in B cell development as a function of age. Expression of AID, an enzyme crucial to class switch recombination (CSR) and SHM, is noted in lymph node, spleen and thymus samples from one-day-old calf (Verma et al., 2010), consistent with significant role of SHM in Ab diversification (Kaushik et al., 2009; Koti et al., 2010).

TABLE 2   Appearance of B cells and immunoglobulins during cattle gestation.

B Lymphocyte	Fetus Age/Gestation (Days)
IgM$^+$ B lymphocytes (Schultz et al., 1973)	59
CD79α$^+$ IgM$^-$, CD21$^-$ (Pro-/Pre-B cells in IPP, liver) (Ekman et al., 2010)	60–85
CD79α$^+$, IgM$^+$, CD21$^-$ cells in thymus (Ekman et al., 2010)	60–85
CD79α$^+$, IgM$^+$, CD21$^+$ cells in spleen (Ekman et al., 2010)	60–85
B and T cells in peripheral blood (Ishino et al., 1991)	70
IgM$^+$ B cells in lymph nodes (Ishino et al., 1991)	90
CD79α$^+$ IgM$^-$, CD21$^-$ (Pro-/Pre-B cells in bone marrow)	95–135
RAG1/RAG2 expression in bone marrow, spleen, liver and IPP (Ekman et al., 2010)	115–175
VDJ and/or VJ recombination in splenocytes (Saini and Kaushik, 2002)	125
Serum IgM (Schultz et al., 1971)	130
IgG$^+$ B lymphocytes (Schultz et al., 1973)	145
Serum IgG (Schultz et al., 1971)	145
IGLL1$^+$ Pre-B cells (Ekman et al., 2010)	180–285
IgA$^+$ B lymphocytes (Ishino et al., 1991)	180
Ig$^+$ B lymphocytes in Peyer's Patches (Ishino et al., 1991)	180
IgM$^+$ and IgG$^+$ B Lymphocytes in tonsils (Ishino et al., 1991)	240

8.2.3   IMMUNOGLOBULIN GENE ELEMENTS

8.2.3.1   LIGHT CHAINS

The jawed vertebrates, with the exception of avian species with single lambda light chain only, express Abs with two light chain isotypes: kappa (κ) and lambda (λ). Relative distribution of each of these isotypes in the Ab repertoire varies across species. In ruminants, such as cattle, λ-light chain is predominantly expressed (>90%) (Arun et al., 1996) whereas mice mainly express κ-light chain (>95%). By contrast, species like camel produce some Abs devoid of light chains altogether (Hamers-Casterman et al., 1993). *IGKV* and *IGLV* genes encoding and κ and λ light chains, respectively, can be identified based on cladistic markers whose function is not understood. While κ and λ light chains provide adequate Ab repertoire for host protection, each isotype may have an important role given conservation of their specific markers since 350 million years (Das et al., 2008). Three surrogate light chains genes, V*preb1*, V*preb3* and *IGLL1*, are identified on chromosome 17, close to the λ-locus, in the bovine genome (Ekman et al., 2009).

8.2.3.1.1   κ-LIGHT CHAIN GENES

Analysis of κ-light chain (IGK) locus on bovine Hereford genome sequence (Elsik et al., 2009; Zimin et al., 2009; Drummond et al., 2011; Lefranc and Lefranc, 2001; Altschul et al., 2009) led to annotation of 22 *IGKV*, 3 *IGKJ* and 1 *IGKC* genes on chromosome 11 (Ekman et al., 2009). However, 17 *IGKV* genes are identified on chromosome 11 in the current reference assembly UMD 3.1 (Zimin et al., 2009). The *IGKV* genes are spread over 150 kbp, approximately 9 kbp 3' of *IGKJ* gene cluster (Fig. 1). Similar to human and mice, the *IGKV* genes, present in both transcriptional orientations, are interspersed (Sitnikova and Nei, 1998) and spread evenly with intervening 4–11 kbp introns. Phylogenetically, the *IGKV* genes are grouped into four subfamilies closely related to the four sheep *IGKV* families designated by roman numerals that are yet to be annotated in the IMGT database (Table 3). Eight of the *IGKV* genes are potentially functional (Ekman et al., 2009) where members of *IGVK2* gene family are mainly expressed (unpublished). Preferentially expressed *IGKV2* gene family is closest to sheep (91%), followed by killer whale 84%, and dolphin 84%. The *IGKV* coded CDR1L size varies (6, 10 or 11 codons) while CRD2L is restricted to 3 codons. While identical for CDR2L, such a pattern differs for CDR1L from humans (6–12 codons) and mice (5–12 codons) (Ekman et al., 2009). However, the *IGKV* encoded CDR1L and CDR2 consists of 11 and 3 codons, respectively, in sheep (Ehrenmann et al., 2010).

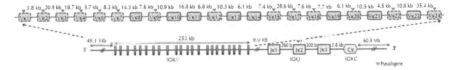

FIGURE 1 Schematic diagram of bovine IGK locus on chromosome 11 adapted from Ekman et al. (2009). The IGK locus is identical both in BTAU 4.6 and UMD 3.1 assembly of Hereford cow genome.

TABLE 3 Phylogenetic relationship of bovine *IGKV* gene families across species.

Cattle	Sheep*	Human*	Mouse*	Pig*	Rabbit*
IGKV1	*IGKVI* (85%)	*IGKV1* (78%)	*IGKV1* (75%)	*IGKV1* (75%)	*IGKV1* (70%)
IGKV2	*IGKVII* (91%)	*IGKV2* (73%)	*IGKV2* (77%)	*IGKV2* (78%)	*IGKV1* (62%)
IGKV3	*IGKVIII* (93%)	*IGKV3* (65%)	*IGKV3* (65%)	*IGKV1* (62%)	*IGKV1* (60%)
IGKV4	*IGKVIV* (91%)	*IGKV2* (74%)	*IGKV2* (80%)	*IGKV2* (81%)	*IGKV1* (60%)

*Reference genes from IMGT database [124] aligned using CLUSTALW [100]. *IGKV* groups and their closest families: human 98 *IGKV* genes grouped into six families—*IGKV1–6*; pig 25 *IGKV* genes grouped in four families—IGKV1,2,3 and 5; rabbit 68 *IGKV* genes grouped into one family—*IGKV1* (IMGT/GENE-DB (Giudicelli et al., 2005); ovine *IGKV* gene families (Genbank Reference Oar_v3.1 Primary Assembly chromosome 3 (Hein and Dudler, 1998) in Roman numerals indicate published designations.

Three *IGKJ* genes, *IGKJ1, IGKJ2* and *IGKJ3,* are clustered closely together within 800 bp followed by one *IGKC* gene. Though, all *IGKJ* genes are functional, *IGKJ1* with classical 23 base pair RSS is preferentially expressed. A lack of *IGKJ2* gene expression seems to be influenced by one-nucleotide short spacer (22 base pair) in its RSS, though it is transcribed

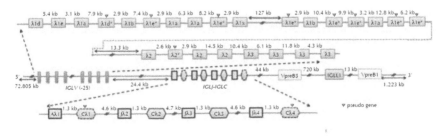

FIGURE 2 Schematic diagram of bovine IGL locus on chromosome 17 adapted from Pasman et al.(Pasman et al., 2010)..

(Stein et al., 2012). The *IGKJ3* gene has distinct cladistics protein signature 'EIN' as compared to 'EIK,' at position 10–12, conserved in most species (Das et al., 2008) with an unknown function.

The *IGKC* gene has at least three alleles that code for two allotypes and these alleles are unequally distributed in four cattle breeds tested. All the alleles are identified in three breeds (Holstein Friesen, German Simmental and Aubrac) whereas *IGKC*[a] allele was noted only in German Pied breed (Stein et al., 2012). Both junctional flexibility, involving N or P nucleotide additions and deletions, together with somatic hypermutations compensate for limited combinatorial diversity at IgK locus. There is no indication to suggest that gene conversion is involved in diversification of the κ-light chain repertoire. Overall, IGK locus comprises eight functional *IGKV* genes, three *IGKJ* genes and single *IGKC* gene. The predominant *IGVK2-IGKJ1-IGKC* recombination encodes most κ-light chains in the Ab repertoire.

8.2.3.1.2 λ-LIGHT CHAIN GENES

The bovine λ-light chain (IGL) locus, spanning 412 kbp on chromosome 17, has 25 to 31 *IGLV* genes (Fig. 2) of which 14 to 17 are potentially functional (Ekman et al., 2009). However, Ekman et al., (2009) describes a total of 63 *IGLV* genes, 32 being unplaced in the genome, of which 11 are potentially functional (Ekman et al., 2009). In the current genome assembly (UMD 3.1) 34 *IGLV* genes are identified in both transcriptional

TABLE 4 Phylogenetic relationship of bovine *IGLV* gene families across species.

Cattle	Sheep*	Human*	Mice*	Rabbit*
IGLV1	*IGLVI* (94.0%)	*IGLV1* (74.8%)	*IGLV* 4 (60.4%)	*IGLV* 2 (70.1%)
IGLV2	*IGLVII* (92.0%)	*IGLV2* (79.3%)	*IGLV* 2 (62.8%)	***IGLV* 2 (76.4%)**
IGLV3	*IGLVIII* (92%)	*IGLV3* (73.8%)	ND	*IGLV* 3 (80.2%)

*Reference genes from IMGT DB (Lefranc, 2001); Bovine *IGLV* families (Pasman et al., 2010) and the closest families across species: human 86 *IGLV* genes grouped into nine families—IGLV1–9; mouse 19 *IGLV* grouped into eight families—*IGLV1–8*; rabbit 31 *IGLV* genes grouped into six families *IGLV1–6* (IMGT/GENE-DB (Giudicelli et al., 2005) ovine *IGLV* groups (Genbank Oar_ v3.1 Primary Assembly aligned by MBLAST (Hein and Dudler, 1998)) in Roman numerals indicate published designations.

orientations, however. Three *IGLV* gene families are organized in three subclusters that are separated by two intervening introns of 126.8 and 138.3 kbp. The predominantly expressed *IGLV1* genes are present in the two 5' subclusters, while *IGLJ*-proximal *IGLV* subcluster comprises rarely expressed *IGLV2* and *IGLV3* genes (Pasman et al., 2010). Of four *IGLJ-IGLC* cassettes (Chen et al., 2008), only *IGLJ2- IGLC2* and *IGLJ3-IGLC3* are functional where *IGLJ3-IGLC3* is preferentially expressed with a minor role for *IGLJ2- IGLC2* cassette (Pasman et al., 2010). Three allotypic variants of *IGLC2* and five of *IGLC3* are described in cattle breeds but their clinical relevance is unknown (Diesterbeck et al., 2012).

The *IGLV* genes are categorized in three families, *IGLV1, IGLV2 and IGLV3*, but only *IGLV1* gene family is predominantly expressed in the antibody repertoire. The role of local methylation and transcriptional elements in preferential gene expression is not determined. The bovine *IGLV1* and *IGLV2* families are closely related with sheep IGLVI and *IGLVII* with a sequence identity of 92.6% and 88.9%, respectively (Table 4). However, bovine *IGLV3* gene family is closely related to an unclassified sheep *IGLV* gene with 75% sequence identity (Pasman et al., 2010). MBLAST searches of reference genomic sequences show closest relation of bovine *IGLV* genes with sheep (94%) followed by walrus (85%) and giant panda (83%). The *IGLV* coded CDR1L consists of 6, 8 or 9 codons whereas CRD2L is restricted to 3 or 7 codons, similar to humans and mice (Ekman et al., 2009). Within the *IGLV1* family, five subfamilies are defined, *IGLV1a, IGLV1b, IGLV1d, IGLV1e* and *IGLV1x* where *IGLV1a* and *IGLV1b*

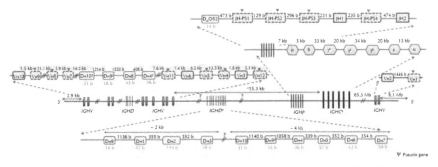

FIGURE 3   Schematic diagram of IGH locus (3' to 5') on chromosome 21 adapted from Niku et al. (2012), Walther et al. (2013), Zimin et al. (2009), Koti et al. (2010) and Zhao et al. (2003) that takes in to consideration UMD3.1 cow genome assembly. Ψ-pseudogene.

genes are mostly expressed. By contrast, *IGLV1d*, *IGLV1e* and *IGLV1x* genes code for λ-light chains that specifically pair with heavy chains expressing exceptionally long CDR3H (>50 amino acids) (Saini et al., 1999, 2003). Based on *in silico* analysis using *EST*-database only eight *IGLV* genes are found expressed in the Ab repertoire. Among four functional *IGLV1a* genes, *IGLV1a.3* is mainly used. While gene conversion has been suggested to be involved in λ-light chain diversification in cattle based on limited analysis (Parng et al., 1996), but this needs to be confirmed (Lucier at al., 1998). Despite seemingly more complexity, restricted Vλ-Jλ3-Cλ3 recombinations encode most of the λ-light chain antibody repertoire.

8.2.3.2   HEAVY CHAIN IMMUNOGENETICS

8.2.3.2.1   HEAVY CHAIN VARIABLE (IGHV) GENES

The Ig heavy chain (IGH) locus, located on chromosome 21q24 (Niku et al., 2012; Tobin-Janzen and Womack, 1992), spans approximately 250 kbp (Fig. 3) but is yet to be fully assembled and annotated. Ten functional *IGHV* genes map to either chromosome 21 or another chromosome 11q23, now assigned as chromosome 8 (Hayes and Petit, 1993). Given two rounds of whole genome duplication events in the evolution of mammals (Flajnik and Kasahara, 2010), presence of two IGH loci in cattle should not be surprising. In this context, it should be noted that V_H and D_H genes are located on multiple chromosomes in humans (Tomlinson et al.,

TABLE 5   Phylogenetic relationship of bovine *IGHV* gene families across species.

Cattle	Sheep*	Human*	Mice*	Rabbit*
IGHV1	*IGHV1* (91.6%)	*IGHV4* (69.5%)	*IGHV2* (80.0%)	*IGHV1* (68.4%)
IGHV2	None	*IGHV4* (71.4%)	*IGHV12* (58.6%)	*IGHV1* (55.9%)
IGHV3	None	*IGHV1* (52.8%)	None	None

*Reference genes IMGT DB (Lefranc, 2001); Bovine *IGHV* groups (Niku et al., 2012) and their closest families across species: sheep 10 *IGHV* genes grouped into one *IGHV1* family; human 341 *IGHV* genes grouped into seven families (*IGHV1–7*); mouse 406 *IGHV* genes grouped into 16 families (IGHV1–16); rabbit 49 *IGHV* genes grouped into one family (*IGHV1*); Source: IMGT/GENE-DB (Giudicelli et al., 2005), Alignment by CLUSTALW (Larkin et al., 2007).

1994) as well. A total of 36 *IGHV* genes are identified in the current cow genome assembly (UMD3.1), though some of the identified *IGHV* genes may be allelic variants. The bovine *IGHV1* gene family is polymorphic given the genomic complexity of 13–15 genes in four cattle breeds (Holstein, Jersey, Hereford and Charolais) in a Southern analysis (Saini et al., 1997). Another study reported 11 functional and 6 pseudogenes in the cattle genome (Das et al., 2008) that originated from gene duplications. The *IGHV* genes are classified into single bovine *IGHV1* (designated earlier as $BovV_H1$) gene family with most sequence identity (67.4–69.8%) to human *IGHV4* (Saini et al., 1997; Berens et al., 1997; Sinclair et al., 1997). Consistent with the presence of other genes in a southern (Saini et al., 1996), another $BovV_H2$ gene family has been identified mostly comprising V_H pseudogenes (Walther et al., 2013). Bovine *IGHV1* family is closest to sheep *IGHV1* (89.8–91.6%) (Table 5) and belongs to less conserved mammalian group I, clan II *IGHV* genes. Though, cross-species hybridization in a Southern revealed the presence of murine *IGHV11* gene homolog in cattle (Saini et al., 1996), but these are not expressed in the Ab repertoire. The less conserved clan I genes that are expressed in 50% of the adult murine primary Ab repertoire (Kofler et al., 1992; Kaushik and Lim, 1996) are present as pseudogenes in the cattle IGH locus, however. The clan I and III genes may reflect a random loss (Das et al., 2008) in cattle similar to other species, for example, loss of clan I and II but retention of clan III *IGHV* genes in swine (Butler et al., 2009). Three distinct restriction fragment length polymorphism (RFLP) patterns are evident in Holstein, Jersey, Hereford and Charolais breeds that involve either deletion or addition of *IGHV* genes (Hamers-Casterman et al., 1993), likely associated with inter or intrabreed recombination due to contemporary cattle breeding practices. Such a polymorphism at bovine IGH locus is a common phenomenon as it is seen across species including mice and humans. The bovine *IGHV1* encoded CDR1H is short (5 codons) and conserved as compared to rabbit, sheep, horse and humans (Table 6). Majority of CDR2H (91%) are long and composed of 16 codons, as in camel (Kabat and Wu, 1991; Wu et al., 2012), but a small proportion (9%) vary in size ranging from 13 to 21 codons (Larsen and Smith, 2013). By contrast, human CDR1H and CDR2H size are restricted to 7 and 19 codons, respectively. Nevertheless, long CDR2H are noted in pigs and horses where these can extend up to 23 and 27 codons, respectively.

TABLE 6 Complementarity-determining region (CDR) size diversity of variable heavy-region of antibodies across species

Species	V_H encoded CDR Size Diversity (codons)				Mechanism of CDR3H diversification					
	V_H Gene Families	CDR 1H	CDR 2H	Reference	CDR 3H Size	CSNS	N*	P**	D-D fusion	Reference
Human	7	7	19	(Matsuda et al., 1998)	2–26	—	+	+	+	(Wu et al., 1993)
Mouse	14	5	17	(Kofler et al., 1992)	2–19	—	+	+	+	(Wu et al., 1993)
Rabbit	1	5–6	13–19	(Knight and Winstead, 1997)	4–19	—	+	+	?	(Knight, 1992; Friedman et al., 1994)
Sheep	1 or 9	5–7	16–18	(Dufour et al., 1996; Charlton et al., 2000)	3–23	—	+	+	?	(Charlton et al., 2000)
Cattle	1	5	13–21***	(Saini et al., 1997; Berens et al., 1997; Sinclair et al., 1997)	3–66	+	+	+	?	(Saini and Kaushik, 2002; Koti et al., 2010; Saini et al., 1999; Saini et al., 1997; Wang et al., 2013)
Pig	1	4–5	16–23	(Sun et al., 1994)	3–25	—	+	+	?	(Butler, 2000; Sun et al., 1994)
Camel	1	5	16	(Nguyen et al., 1998)	10–24	—	+	+	?	(Muyldermans et al., 1994)
Horse	2	7 or 8	2–27	(Almagro et al., 2006; Wagner, 2006)	7–24	—	?	?	?	(Almagro et al., 2006; Wagner, 2006)
Chicken	1	5	17	(Reynaud et al., 1985)	15–30	—	?	+	+	(Reynaud et al., 1985; Reynaud et al., 1991)

* – N nucleotide; ** – P nucleotide; ? – Unknown; ***Mostly (91%) 16 codons.

The VDJ encoded CDR3H size ranges from 3 to 66 codons comprising characteristic GGT and TAT repetitive codons in cattle antibodies (Saini et al., 1999; Wang et al., 2013). Such an exceptionally long CDR3H (>50 codons) is the first to be reported in a species to date (Table 6), which has multiple cysteine residues (Saini et al., 1999) that permit inter-CDRH and intra-CDR3H disulfide bridging. Such an exceptional CDR3H is noted in all antibody isotypes including IgG, IgA and IgE (Walther et al., 2013; Larsen and Smith, 2012). The exceptionally long CDR3H is encoded by the single *IGHV* (*gI.110.20; IGHV10* in Fig. 3) gene (Wang et al., 2013) that may encode up to 5 codons in the CDR3H, unlike other bovine *IGVH* genes. An insertion of conserved short nucleotide sequence (CSNS), 13–18 amino acids long and high in alanine content of unknown origin, specifically at the V-D junction further extend CDR3H size (Koti et al., 2010). These additional amino acids are an essential component of the "stalk" supporting the "knob" structure of these unique CDR3H (Wang et al., 2013). Similar to other species, N or P nucleotide additions add to junctional diversity (Table 6). Overall, limited germline *IGHV* gene sequence divergence restricts Ab diversity in cattle (Table 7), unlike humans and rodents.

TABLE 7 Bovine antibody combinatorial and mutational diversification mechanisms.

Germline Genes	Heavy Chain*	Light Chain	
		Kappa	Lambda
Variable (V)	36 (10 Functional)	22 (8 Functional)	25 (17 Functional)
Diversity (D)	10–13	—	—
Joining (J)	6 (2 Functional)	3	4 (2 Functional)
Potential Recombinational diversity	260	24	34
Junctional diversity			
Nucleotide loss:	+	?	+
Neonate Adult	+	+	+
CSNS additions ($V_H D_H$ only):	—	—	—
Neonate Adult	+	—	—
N additions:	+	?	?
Neonate Adult	+	+	+
Antigen independent SHM in neonates	+	?	?
Potential H+L Pairings	$260\times(24+34) = 0.15\times10^5$		
SHM upon antigen exposure in periphery	+	?	+

*Total genes identified on chromosomes 8 and 21.

TABLE 8 Percent nucleotide identity of bovine germline *IGHD* genes with other species.

Species	Bovine germline *IGDH* genes								
	IGDH1 (Shojaei et al., 2003)	*IGDH2* (Shojaei et al., 2003)	*IGHD3* (Shojaei et al., 2003)	*IGHD4/4-2** (Koti et al., 2010)	*IGHD5* (Koti et al., 2010)	*IGHD6* (Koti et al., 2010)	*IGHD7* (Koti et al., 2010)	*IGHD8* [60]	*IGHDQ52* (Hosseini et al., 2004)
Chicken (Reynaud et al., 1991)	**DY** **(69%)**	D6 (63.3%)	D6 (69.0%)	D6 (63.3%)	DY (69.0%)	**DY (69.0%)**	**D6** **(69.0%)**	D6 (65.4%)	D1/D6 (35.7%)
Rabbit (Friedman et al., 1994)	D5 (60.0%)	**D2B** **(82.9%)**	**D2B** **(73.3%)**	**D5** **(72.0%)**	**D2B** **(71.4%)**	D5 (60.0%)	D5 (66.7%)	**D2B (77.8%)**	D6 (57.1%)
Shark (Hinds and Litman, 1986)	801 (46.2%)	801 (53.8%)	801 (61.5%)	HXIA (60.0%)	HXIA (46.7%)	801 (46.2%)	801 (61.5%)	801 (61.5%)	**801 (72.7%)**

*Bovine genome, clone accession number NW_001504477.1.

8.2.3.2.2 HEAVY CHAIN DIVERSITY (IGHD) GENES

Characterization of bovine *IGHD* genes in Holstein cattle has led to the identification of 10–15 *IGHD* genes (Koti et al., 2008, 2010; Shojaei et al., 2003) varying in size from 14 to 154 bp that are probably organized in several clusters (Koti et al., 2008, 2010). But these *IGHD* gene clusters are spread over three chromosomes in UMD 3.1 assembly of Hereford cow genome due to incorrect assembly (Niku et al., 2012; Walther et al., 2013). Bovine *IGHD* genes are classified into four *IGHD* gene families: *IGHD-A* (*IGHD1* and IGHD6), *IGHD-B* (*IGHD2*, *IGHD3*, *IGHD5*, *IGHD7* and *IGHD8*), *IGHD-C* (*IGHD4*) and *IGHD-D* (*IGHDQ52*). Two more *IGHD* genes, called *IGHD16* (*IGHD 9* in Fig. 3) and *IGHD31* (*IGHD10* in Fig. 3) are identified outside these clusters but their expression is uncertain (unpublished data). Similar to other species, polymorphism exists at the *IGHD* locus which is evident across various cattle breeds (Zimin et al., 2009). The *IGHD* genes likely originated from gene duplication (Das et al., 2008) given high sequence identity between *IGHD* genes, for example, *IGHD1* and *IGHD6* (97.6%), *IGHD3* and *IGHD7* (94.8%). Phylogenetically, *IGHD1*, *IGHD3*, *IGHD6* and *IGHD7* genes are closest to chicken *IGHD-DY* and *IGHD-D6* genes (Table 8), while *IGHD2*, *IGHD4*, *IGHD5* and *IGHD8* genes are closest to rabbit *IGHD-D2B* and *IGHD-D5* genes. As would be expected, the conserved *IGHDQ52* gene is closest to conserved shark *IGHDH01* gene. The bovine *IGHD* genes are flanked by classical RSS comprising nonamer and heptamer sequences separated by a 12 bp spacer. The $V_H D_H J_H$ encoded CDR3H region in cattle antibodies varies from 3 to 66 codons. In general, *IGHD* encode three categories of CDR3H: short (3–10 codons), mid-sized (11–29 codons) and long (≥46 codons) (Walther et al., 2013). The single longest *IGHD2* gene present in cattle, unlike other species, is capable of potentially encoding 49 codons. In chicken, mice, horse and humans, *IGHD-IGHD* gene fusions result in increased CDR3H size (Meek et al., 1989), but no evidence for *IGHD-IGHD* fusion exists in cattle despite the presence of cryptic RSS (Pasman and Kaushik, 2012).

8.2.3.2.3   HEAVY-CHAIN JOINING (IGHJ) GENES

Six bovine *IGHJ* genes, 130–500 bp apart, span 18 kB and lie 7 kB upstream of the *IGHM* genes on chromosome 21 (Zhao et al., 2003).
Duplication of *IGHJ* genes together with *IGHDQ52* genes is noted on
chromosome 11 (Hosseini et al., 2004), reassigned to chromosome 8
(Zimin et al., 2009). This duplicated "low" locus (Hosseini et al., 2004) is
similar to the "high" locus where *IGHJ4 and IGHJ6* genes are functional.
Only two bovine *IGHJ* genes, *IGHJ1* and *IGHJ2*, are expressed as others either lack RSS or splice site. A very low expression of *IGHJ6* gene
in bovine Abs has been reported (Hosseini et al., 2004). Similar to other
mammals, *IGHJ* genes characteristically encode "VTVSS" motifs at 3'
end. Sheep also have six *IGHJ* genes with the *IGHJ4* and *IGHJ6* genes
being functional, with a corresponding high sequence identity with bovine
IGHJ1 (86.7%) and *IGHJ2* (84.7%) genes (global alignment ClustalW
(Larkin et al., 2007). This is also evident in a BLAST 2.2.28 (Altschul
et al., 1997) search for local alignments of reference genomic databases
show (nucleotide identity %, E-value) that confirms bovine *IGHJ1* gene
being closely related to sheep *IGHJ4* (95%, 1e-06). Given close phylogenetic relationship between bovidae and cetacea within the artiodactyla,
bovine *IGHJ1* gene is also closely related to bottlenose dolphin (94%, 3e-
04), killer whale (94%, 3e-04) and baboon (92%, 1e-04).

8.2.3.2.4   HEAVY CHAIN CONSTANT-REGION GENES

Bovine Ig heavy chain (IGH) locus is organized (5'-JH-7 kB-µ-5 kB-δ-
33 kB-γ3–20 kB-γ1–34 kB-γ2–20 kB-ε-13 kB-α-3') and spans approximately 150 kB on chromosome 21 (Zhao et al., 2003). Alignment of the
heavy chain *IGHJ* and *IGHC* gene cluster using BLAST shows a 95% ID
on the +/– strand of chromosome 21 of aligned contigs AY221098 and
AY158087 containing the bovine constant regions and the IGHJ "high"
expressed locus (Zhao et al., 2003; Hosseini et al., 2004). An additional
IGH loci with a functional *IGHM* and a *IGHD* pseudogene was identified
on chromosome 11q23 (Hayes and Petit, 1993), currently assigned to chromosome 8 (Zimin et al., 2009). These two loci are apparently functional

(Hosseini et al., 2004) where trans-chromosomal recombinations might occur (Kuroiwa et al., 2009). Other ruminant species, goat and sheep, are also known to have two IGH loci. In sheep, the locus is apparently located on chromosome 3, corresponding to chromosome 11 of goat and cattle (Hayes et al., 1993). In contrast to humans and mice, both IGH loci with *IGHM* genes are functional and both need to be disrupted for inducing B-cell deficiency in cattle (Kuroiwa et al., 2009). Whether allelic exclusion occurs at the two functional IGH loci in cattle needs to be understood.

The IgM constant gene (*IGHM*) comprises four constant exons (*IGHM 1–4*) encoding each of the four domains together with two other exons (*M1* and *M2*) encoding the transmembrane domains. The *M1* exon is spliced to the *IGHM4* exon, as in other species (Mousavi et al., 1998), resulting in membrane form transcript of IgM. Three bovine IgM allotypes are described (IgMa, IgMb and IgMc) (Saini and Kaushik, 2001), though other IgM variants may be derived via alternative splicing, for example, insertion of three in-frame codons at the *IGHM1* and *IGHM2* junction (Saini and Kaushik, 2001). The antigen binding ability of bovine IgM is influenced by relative inflexibility of *IGHM2* due to fewer prolines as it acts as a hinge (Saini and Kaushik, 2001).

The bovine germline IgD (*IGHD*) gene is transcriptionally active [105] but at a low level. The *IGHD1* exon is highly similar to *IGHM1* (96.6% at nucleotide and 93.5% at protein levels) (Zhao et al., 2002). The *IGHD* gene has a short switch region, $S\delta$, that may permit class switch recombination [106], unlike other species.

Three subclasses of IgG (IgG1, IgG2, IgG3) (Knight et al., 1988; Kacskovics and Butler, 1996; Rabbani et al., 1997) are identified in cattle, unlike four in humans, two in sheep and one in rabbit. Bovine *IGHG1* gene is most likely the homologue of both *IGHG2* and *IGHG3* genes, as gene duplication first led to *IGHG2* gene followed by the second event to *IGHG3* gene. A high sequence similarity exists between *IGHG3* and *IGHG1* genes (85.1%) as compared to *IGHG2* gene (83.4%) (Zhao et al., 2003). Allelic differences exist across all the IgG subclasses of cattle. Four allotypic variants of IgG1 (IgG1a, IgG1b, IgG1c and IgG1d) have been described (Symons et al., 1989; Saini et al., 2007). The unique *Pro-Ala-Ser-Ser* motifs in the CH1 (positions 189–192 and 205–208) domain of IgG1c seem to confer a novel cellular adhesion and migration function

(Saini et al., 2007). The role of IgG1 isotype in protection of mucosal surfaces needs to be understood from a functional perspective. Nucleotide sequences describing two IgG2 allotypic variants (IgG2a and IgG2b) have been described (Kacskovics and Butler, 1996). Two allotypes, IgG3a and IgG3b, of IgG3 subclass differ by six amino acids in the coding region and 84 base pair insertion in the intron between the CH2 and CH3 exons (Rabbani et al., 1997).

A single copy of Bovine epsilon (*IGHE*) gene is identified (Knight et al., 1988) with four exons (CH1–4) with 87% sequence similarity to sheep *IGHE* gene. Bovine IgE has heat labile skin sensitizing ability analogous to human IgE (Hammer et al., 1971).

A single *IGHA* gene is identified in bovine genome (Knight et al., 1988) where nucleotide sequence of *IGHA* reveals three bovine *IGHA* exons separated by two introns (Brown et al., 1997). Cattle IgA, though closest to IgA of another artiodactyl swine at protein level, shares an additional N-linked glycosylation site at position 282 with rabbit IgA3 and IgA4. Restriction fragment length polymorphism (Brown et al., 1997) and serological (De Benedictis et al., 1984) analysis have revealed two allelic variants of bovine IgA, though it could not be confirmed from genomic DNA analysis of 50 Swedish cattle.

8.2.4 DEVELOPMENT OF ANTIBODY REPERTOIRE

8.2.4.1 DEVELOPMENT OF NEONATAL VARIABLE-REGION REPERTOIRE

The *VDJ* and *VJ* recombinations appear as early as 125 days of gestation in splenic B-cells followed by serum Ig in 145-days-old fetus (Saini and Kaushik, 2002). At this developmental stage, some splenic B-cells may express *VDJ* but not *VJ* recombinations. At the same time, however, some B cells may secrete λ-light chain only because of nonproductive *VDJ* recombinations. Two *IGHV* genes *IGHV(gI.110.20)* and *IGHV1S3(BF2B5)* (Saini and Kaushik, 2002) are preferentially used in the fetal *VDJ* recombinations. In contrast to J-proximal conserved *IGHDQ52* gene, *IGHD7* and *IGHD5* genes are most expressed in fetal B cells similar to adults (Koti et al., 2010). The bovine *IGHJ1* gene (pB7S2) expression is predominant in both fetal and adult *VDJ* recombinations (Saini et al., 1997). Both N and P additions as well as junctional flexibility contribute to fetal *VDJ* recombination diversity. Extensive CDR3H size heterogeneity (9 to 56 codons) and somatic mutations in the absence of Ag exposure characterize the developing Ab repertoire (Saini and Kaushik, 2002). No evidence for gene conversion has been noted in the diversification of variable-heavy chain region repertoire both in neonatal and adult B cells (Kaushik et al., 2009). The fetal Abs with exceptionally long CDR3H originate from unique recombinations of the germline *IGHV(gI.110.20)*, longest *IGHD2* and *IGHJ1(pB7S2)* genes (Saini and Kaushik, 2002). However, CSNS insertions at *V-D* junction seen in adult *VDJ* recombinations (Koti et al., 2010) that contribute to the stalk structure of the antigen-combining site (Wang et al., 2013) are absent. Thus, the structure of the antigen-combining site encoded by fetal *VDJ* recombinations is likely to be different because of a shorter or nonexistent stalk. Somatic hypermutations are evident in the CDR1H and CDR2H of 125-days-old fetal *VDJ* recombinations in the absence of exposure to exogenous Ag. The biased 'hot spot' triplets in the CDRs of bovine *VDJ* recombinations predispose them to SHMs (Kaushik et al., 2009) similar to other species. The untemplated somatic hypermutations (Lucier et al., 1998) are also involved in diversifying the *VJ* recombinations encoding cattle λ-light-chains. Overall, intrinsic nonantigen dependent somatic hypermutations and CDR3H size heterogeneity diversify the developing bovine neonatal antibody repertoire, given the restricted germline sequence divergence and combinatorial diversity.

8.2.4.2   DEVELOPMENT OF ADULT VARIABLE-REGION REPERTOIRE

Most bovine *IGHV* and *IGHD* genes are expressed in adult VDJ recombinations with the exception of two unclassified *IGHD* (*IGHD16* and *IGHD31*) genes. However, conserved *IGHDQ52* is expressed at very low levels. Predominant expression of *IGHJ1* gene, notable in fetal VDJ recombinations, persists in the adulthood. As expected, somatic hypermutations in the CDRs occur during affinity maturation where transition nucleotide substitutions predominate over transversions in the adult VDJ recombinations (Kaushik et al., 2009). The exceptionally long CDR3H in circulating B cells, (8–10%) of B cells initially observed in IgM, extends to IgG (Larsen and Smith, 2012), IgA and IgE isotypes (Walther et al., 2013). Similar to fetal Abs, *IGHV1-IGHD2-IGHJ1* gene recombinations, together with junctional flexibility and/or N or P additions, encode Abs with exceptionally long CDR3H in the adult Ab repertoire. Most remarkably, non-N or non-P insertion of 13–18 conserved short nucleotide sequence (CSNS), specifically at $V_H.D_H$ junctions, increases the CDR3H size (~61 codons) upon encounter with Ag in the periphery (Koti et al., 2010). Recent bovine antibody crystallization has revealed that the CSNS encode the 'stalk' displaying the 'knob' structure where minidomains, created by intraCDR3H disulfide bridges between the cysteines (Wang et al., 2013), provide configurational diversity.

The B cells expressing immunoglobulin with unusually long CDR3H undergo affinity maturation via somatic mutations upon antigen encounter (Kaushik et al., 2002, 2009; Verma and Aitken, 2012). Given the restricted germline combinatorial diversity both at the heavy and light chain in cattle, the adult antibody repertoire is diversified by somatic hypermutations and generation of exceptionally long CDR3H beyond the germline potential via novel CSNS insertion specifically at the V_H-D_H junction.

8.2.5   MECHANISMS OF BOVINE ANTIBODY DIVERSIFICATION

The primary antibody repertoire of cattle is composed of limited combinatorial diversity (0.15×10^5) because of restricted sequence divergence and complexity both at $BovV_H$ and $BovV_\lambda$ loci (Table 6). No evidence exists for gene conversion at the variable heavy chain region (Kaushik et al., 2009), though it requires confirmation for λ light chain variable region (Lucier et al., 1998; Parng et al., 1996). Nevertheless, somatic mutations contribute significantly to diversification of bovine Ab repertoire (Kaushik et al., 2002, 2009). In this context, AID enzyme crucial to somatic hypermutations has been characterized in cattle (Verma et al., 2010). Essentially, cattle use two antibody diversification strategies during B cell development: (a) Somatic hypermutations without exposure to exogenous

TABLE 9   Characteristics of bovine antibody mediated humoral immune system.

- Bovine IgM is less flexible due to few prolines in the $C\mu2$ region that functions as hinge. In addition to IgM allotypes, additional variants originate via alternative splicing (Saini and Kaushik, 2001).

- IgG1 isotype, in addition to of IgA, is involved in mucosal protection (Newby and Bourne, 1976; Butler and Kerli , 2004). The Pro-Ala-Ser-Ser motifs in $C\gamma1$ domain of IgG1c allotype may be involved in cell adhesion and migration function (Saini et al., 2007).

- IgD is transcriptionally active at low level (Zhao et al., 2002) and has a short switch region between μ and δ exons but it is not yet known if it is involved in class switch recombination (Sun et al., 2012).

- Lambda light chains are mostly expressed in cattle antibodies with limited role in antigen recognition (Butler, 1998).

- Antigen independent somatic hypermutations and extensive CDR3H size heterogeneity provide mechanisms of antibody diversification in B-cell ontogeny (Saini and Kaushik, 2002; Koti et al., 2010).

- A relatively less conserved single polymorphic immunoglobulin $BovV_H1$ gene family, related to mammalian group, I, clan, II, is predominantly expressed in cattle (Saini et al., 1997). Thus, limited germline sequence divergence of both variable region heavy and λ-light chain genes restricts combinatorial diversity.

- Restricted combinatorial diversity is compensated via novel antibody diversification mechanism of exceptionally long CDR3H generation (51-66 codons) where multiple even numbered cysteine residues possibly permit inter or intra CDR3H disulfide bridging giving rise to new configurational diversity to antigen-combining site (Saini and Kaushik, 2002; Saini et al., 1999). These Igs are expressed by 8–10% of circulating B cells and are the largest known to exist in a species.

- While exceptionally long CDR3H (>50 codons) is encoded by the single known D_H2 gene (Koti et al., 2010; Shojaei et al. ,2003) in fetal VDJ recombinations, novel conserved short nucleotide sequence (CSNS) are specifically inserted at the V_H-D_H junction in adults further extending CDR3H upon antigen exposure in the periphery (Koti et al., 2010).

- Restricted $V_\lambda + V_H$ pairs characterize antibodies with the atypical CDR3H occurs (Saini et al., 2003).

- Somatic hypermutations are mainly involved in antibody diversification during affinity maturation in the periphery (Kaushik et al., 2009; Koti et al., 2010).

Ag that diversify the developing antibody repertoire during B cell ontogeny (Koti et al., 2010); and (b) Extensive CDR3H size heterogeneity (3 to 66 codons) in the heavy-chain variable region leading to significant configurational diversity of the Ag-combining site (Saini and Kaushik, 2002). Most remarkably, cattle Abs express an exceptionally long CDR3H (>50 to 66 amino acids; Table 7) with multiple even numbered cysteine residues, both in fetal and adult B cells (Saini and Kaushik, 2002; Saini et al., 1999), not yet known to exist in other species. In general, however, CDR3H size of cattle Abs is relative long with an average length of 22.7±3.2 amino acids (Almagro et al., 2006) that varies between IgM (21.7±1.8) and IgG (18.2±1.3) isotypes (Kaushik et al., 2009). Further, higher diversity indices are observed in the third framework region of IgG as compared to IgM Abs of cattle (Kaushik et al., 2009). The Abs with unusually long CDR3H exclusively pair with V_λ light chains with *Ser90* conserved in the CDR3L (Saini et al., 1999) that provide minimal structural support without contact with an epitope (Saini et al., 2003). Both N and/ or P nucleotide additions, together with junctional flexibility, contribute to antibody diversity in developing and adult B cells. Addition of conserved short nucleotide sequences (CSNS; 13 to 18 'A' rich nucleotides) of unknown origin, specifically at *V-D* junctions of adult *VDJ* recombinations, provides a novel mechanism of antibody diversification upon encounter with Ag in the periphery (Koti et al., 2010). Recent crystallization of bovine antibodies with large CDR3H has revealed a unique 'stalk and knob' structure where configurational diversity is generated via creation of minidomains via intraCDR3H disulfide bridges between the cysteine amino acids (Wang et al., 2013). Thus, exceptionally long CDR3H in all bovine antibody isotypes provides a distinct novel mechanism of bovine antibody diversification where diverse cysteine intra-CDR3H disulfide bridging provides a configurational diversity to the antigen-combining site.

8.2.6   FUTURE DIRECTIONS

Some unique features of the bovine immunoglobulin repertoire and its development (Table 9) have emerged that advance our understanding of the humoral immunity. The bovine B cells are not yet fully characterized, similar to delineation of B-1a, B-1b and B-2 cells in mice and humans, in the context of CD5 antigen being a lineage or activation marker. Advances in the knowledge of the bovine immunoglobulin genetic elements, genomic organization and expression have provided novel insights into the origin of Ab based immunity from a phylogenetic perspective. Some gaps in the current knowledge would be filled once bovine genome from several cattle breeds is accurately assembled, annotated and analyzed. For example, relative role of partially duplicated Ig locus on chromosome 8 needs to be understood in the context of construction of humoral immunity, allelic exclusion and B cell development. The molecular origin of exceptionally long CDR3H is now known (Koti et al., 2010), but the mechanism of CSNS addition specifically at the *V-D* junction after Ag stimulation needs to be determined. The structure of antibodies with unusually long CDR3H with multiple even numbered cysteine amino acids capable of forming intra or interCDR di-sulfide bridges needs to be further studied to understand the extent of unconventional configurational diversity of the antigen binding site. Whether IgD is an outcome of class switch recombination in cattle, given the presence of switch site between *IGHM* and *IGHD* unlike other species, is not yet known. How bovine IgG1 isotype protects mucosal surfaces in cattle in the context of IgA needs to be examined? As for light chains, it is unclear why λ-light chains dominate in cattle antibodies despite significant complexity of the IGK locus.

An understanding of the bovine immune system is economically relevant for raising healthier beef and dairy cattle by preventing disease and, also, developing novel vaccines, therapeutic antibodies and immunodiagnostics. Such novel antibody based therapeutics and vaccines could be harvested via milk for pharmaceutical applications. Knowledge gained from studies of bovine Ig genetics will find application in preventing disease and raising healthier cattle by incorporating Ig and related host defense genes as genetic biomarkers in cattle breeding strategies. This is especially important because of decreasing antibody gene pool, including other relevant genes, in various cattle breeds because of skewed breeding strategies. Similarly, distribution of IgM and IgG allotypes across cattle breeds in correlation with disease resistance and susceptibility would help select healthier cattle. The cloning methods have permitted development of transgenic cattle that express and produce human Ig (Kuroiwa et al.,

2002) and open opportunities for the development of novel pharmaceuticals. The unique bovine antibodies with exceptionally long CDR3H (up to 66 amino acids) permit engineering of antibodies against a desired infectious or noninfectious agent and, also, development of novel vaccines via antigenization. In this context, engineered antibody fragments have been developed that recognize and neutralize Bovine Herpes Virus-1 (Koti et al., 2010, 2011; Pasman et al., 2012). The significance of engineering bovine Igs extends beyond cattle for disease prevention to other species, including humans where these are likely to be used in preventing enteric infections via oral immunization.

ACKNOWLEDGEMENTS

Studies on bovine immunoglobulin genetics described in this chapter were supported by NSERC Canada Discovery grants to Azad K. Kaushik.

KEYWORDS

- antibody
- bovine
- cattle antibody repertoire
- CSNS
- exceptionally long CDR3H
- immunoglobulin
- immunoglobulin Genes
- VDJ recombination

REFERENCES

Agrawal, A., Eastman, Q.M., Schatz, D.G., *Transposition mediated by RAG1 and RAG2 and its implications for the evolution of the immune system.* Nature, (1998): 394(6695), 744–751.

Alitheen, N.B., McClure, S., McCullagh, P., *B-cell development: one problem, multiple solutions.* Immunol Cell Biol, (2010): 88(4), 445–450.

Almagro, J.C., et al., *Analysis of the horse V(H) repertoire and comparison with the human IGHV germline genes, and sheep, cattle and pig V(H) sequences.* Mol Immunol, (2006): 43(11), 1836–1845.

Altschul, S.F., et al., *Gapped BLAST and PSI-BLAST: a new generation of protein database search programs* Nucleic acids research, (1997): 25(17), 3389–3402.

Altschul, S.F., et al., *PSI-BLAST pseudocounts and the minimum description length principle.* Nucleic acids research, (2009): 37(3), 815–824.

Anderson, C.L., et al., *Perspective-- FcRn transports albumin: relevance to immunology and medicine.* Trends Immunol, (2006): 27(7), 343–348.

Arun, S.S., Breuer, W., Hermanns, W., *Immunohistochemical examination of light-chain expression (lambda/kappa ratio) in canine, feline, equine, bovine and porcine plasma cells.* Zentralbl Veterinarmed A, (1996): 43(9), 573–576.

Bailey, M., Christoforidou, Z., Lewis, M., *Evolution of immune systems: Specificity and autoreactivity.* Autoimmun Rev, (2013): 12(6), 643–647.

Berens, S.J., Wylie, D.E., Lopez, O.J., *Use of a single VH family and long CDR3s in the variable region of cattle Ig heavy chains.* Int Immunol, (1997): 9(1), 189–199.

Brambell, F.W., Hemmings, W.A., Morris, I.G., *A Theoretical Model of Gamma-Globulin Catabolism.* Nature, (1964): 203: 1352–1354.

Brandon, M.R., Watson, D.L., Lascelles, A.K., *The mechanism of transfer of immunoglobulin into mammary secretion of cows.* Aust J Exp Biol Med Sci, (1971): 49(6), 613–623.

Brown, W.R., et al., *Characterization of the bovine C alpha gene.* Immunology, (1997): 91(1), 1–6.

Butler, J., Kerli ME, *Immunocytes and immunoglobulins in milk,* in *Mucosal Immunology*, O.P. et al, Editor (2004): Academic Press: New York. p. 1763–1793.

Butler, J.E. Kerli, M.E., *Immunocytes and immunoglobulins in milk,* in *Mucosal Immunology*, O.P.e. al, Editor (2004): Academic Press: New York. p. 1763–1793.

Butler, J.E., et al., *Antibody repertoire development in fetal and neonatal piglets. II. Characterization of heavy chain complementarity-determining region 3 diversity in the developing fetus.* J Immunol, (2000): 165(12), 6999–7010.

Butler, J.E., et al., *Immunoglobulins, antibody repertoire and B cell development.* Dev Comp Immunol, (2009): 33(3), 321–333.

Butler, J.E., *Immunoglobulin diversity, B-cell and antibody repertoire development in large farm animals.* Rev Sci Tech, (1998): 17(1), 43–70.

Butler, J.E., Maxwell, C.F., Pierce, C.S., Hylton, M.B., Asofsky, R., Kiddy, C.A., *Studies on the relative synthesis and distribution of IgA and IgG1 in various tissues and body fluids of the cow.* J Immunol, (1972): 109: 38–46.

Butler, J.E., *Why I agreed to do this.* Dev Comp Immunol, (2006): 30: 1–17.

Cannon, J.P., et al., *Recognition of additional roles for immunoglobulin domains in immune function.* Semin Immunol, (2010): 22(1), 17–24.

Cervenak, J. Kacskovics, I., *The neonatal Fc receptor plays a crucial role in the metabolism of IgG in livestock animals.* Vet Immunol Immunopathol, (2009): 128(1–3): 171–177.

Charlton, K.A., et al., *Analysis of the diversity of a sheep antibody repertoire as revealed from a bacteriophage display library.* J Immunol, (2000): 164(12), 6221–6229.

Chen, L., et al., *Characterization of the bovine immunoglobulin lambda light chain constant IGLC genes.* Vet Immunol Immunopathol, (2008): 124(3–4): 284–294.

Cohn, M. Langman, R.E., *The protection: the unit of humoral immunity selected by evolution.* Immunol Rev, (1990): 115, 11–147.

Cooper, M.D. Alder, M.N., *The evolution of adaptive immune systems.* Cell, (2006): 124(4), 815–822.

Criscitiello, M.F. Flajnik, M.F., *Four primordial immunoglobulin light chain isotypes, including lambda and kappa, identified in the most primitive living jawed vertebrates.* Eur J Immunol, (2007): 37(10), 2683–2694.

Das, S., et al., *Evolutionary dynamics of the immunoglobulin heavy chain variable region genes in vertebrates.* Immunogenetics, (2008): 60(1), 47–55.

Das, S., et al., *Evolutionary redefinition of immunoglobulin light chain isotypes in tetrapods using molecular markers.* Proc Natl Acad Sci USA, (2008): 105(43), 16647–16652.

David, C.W., et al., *Cell proliferation, apoptosis, and B- and T-lymphocytes in Peyer's patches of the ileum, in thymus and in lymph nodes of preterm calves, and in full-term calves at birth and on day 5 of life.* J Dairy Sci, (2003): 86(10), 3321–3329.

De Benedictis, G., Capalbo, P., Dragone, A., *Identification of an allotypic IgA in cattle serum.* Comp Immunol Microbiol Infect Dis, (1984): 7(1), 35–42.

Diesterbeck, U.S., et al., *Detection of new allotypic variants of bovine lambda-light chain constant regions in different cattle breeds.* Developmental and comparative immunology, (2012): 36(1), 130–139.

Drummond AJ, et al., *Geneious v5.4,* in *Genious* 2011.

Dufour, V., Malinge, S., Nau, F., *The sheep Ig variable region repertoire consists of a single VH family.* J Immunol, (1996): 156(6), 2163–2170.

Ehrenmann, F., Kaas, Q., Lefranc, M.P., *IMGT/3Dstructure-DB and IMGT/DomainGapAlign: a database and a tool for immunoglobulins or antibodies, T cell receptors, MHC, IgSF and MhcSF.* Nucleic Acids Res, (2010): 38(Database issue): D301–307.

Ekman, A., et al., *B-cell development in bovine fetuses proceeds via a pre-B like cell in bone marrow and lymph nodes.* Dev Comp Immunol, (2010): 34(8), 896–903.

Ekman, A., et al., *Bos taurus genome sequence reveals the assortment of immunoglobulin and surrogate light chain genes in domestic cattle.* BMC Immunol, (2009): 10(1), 22.

Ekman, A., Ilves, M., Iivanainen, A., *B lymphopoiesis is characterized by pre-B cell marker gene expression in fetal cattle and declines in adults.* Dev Comp Immunol, (2012): 37(1), 39–49.

Elsik, C.G., et al., *The genome sequence of taurine cattle: a window to ruminant biology and evolution.* Science, (2009): 324(5926): 522–528.

Farrell, H.M., Jr., et al., *Nomenclature of the proteins of cows' milk--sixth revision.* J Dairy Sci, (2004): 87(6), 1641–1674.

Flajnik, M.F. L. Du Pasquier, *Evolution of innate and adaptive immunity: can we draw a line?* Trends Immunol, (2004): 25(12), 640–644.

Flajnik, M.F. Kasahara, M., *Origin and evolution of the adaptive immune system: genetic events and selective pressures.* Nat Rev Genet, (2010): 11(1), 47–59.

Friedman, M.L., et al., *Neonatal VH, D, and JH gene usage in rabbit B lineage cells.* J Immunol, (1994): 152(2), 632–641.

Gapper, L.W., et al., *Analysis of bovine immunoglobulin G in milk, colostrum and dietary supplements: a review.* Anal Bioanal Chem, (2007): 389(1), 93–109.

Giudicelli, V., Chaume, D., Lefranc, M.P., *IMGT/GENE-DB: a comprehensive database for human and mouse immunoglobulin and T cell receptor genes.* Nucleic acids research, (2005): 33(Database issue): D256–61.

Hackney, J.A., et al., *DNA targets of AID evolutionary link between antibody somatic hypermutation and class switch recombination.* Adv Immunol, (2009): 101: 163–189.

Hamers-Casterman, C., et al., *Naturally occurring antibodies devoid of light chains.* Nature, (1993): 363(6428): 446–448.

Hammer, D.K., Kickhofen, B., Schmid, T., *Detection of homocytotropic antibody associated with a unique immunoglobulin class in the bovine species.* Eur J Immunol, (1971): 1(4), 249–257.

Hayes, H.C. Petit, E.J., *Mapping of the beta-lactoglobulin gene and of an immunoglobulin M heavy chain-like sequence to homoeologous cattle, sheep, and goat chromosomes.* Mammalian genome: official journal of the International Mammalian Genome Society, (1993): 4(4), 207–210.

Hayes, H.C. Petit, E.J., *Mapping of the beta-lactoglobulin gene and of an immunoglobulin M heavy chain-like sequence to homoeologous cattle, sheep, and goat chromosomes.* Mamm Genome, (1993): 4(4), 207–210.

Hein, W.R. Dudler, L., *Diversity of Ig light chain variable region gene expression in fetal lambs.* Int Immunol, (1998): 10(9), 1251–1259.

Hinds, K.R. Litman, G.W., *Major reorganization of immunoglobulin VH segmental elements during vertebrate evolution.* Nature, (1986): 320(6062), 546–549.

Hosseini, A., et al., *Duplicated copies of the bovine JH locus contribute to the Ig repertoire.* International immunology, (2004): 16(6), 843–852.

Hurley, W., *Proteins*, in *Advanced dairy chemistry* 2003, Kluwer Academic: New York. p. 421–447.

Ishino, S., et al., *Immunohistochemical studies on ontogeny of bovine lymphoid tissues.* J Vet Med Sci, (1991): 53(5), 877–882.

Jones, J.M. Simkus, C., *The roles of the RAG1 and RAG2 "non-core" regions in V(D)J recombination and lymphocyte development.* Arch Immunol Ther Exp (Warsz), (2009): 57(2), 105–116.

Kabat, E.A. Wu, T.T., *Identical V region amino acid sequences and segments of sequences in antibodies of different specificities. Relative contributions of VH and VL genes, minigenes, and complementarity-determining regions to binding of antibody-combining sites.* J Immunol, (1991): 147(5), 1709–1719.

Kacskovics, I. Butler, J.E., *The heterogeneity of bovine IgG2--VIII. The complete cDNA sequence of bovine IgG2a (A2) and an IgG1.* Mol Immunol, (1996): 33(2), 189–195.

Kacskovics, I., et al., *FcRn mediates elongated serum half-life of human IgG in cattle.* Int Immunol, (2006): 18(4), 525–536.

Kacskovics, I., *Fc receptors in livestock species.* Vet Immunol Immunopathol, (2004): 102(4), 351–362.

Kaushik, A. Lim, W., *The primary antibody repertoire of normal, immunodeficient and autoimmune mice is characterized by differences in V gene expression.* Res Immunol, (1996): 147(1), 9–26.

Kaushik, A. Lim, W., *The primary antibody repertoire of normal, immunodeficient and autoimmune mice is characterized by differences in V gene expression.* Research in immunology, (1996): 147(1), 9–26.

Kaushik, A., Shojaei, F., Saini, S.S., *Novel insight into antibody diversification from cattle.* Vet Immunol Immunopathol, (2002): 87(3–4): 347–350.

Kaushik, A.K., et al., *Somatic hypermutations and isotype restricted exceptionally long CDR3H contribute to antibody diversification in cattle.* Vet Immunol Immunopathol, (2009): 127(1–2): 1061–13.

Knight, K.L. Winstead, C.R., *Generation of antibody diversity in rabbits.* Curr Opin Immunol, (1997): 9(2), 228–232.

Knight, K.L., Suter, M., Becker, R.S., *Genetic engineering of bovine Ig. Construction and characterization of hapten-binding bovine/murine chimeric IgE, IgA, IgG1, IgG2, and IgG3 molecules.* J Immunol, (1988): 140(10), 3654–3659.

Knight, K.L., *Restricted VH gene usage and generation of antibody diversity in rabbit.* Annu Rev Immunol, (1992): 10, 593–616.

Kofler, R., et al., *Mouse variable-region gene families: complexity, polymorphism and use in non-autoimmune responses.* Immunological reviews, (1992): 128, 5–21.

Kofler, R., et al., *Mouse variable-region gene families: complexity, polymorphism and use in non-autoimmune responses.* Immunol Rev, (1992): 128, 5–21.

Koti, M., Nagy, E., Kaushik, A.K., *A single point mutation in framework region 3 of heavy chain affects viral neutralization dynamics of single-chain Fv against bovine herpes virus type 1.* Vaccine, (2011): 29(45), 7905–7912.

Koti, M., et al., *Construction of single-chain Fv with two possible CDR3H conformations but similar inter-molecular forces that neutralize bovine herpesvirus 1.* Mol Immunol, (2010): 47(5), 953–960.

Koti, M., Kataeva, G., Kaushik, A.K., *Novel atypical nucleotide insertions specifically at VH-DH junction generate exceptionally long CDR3H in cattle antibodies.* Mol Immunol, (2010): 47(11–12), 2119–2128.

Koti, M., Kataeva, G., Kaushik, A.K., *Organization of D(H)-gene locus is distinct in cattle.* Dev Biol (Basel), (2008): 132, 307–313.

Kuroiwa, Y., et al., *Antigen-specific human polyclonal antibodies from hyperimmunized cattle,* in *Nature biotechnology* 2009. p. 173–181.

Kuroiwa, Y., et al., *Cloned transchromosomic calves producing human immunoglobulin.* Nat Biotechnol, (2002): 20(9), 889–894.

Laegreid, W.W., et al., *Association of bovine neonatal Fc receptor alpha-chain gene (FC-GRT) haplotypes with serum IgG concentration in newborn calves.* Mamm Genome, (2002): 13(12), 704–710.

Larkin, M.A., et al., *Clustal W and Clustal X version 2.0.* Bioinformatics, (2007): 23(21), 2947–298.

Larsen, P.A. Smith, T.P., *Application of circular consensus sequencing and network analysis to characterize the bovine IgG repertoire.* BMC Immunol, (2012): 13, 52.

Larsen, P.A. Smith, T.P.L., *Application of circular consensus sequencing and network analysis to characterize the bovine IgG repertoire.*

Leach, J.L., et al., *Isolation from human placenta of the IgG transporter, FcRn, and localization to the syncytiotrophoblast: implications for maternal-fetal antibody transport.* J Immunol, (1996): 157(8), 3317–3322.

Lefranc, M.P. Lefranc, G., *The Immunoglobulin FactsBook* 2001: Academic Press. 458.

Lefranc, M.P., *Nomenclature of the human immunoglobulin genes.* Current protocols in immunology / edited by John E. Coligan ... [et al.], (2001): Appendix 1: Appendix 1P.

Litman, G.W., Rast, J.P., Fugmann, S.D., *The origins of vertebrate adaptive immunity.* Nat Rev Immunol, (2010): 10(8), 543–553.

Lucier, M.R., et al., *Multiple sites of V lambda diversification in cattle.* J Immunol, (1998): 161(10), 5438–5444.

Matsuda, F., et al., *The complete nucleotide sequence of the human immunoglobulin heavy chain variable region locus.* J Exp Med, (1998): 188(11), 2151–2162.

Mayer, B., et al., *Redistribution of the sheep neonatal Fc receptor in the mammary gland around the time of parturition in ewes and its localization in the small intestine of neonatal lambs.* Immunology, (2002): 107(3), 288–296.

Mayer, B., et al., *The neonatal Fc receptor (FcRn) is expressed in the bovine lung.* Vet Immunol Immunopathol, (2004): 98(1–2): 85–89.

Meek, K.D., Hasemann, C.A., Capra, J.D., *Novel rearrangements at the immunoglobulin D locus. Inversions and fusions add to IgH somatic diversity.* J Exp Med, (1989): 170(1), 39–57.

Mousavi, M., et al., *Characterization of the gene for the membrane and secretory form of the IgM heavy-chain constant region gene (C mu) of the cow (Bos taurus).* Immunology, (1998): 93(4), 581–588.

Muyldermans, S., et al., *Sequence and structure of VH domain from naturally occurring camel heavy chain immunoglobulins lacking light chains.* Protein Eng, (1994): 7(9), 1129–1135.

Naessens, J., *Surface Ig on B lymphocytes from cattle and sheep.* Int Immunol, (1997): 9(3), 349–354.

Neuberger, M.S. Scott, J., *Immunology. RNA editing AIDs antibody diversification?* Science, (2000): 289(5485), 1705–1706.

Newby, T.J. Bourne, F.J., *Relative resistance of bovine and porcine immunoglobulins to proteolysis.* Immunol Commun, (1976): 5(7–8): 631–635.

Nguyen, V.K., Muyldermans, S., Hamers, R., *The specific variable domain of camel heavy-chain antibodies is encoded in the germline.* J Mol Biol, (1998): 275(3), 413–418.

Niku, M., et al., *The bovine genomic DNA sequence data reveal three IGHV subgroups, only one of which is functionally expressed.* Developmental and comparative immunology, (2012):

Pancer, Z. Cooper, M.D., *The evolution of adaptive immunity.* Annu Rev Immunol, (2006): 24: 497–518.

Parng, C.L., et al., *Gene conversion contributes to Ig light chain diversity in cattle.* J Immunol, (1996): 157(12), 5478–5486.

Pasman, Y. Kaushik, A.K., *Partial organization of bovine variable-heavy chain gene locus and influence of recombination signal sequences (RSS) on various variable region gene expression.* Journal of Immunology, (2012): 188: 42–46.

Pasman, Y., Nagy, E., Kaushik, A.K., *Enhanced bovine herpesvirus type 1 neutralization by multimerized single-chain variable antibody fragments regardless of differential glycosylation.* Clin Vaccine Immunol, (2012): 19(8), 1150–1507.

Pasman, Y., et al., *Organization and genomic complexity of bovine lambda-light chain gene locus.* Vet Immunol Immunopathol, (2010): 135(3–4): 306–313.

Pink, J.R., Vainio, O., Rijnbeek, A.M., *Clones of B lymphocytes in individual follicles of the bursa of Fabricius.* Eur J Immunol, (1985): 15(1), 83–87.

Rabbani, H., et al., *Polymorphism of the IGHG3 gene in cattle.* Immunogenetics, (1997): 46(4), 326–31.

Reynaud, C.A., et al., *A single rearrangement event generates most of the chicken immuno-globulin light chain diversity.* Cell, (1985): 40(2), 283–291.

Reynaud, C.A., Anquez, V., Weill, J.C., *The chicken D locus and its contribution to the immuno-globulin heavy chain repertoire.* Eur J Immunol, (1991): 21(11), 2661–2670.

Saini, S., et al., *Homologues of murine Vh11 gene are conserved during evolution.* Exp Clin Im-munogenet, (1996): 13(3–4): 154–60.

Saini, S.S. Kaushik, A., *Extensive CDR3H length heterogeneity exists in bovine foetal VDJ rear-rangements.* Scand J Immunol, (2002): 55(2), 140–148.

Saini, S.S. Kaushik, A., *Origin of bovine IgM structural variants.* Mol Immunol, (2001): 38(5), 389–396.

Saini, S.S., et al., *Bovine IgM antibodies with exceptionally long complementarity-determining region 3 of the heavy chain share unique structural properties conferring restricted VH + Vlambda pairings.* Int Immunol, (2003): 15(7), 845–853.

Saini, S.S., et al., *Exceptionally long CDR3H region with multiple cysteine residues in func-tional bovine IgM antibodies.* Eur J Immunol, (1999): 29(8), 2420–2426.

Saini, S.S., et al., *Structural evidence for a new IgG1 antibody sequence allele of cattle.* Scand J Immunol, (2007): 65(1), 32–38.

Saini, S.S., Hein, W.R., Kaushik, A., *A single predominantly expressed polymorphic immuno-globulin VH gene family, related to mammalian group, I, clan, II, is identified in cattle.* Mol Immunol, (1997): 34(8–9): 641–651.

Schultz, R.D., Confer, F., Dunne, H.W., *Occurrence of blood cells and serum proteins in bovine fetuses and calves.* Can J Comp Med, (1971): 35(2), 93–98.

Schultz, R.D., Dunne, H.W., Heist, C.E., *Ontogeny of the bovine immune response.* Infect Im-mun, (1973): 7(6), 981–991.

Schultz, R.D., Dunne, H.W., Heist, C.E., *Transport, distribution and synthesis of bovine immu-noglobulins. Ontogeny of the bovine immune response.* J Dairy Sci, (1971): 54(9), 1321–1322.

Senogles, D.R., et al., *Ontogeny of circulating B lymphocytes in neonatal calves.* Res Vet Sci, (1978): 25(1), 34–36.

Shojaei, F., Saini, S.S., Kaushik, A.K., *Unusually long germline DH genes contribute to large sized CDR3H in bovine antibodies.* Mol Immunol, (2003): 40(1), 61–67.

Sinclair, M.C., Gilchrist, J., Aitken, R., *Bovine IgG repertoire is dominated by a single diversi-fied VH gene family.* J Immunol, (1997): 159(8), 3883–3889.

Sitnikova, T. Nei, M., *Evolution of immunoglobulin kappa chain variable region genes in verte-brates.* Mol Biol Evol, (1998): 15(1), 50–60.

Stein, S.K., et al., *Comparison of joining and constant kappa-light chain regions in different cattle breeds.* Animal genetics, (2012):

Story, C.M., Mikulska, J.E., Simister, N.E., *A major histocompatibility complex class I-like Fc receptor cloned from human placenta: possible role in transfer of immunoglobulin G from mother to fetus.* J Exp Med, (1994): 180(6), 2377–2381.

Sun, J., et al., *Expressed swine VH genes belong to a small VH gene family homologous to hu-man VHIII.* J Immunol, (1994): 153(12), 5618–5627.

Sun, Y., et al., *Immunoglobulin genes and diversity: what we have learned from domestic ani-mals.* J Anim Sci Biotechnol, (2012): 3(1), 18.

Symons, D.B., Clarkson, C.A., Beale, D., *Structure of bovine immunoglobulin constant region heavy chain gamma 1 and gamma 2 genes.* Mol Immunol, (1989): 26(9), 841–580.

Tobin-Janzen, T.C. Womack, J.E., *Comparative mapping of IGHG1, IGHM, FES, and FOS in domestic cattle.* Immunogenetics, (1992): 36(3), 157–165.

Tomlinson, I.M., et al., *Human immunoglobulin VH and D segments on chromosomes 15q11.2 and 16p11.2.* Human molecular genetics, (1994): 3(6), 853–60.

Tonegawa, S., *Somatic generation of antibody diversity.* Nature, (1983): 302(5909): 575–581.

Verma, S. Aitken, R., *Somatic hypermutation leads to diversification of the heavy chain immunoglobulin repertoire in cattle.* Vet Immunol Immunopathol, (2012): 145(1–2): 14–22.

Verma, S., Goldammer, T., Aitken, R., *Cloning and expression of activation induced cytidine deaminase from Bos taurus.* Vet Immunol Immunopathol, (2010): 134(3–4): 151–159.

Wagner, B., *Immunoglobulins and immunoglobulin genes of the horse.* Dev Comp Immunol, (2006): 30(1–2): 155–164.

Walther, S., Czerny, C.P., Diesterbeck, U.S., *Exceptionally Long CDR3H Are Not Isotype Restricted in Bovine Immunoglobulins.* PLoS One, (2013): 8(5), e64234.

Wang, F., et al., *Reshaping Antibody Diversity.* Cell, (2013): 153(6), 1379–1393.

Weinstein, P.D.,erson, A.O., Mage, R.G., *Rabbit IgH sequences in appendix germinal centers: VH diversification by gene conversion-like and hypermutation mechanisms.* Immunity, (1994): 1(8), 647–659.

Wu, L., et al., *Fundamental characteristics of the immunoglobulin VH repertoire of chickens in comparison with those of humans, mice, and camelids.* Journal of immunology, (2012): 188(1), 322–333.

Wu, T.T., Johnson, G., Kabat, E.A., *Length distribution of CDRH3 in antibodies.* Proteins, (1993): 16(1), 1–7.

Yasuda, M., et al., *Histological studies on the ontogeny of bovine gut-associated lymphoid tissue: appearance of T cells and development of IgG+ and IgA+ cells in lymphoid follicles.* Dev Comp Immunol, (2004): 28(4), 357–369.

Yasuda, M., et al., *The sheep and cattle Peyer's patch as a site of B-cell development.* Vet Res, (2006): 37(3), 401–415.

Zhao, Y., et al., *Artiodactyl IgD: the missing link.* J Immunol, (2002): 169(8), 4408–4416.

Zhao, Y., et al., *Physical mapping of the bovine immunoglobulin heavy chain constant region gene locus.* J Biol Chem, (2003): 278(37), 35024–35032.

Zhao, Y., Jackson, S.M., Aitken, R., *The bovine antibody repertoire.* Dev Comp Immunol, (2006): 30(1–2), 175–186.

Zimin, A.V., et al., *A whole-genome assembly of the domestic cow, Bos taurus.* Genome biology, (2009): 10(4), R42.

CHAPTER 9

INFORMATIC TOOLS FOR IMMUNOGLOBULIN GENE SEQUENCE ANALYSIS

HELENA HAZANOV, MIRI MICHAELI, GITIT LAVY-SHAHAF, and
RAMIT MEHR

CONTENTS

Some part of the text is reprinted from *Journal of Autoimmunity*, Vol. 35, Neta S.
Zuckerman, Helena Hazanov, Michal Barak, Hanna Edelman, Shira Hess, Hadas Shcolnik,
Deborah Dunn-Walters, Ramit Mehr, Somatic hypermutation and antigen-driven selection
of B cells are altered in autoimmune diseases, 325–335, Dec. 2010, with permission from
Elsevier Limited.

ABSTRACT

Analyzing immunoglobulin gene sequences, especially in the high throughput sequencing age, raises many challenges. The diverse repertoire and somatic hypermutation they undergo differ the immunoglobulin sequences from other genes, making the commonly used tools unfit for their analysis. Unlike the other genes, immunoglobulins lack a reference gene, raising problems in cleaning the high throughput sequences and defining the germline sequence that will be used as such. Clustering into clones and repertoire representation are nonexistent issues when dealing with uniform genes, but are key analyzes while dealing with immunoglobulin's. This chapter is a thorough review of the informatics tools that were designed to address the unique nature of the immunoglobulins.

9.1   INTRODUCTION

The diverse repertoire of T and B lymphocytes within each individual is constantly changing. While T cell receptor (TCR) and B cell receptor (BCR) diversification endows the system with the ability to produce receptors recognizing any possible biological molecule or pathogen, the staggering receptor diversity—up to 10^{11} different B or T cell clones in each human, for example, makes it very difficult to study how the lymphocyte repertoire changes under various conditions. The huge diversity is achieved by V(D)J rearrangement and, in B cells, by accumulation of point mutations in the immunoglobulin (Ig) gene sequences to improve the BCRs affinity to antigens.

Studying the generation, development and selection of lymphocyte repertoires, and their functions during immune responses, as well as tracking of mutation accumulation in the BCRs, is essential for understanding the function of the immune system in healthy individuals, and in monitoring and intervening with the immune system in immune deficient, autoimmune disease or cancer patients.

Such studies are very important, for example, understanding how the immune system copes with complex infections such as those with the human immunodeficiency virus (HIV) or hepatitis B virus, and finding the best neutralizing antibodies (Scheid et al., 2009); for elucidating the changes in immune function during natural aging (Ademokun et al., 2011); or for correctly classifying lymphocyte cancers (Boyd et al., 2009). In order to analyze the Ig gene repertoire and the mutations that have accumulated in these genes, several preliminary steps must be taken. The high throughput sequencing (HTS) data should be cleaned, the component segments of each gene (germline (GL) segments) must be identified, sequences should be grouped into clonally related sets, alignments and lineage tree analysis should be performed to infer the junction regions between segments, and then one needs to correctly identify the mutations and their most likely history in each clone.

The rearrangements and the somatic hypermutation (SHM) they undergo make the Ig genes unique in their diversity; they lack the uniformity of most other genes. Therefore, most of the general bioinformatical tools that are designed for dealing with uniform, unmutated genes are not useful for analyzing Ig genes. The community of researchers focusing on BCR bioinformatics has developed various software packages that address the special needs of Ig gene research, and these tools will be reviewed here.

9.2 HIGH-THROUGHPUT SEQUENCING DATA CLEANING TOOLS

The recent development of high HTS enables researchers to obtain large numbers of sequences from several samples simultaneously (Galan et al., 2010). HTS has a great advantage over classical sequencing methods in the field of Ig gene research, as it enables us to extract more sequences per sample and it is sensitive enough so we can identify different unique sequences. HTS presents us now, for the first time, with the ability to analyze and compare large samples of mutated Ig gene repertoires in health, aging and disease (Scheid et al., 2009; Boyd et al., 2009; Campbell et al., 2008; Ademokun et al., 2010; Gibson et al., 2009; Dunn-Walters et al., 2010. However, the huge numbers of sequences obtained require a large amount of preprocessing work to clean out artifacts, sort sequences according to sample according to their molecular identification (MID) tags, identify primers, and discard sequences that do not contain enough information, such as sequences much shorter or longer than the expected length of an Ig variable region gene, or sequences with average quality scores below a defined threshold.

In order to receive reliable results that are not affected by sequencing artifacts while analyzing Ig sequences, one must first make sure that all such artifacts are cleaned out of the input data. Although HTS has already been available for several years, there are very few such cleaning programs available for users, and none that can deal with the cleaning of Ig genes (reviewed in Michaeli, 2012. Ig-HTS-Cleaner Michaeli, 2012 is a program that can clean the sequences of artifacts, and would be suitable for use with Ig genes in spite of their unique characteristics. The program enables the user to give the ends of the genes (primers and MID tags) as input no matter what their origin is, it can handle multiple tags, and does not require any additional programs to run. The Ig-HTS-Cleaner program does not require any knowledge in programming nor complicated installation, only a simple input file which contains the parameters for run.

This program performs the following tasks. First, it assigns the sequences to samples according to their MID tags, and discards sequences in which MID tags cannot be identified—which is useful in case samples are coded not by a single MID tag but by a combination of MID tags, or in cases where different samples were sequenced in the same lanes. It also discards sequences in which the MID tag combination is identifiable but does not appear in the list of sample codes, because these sequences are most probably artifactual chimeric (hybrid) sequences created during polymerase chain reaction (PCR) amplification or sequencing. Second, Ig-HTS-Cleaner identifies the primers at both ends of each read, using dynamic programming with the user-defined limit to the number of mismatches allowed, in cases where an exact match cannot be found. Primers need to be identified to be removed from the read, because mismatches in these segments may be PCR errors and thus should not be counted as bona fide somatic mutations. Third, the program discards all reads that do not conform with the defined length range of the sequenced genes (and thus may be irrelevant genes or chimeric sequences), and those that have quality scores below the user-defined threshold. All discarded read are counted and stored in separate files for quality control. This enables the user to study the effects of changing the program's parameters (such as the maximum number of allowed mismatches in primer search), and thus optimize the parameters for the dataset at hand. Moreover, the FASTA output files enable easy downstream analyzes of the sequences.

One of the shortcomings of pyrosequencing is that during the sequencing of homopolymer tracts (HPTs, repeats of the same nucleotide), the polymerase can add or delete one or more nucleotides from these repeats, or alternatively, the signal of poly nucleotide incorporation can be misread (Huse et al., 2007). These errors may result in insertions/ deletions (indels) that are a result of the sequencing and therefore are considered as artifacts (11). This problem is more severe in Ig gene analysis due to the lack of template or reference genes. In Ig gene research, it is very important to distinguish between artifact indels and legitimate indels that are a result of normal SHM and affinity maturation of B cells, although naturally occurring indels are very rare. Ig-Indel-Identifier Michaeli, 2012 is a program that identifies legitimate and artifact indels and does not discard sequences that contain uncertain indels, allowing maximal information utilization by keeping these uncertain sequences. This program manages to identify many of these cases, so that manual examination of the sequences is only needed in very few cases.

9.3   GL SEGMENT IDENTIFICATION TOOLS AND JUNCTION ANALYSIS

Mutated sequences must be compared to the pre-mutation rearranged sequence to identify mutations. Usually, this sequence is not available, so it is reconstructed by identifying the original gene segments used, based on highest homology to the mutated sequence. There are several programs that researchers use for this purpose, as follows.
- The IMGT/V-QUEST is the most complete algorithm for deciphering Ig and TCR gene segment composition, having the ability to analyze both Ig and TCR for human, mouse and various other organisms (Giudicelli et al., 2004). V-QUEST is based on BLAST algorithm, which is not as sensitive as the dynamic programming methods for sequence alignment and does not guarantee finding the best alignment of two sequences (Altschul et al., 1990).

- JOINSOLVER (Souto-Carneiro et al., 2004) was developed specifically to analyze the complementarity determining region 3 (CDR3) of the Ig genes in human B cells. The strategy of JOINSOLVER™ is to search for D GL sequences flanking VH and JH GL genes. Additionally, it searches for π and N type additions in the IGHV–IGHD and IGHD–IGHJ junctions.
- SoDA (Volpe et al., 2006) uses a variation on the dynamic programming sequence alignment algorithm that takes into account the variation around the IGHV–IGHD and IGHD–IGHJ junctions resulting from the competing effects of nucleotide addition and exonuclease action (Gaëta et al., 2007). The newly developed SoDA2 (Munshaw and Kepler, 2010), is based on a Hidden Markov Model and is used to compute the posterior probabilities of candidate rearrangements and to find those with the highest values among them.
- iHMMune-align is an application that incorporates explicit models of the various antibody generation processes in the form of probability distributions along a hidden Markov model (HMM) of the variable region of the heavy chain gene, and generates an alignment of the rearranged sequence with its most likely component GL genes. Its development was particularly designed to improve IGHD gene identification (Gaëta et al., 2007).

9.4   FINDING CLONES

B cells undergo BCR rearrangement independently of one another, therefore the same V(D)J combination can appear in more than one clone. The difference between clones with identical V(D)J combination lies in the random generation of junctions by P- and N- additions. Ig_Clone_Finder (Michaeli et al., 2013) is a program that clusters all sequences that have the same V, D and J segments into the same clone. However, this method may group together unrelated clones, which means that manual checking and correcting is required. Gaëta et al. (Chen et al., 2010) had developed an algorithm that uses a hierarchical agglomerative clustering method to group Ig gene sequences on the basis of CDR3 sequence similarity as well as IGHV and IGHJ usage. The CDR3 includes the junctions, hence, similarity in that area reduces the chances of wrong clonal ascription.

9.5 ALIGNMENT

When each sequence has an identified GL V(D)J segments, the sequences are sorted into groups (clones) having the same V(D)J segments and similar junction region. The GL junction regions are then deduced from a consensus that is achieved by aligning all clonally related sequences. Later, all sequences in each clone are aligned again, this time, together with their GL sequences to identify the mutated nucleotides in each sequence.

The alignment in both cases can be done by any alignment tool available, however, ClustalW2 (Larkin et al., 2007) is the most commonly used. Since the alignment tools have a limited number of sequences that can be aligned together (500 sequences for ClustalW2), they may be insufficient when analyzing large datasets from HTS. Clustal Omega (Sievers et al., 2011) was specially designed for those datasets (up to 2000 sequences per alignment).

9.6 REPERTOIRE PRESENTATION

T and B cell receptor repertoires are diversified by variable region gene rearrangement and selected based on functionality and non-self reactivity. The study of lymphocyte repertoires will enable clinical immunologists to develop better therapeutic monoclonal antibodies, vaccines, transplantation donor-recipient matching protocols, and other immune intervention strategies. The recent development of high-throughput methods for repertoire data collection—from multicolor flow cytometry through single-cell imaging to deep sequencing—challenges the theoretical immunology community to develop methods for data organization and analysis.

In the last two years, studies using high-throughput sequencing of TCR or BCR genes have yielded several interesting new insights about human TCR and BCR clonal repertoires. First, the overall repertoire size has been estimated as several million clonotypes, and it was recently shown that there are at least 1 million TCR Vβ clones in a single 2 mL human blood sample (Warren et al., 2011). Second, the TCRβ (Warren et al., 2011; Venturi et al., 2011), and BCR heavy chain (Boyd et al., 2010) V and J gene usage frequencies among individuals are similar, but there are intrinsic differences in the likelihood of recombination of individual gene segments. Slightly different rearrangements (in the same or different individuals) often yield the same common nucleic acid sequence, a phenomenon termed "convergent recombination" (Quigley et al., 2010; Venturi et al., 2006). Third, in spite of the high estimated diversity of the TCRβ repertoire, a significant component of the repertoire is shared (especially at the amino acid level) between individuals (Boyd et al., 2009; Warren et al., 2011; Venturi et al., 2011), probably as a result of evolution of the gene segment repertoire towards containing receptors specific for common pathogen-derived peptides. Fourth, it is possible to determine the individual's GL gene segment repertoire from the sampled sequences, even in B cells, and this process reveals new allelic polymorphisms (Boyd et al., 2010). Fifth, some of the relatively large clones are shared between the naïve and memory T cell repertoires, and one can observe the naïve to memory cell differentiation by taking successive blood samples (Warren et al., 2011; Venturi et al., 2011). A study of the repertoire in several memory B cell subsets found that the memory B cell repertoires differ from the transitional and naïve repertoires, and that the IgM memory repertoire is distinct from that of class-switched memory. They concluded that a large proportion of IgM memory cells develop in response to different stimuli than for class-switched memory cell development (Wu et al., 2010). More interesting and potentially surprising insights are bound to be revealed as such high-throughput sequencing studies are conducted by many more groups, and diverge to describe repertoires in various disease situations. The first steps in this direction have been made by showing intraclonal variation in B cell chronic lymphocytic leukemia (CLL) (Campbell et al., 2008) and that the antibody repertoire in HIV infection is larger than previously expected (Scheid et al., 2009). Studying B and T cell repertoires may also help in better understanding subset relationships (Warren et al., 2011; Venturi et al., 2011; Wu et al., 2010); detecting rare clones, such as lymphomas after chemotherapy (Boyd et al., 2009; Campbell et al., 2008); and designing better vaccines.

In spite of the work already done, clonal repertoire analysis still poses several difficult challenges to computational immunologists. How does one present a whole repertoire? One useful way to condense repertoire information is the study of CDR3 length distributions. The CDR3 is the most hyper-variable region in BCR and TCR genes, and the most critical structure in antigen recognition and thereby in determining the fates of developing and responding lymphocytes. There are over 10^6 different CDR3 sequences of the TCR Vβ chain in a human blood sample (Warren et al. 2009), and about the same number of B cell clones. CDR3 length distributions (also called spectratypes) make it possible to get a picture of TCR and Ig repertoire diversity and show variations between individuals and over time, and in different disease situations. BCR spectratypes are relatively straightforward, as PCR primers bind all V and J families, and hence only one spectratype per sample is required. For TCRs, however, the different families cannot be amplified with the same primers, and hence multiple spectratypes per sample are needed. Yet, obtaining spectratype data is, now, still much cheaper, faster and easier than sequencing, and allows to study many samples from each experimental group.

Another option is to present clonotypes. A TCR clonotype was defined by Yassai et al., (*29*) as "a unique nucleotide sequence that arises during the gene rearrangement process for that receptor. The combination of nucleotide sequences for the surface expressed receptor pair would define the T cell clonotype". Similar definitions apply to B cell clonotypes. The numbers of clonotypes can vary between repertoires and samples.

Interesting questions that have been addressed so far include the depth of repertoire coverage in each sample, the number of clonotypes shared between cell subsets within one individual or between individuals, clonotype size distributions, and to which extent these distributions are determined by the rearrangement process versus developmental and antigen-driven selection forces. A very good example of the various analysis methods used to address these questions is the study by Venturi et al. (Venturi et al., 2011).

One way to look at whole repertoires is to present the numbers of clones, or numbers of sequences—or unique sequences—present in the repertoire for each V-J segment combination. Counting clones or unique sequences is preferable to counting all sequences, as different PCR primer efficiencies may result in different numbers of reads for each combination, regardless of their number in the original DNA sample. A variation of this presentation method, which is based on representing each combination by a circle with size corresponding to the number of sequences—and hence can be easily extended to three dimensions to also represent the D segments—was used by several researchers (Boyd et al., 2009; Weinstein et al., 2009).

9.7 LINEAGE TREES

An easy way to track and analyze the relationships between clonally related Ig gene sequences is by using lineage trees. The tree root is the ancestor sequence, usually the rearranged, pre-mutation sequence. Each tree node represents a single mutation (point mutation, insertion or deletion). Since phylogenetic software packages make assumptions that are not necessarily appropriate for lineage trees, lineage tree generation is best performed using the IgTree© program (Barak et al., 2008), which implements a distance method-based algorithm that finds the most likely tree with a high probability. It runs on the aligned clonally related groups of sequences. After the construction of lineage trees, various mutational analysis that rely on tree structure can be performed, such as amino acid (AA) substitution counts (Zuckerman et al., 2010a, 2010b, 2010c), which may determine the effect that mutations have on the final antibody, and analysis of the frequencies of replacement and silent mutations (R:S analysis) (Uduman et al., 2011; Hershberg et al., 200), which provides insights regarding the nature of selection. Lineage trees also enable the investigation of B cell clonal dynamics, such as initial affinity or selection threshold of clones, by measuring their graphical properties, using the MTree© program (Dunn-Walters et al., 2007). A thorough statistical analysis which correlated tree characteristics with B cell response dynamic parameters, such as the mutation rate or the selection threshold, using a computer simulation of the normal immune response (Steiman-Shimony et al., 2006), has concluded that seven specific tree characteristics possess the highest correlation values with the biological parameters and are hence most informative.

9.8 MOTIF ANALYSIS

SHM introduces non-templated point mutations in the variable region of rearranged Ig heavy and light chain genes. Somatic mutations occur mostly in RGYW/WRCY (R=A/G, Y=C/T, W=A/T) hotspot motifs. Understanding the mutation targeting motifs may help understanding the mutational process leading to each mutation. PictoIg© program (Zuckerman et al., 2010) is a program that allows the exploration of the sequence up to 10 nucleotides up—and down—stream of the mutated location. Nucleotides flanking the mutated nucleotides are enumerated per tree for each data group, based on previous work by Spencer and Dunn-Walters et al. (Spencer et al., 2005). The percentage composition of each base at each position flanking a particular mutation, up to ten positions away from the mutated nucleotide in each direction, is then determined. The baseline percentage composition of the GL sequences is subtracted from this to show any differences particular to that mutation. These differences are drawn as sequence logos, where nucleotides that are observed in excess (over-represented) or in paucity (under-represented), are drawn above or below the x axis, respectively. For each nucleotide in each position in each type of mutation, a $\chi 2$ analysis is performed to examine whether the frequency of the nucleotide is significant compared to its theoretical frequency. The F test is then used for comparing the mutational motifs of two samples.

9.9 MUTATION STATISTICS

The spectrum of nucleotide substitutions observed in mutation analyzes is largely dependent on the paths used by the cells to resolve the initial U-G lesion created by activation-induced (DNA-cytosine) deaminase (AID). A simple replication over the lesion results in the transition mutations (purine mutates to a purine or pyrimidine mutates to a pyrimidine) C–>T and G–>A. All other types of mutations, including transversion mutations (purine mutates to a pyrimidine and vice versa), and mutations from A/T nucleotides, depend on recognition of the UG mismatch by proteins involved in the base excision or mismatch repair mechanisms. Indeed, a transition over transversion bias of 3:2 was observed in SHM substitutions (Di Noia et al., 2007), rather than the dominance of transversion mutations that would be expected from a completely random process. Mutations from C/G base pairs are mutated with similar frequencies in reverse complement motifs, implying that the AID machinery acts equally on both DNA strands (Spencer et al., 2009; Dunn-Walters and Spencer, 1998). However, A was found to be more frequently mutated than T, suggesting that there is a bias for generating these mutations on only one strand, during the second phase of SHM (Spencer et al., 2005; Smith et al., 1996; Rogozin et al., 2001). After a list of mutations is established, the fraction of mutations from each nucleotide can be calculated and compared between samples by the $\chi 2$ test. The transition and transversion fractions can also be calculated and the transition over transversion bias compared as well (Zuckerman et al., 2010).

9.10   TESTING FOR SELECTION

Point mutations introduced by SHM anywhere in the IgV gene can be a replacement mutation[®], yielding an amino acid replacement, or a silent mutation (S), not yielding a replacement. Jukes and King (55) have shown that, theoretically, there are 526 possible single base changes (substitution mutations) in the 61 codons of the 20 amino acids. Of these, 392 produce amino acid replacements (R mutations) and 134 are silent (S mutations). They omitted changes that produced 'stop codons' from the calculation because such changes will be rejected. Thus, In the absence of any selection operating on the gene product, a random mutational process would bring about an even distribution of ρ and σ mutations throughout the gene, with ratio of R:S=2.925. Following this logic, a ratio of R:S mutations > 2.9 (or a frequency of ρ mutations significantly different from that expected under random, non-selected processes) would indicate selection for ρ mutations, while an R:S ratio < 2.9 (or a significantly lower frequency of ρ mutations than expected under random mutation and no selection) would indicate selection against ρ mutations. In addition, some codons are more "mutable" than others, that is, the fraction of possible nucleotide changes in those codons that would lead to replacement mutations is high; while other codons are less susceptible to mutations. This is based on codon tables alone, ignoring the concept of "hot spots." Chang and Casali (1994) had extended this idea by applying a binomial test to examine where fractions of ρ mutations were significantly higher or lower than what is expected from a random process. This method has been later corrected by Lossos et al.

(2000), who suggested using a multinomial probability model, instead of the binomial model used by Chang and Casali (1994).. The revised model calculated the probability for excess or scarcity of ρ mutations in the CDRs or frameworks (FRs) occurring by chance. However, all the above methods were shown to yield many false positive indications of selection (Mayorov et al., 2005; Bose et al., 2005). The impact of microsequences on relative mutability and transition bias were included, while ρ mutations outside the region of interest were excluded, thus avoiding the influence of selective forces not being tested for. Moreover, the multinomial test described by et al. (2000), was shown to be equivalent to a binomial test, and thus virtually the same test as proposed by Chang and Casali (1994).

Recently, a correction to these conventional methods, the "focused" binomial test, was offered and verified by Hershberg et al. (2008). A binomial test was used to compare the frequency of ρ and σ mutations found in different regions in mutated IgV gene sequences to their expected frequency based on codon usage of the GL sequence. This method, now normalized by z-score (Uduman et al., 2011), is currently the most accurate method for R:S selection assessment.

9.11   AUTOMATION

The analysis of an Ig sequence dataset is thus composed of between 10 to 20 different steps, each performed by a different program. As long as B cell repertoire research had been based on Sanger sequencing, yielding at most hundreds of sequences in each study, each of these analysis steps could be performed separately and semi-manually for each clone. With the introduction of HTS, however, the enormous number and diversity of Ig gene sequence reads makes it impossible to manually analyze the sequencing results. To address this challenge, an almost completely automated analysis pipeline was developed, which integrates the programs used in each step of the analysis and enables us to analyze large numbers of reads (Michaeli et al., 2013).

9.12   CONCLUDING REMARKS

Analyzing Ig gene sequences in the HTS age is an exciting challenge, with an enormous research potential. The fast accumulation of data, together with the unique characteristics of Ig genes, created an urgent need for the development of special bioinformatical analysis tools. The tools reviewed here are state-of-the-art tools in Ig gene analysis. However, as technologies for HTS and the amounts of sequences generated using them continue to evolve, better concepts and more tools will be required.

KEYWORDS

- **bioinformatics**
- **diversity**
- **high throughout sequencing**
- **immunoglobulin genes**
- **immunoinformatics**
- **lineage trees**
- **lymphocytes**
- **repertoire**
- **somatic hypermutation**

REFERENCES

Ademokun, A., Wu, Y.-C., Dunn-Walters, D.K., "The aging B cell population: composition and function," *Biogerontology*, vol. 11, no. 2, 125–137, Apr. 2010.

Ademokun, A., Y.-Wu, C., Martin, V., Mitra, R., Sack, U., Baxndale, H., Kipling, D., Dunn-Walters, D.K., "Vaccination-induced changes in human B-cell repertoire and pneumococcal IgM and IgA antibody at different ages," *Aging cell*, vol. 10, no. 6, 922–930, Dec. 2011.

Altschul, S.F., Gish, W., Miller, W., Myers, E.W., Lipman, D.J., "Basic local alignment search tool," *J Mol Biol*, vol. 215, no. 3, 403–410, Oct. 1990.

Barak, M., Zuckerman, N.S., Edelman, H., Unger, R., Mehr, R., "IgTree: creating Immuno-globulin variable region gene lineage trees," *J Immunol Methods*, vol. 338, no. 1–2, 67–74, Sep. 2008.

Bose, B., Sinha, S., "Problems in using statistical analysis of replacement and silent mutations in antibody genes for determining antigen-driven affinity selection," *Immunology*, vol. 116, no. 2, 172–183, Oct. 2005.

Boursier, L., Su, W., Spencer, J., "Analysis of strand biased 'G'.C hypermutation in human immunoglobulin Vlambda. Gene segments suggests that both DNA strands are targets for deamination by activation-induced cytidine deaminase," *Molecular immunology*, vol. 40, no. 17, 1273–1278, Mar. 2004.

Boursier, L., Su, W., Spencer, J., "Imprint of somatic hypermutation differs in human immuno-globulin heavy and lambda chain variable gene segments," *Molecular immunology*, vol. 39, no. 16, 1025–1034, Jun. 2003.

Boyd, S.D., Gaëta, B.A., Jackson, K.J., Fire, A.Z., Marshall, E.L., Merker, J.D., et al. "Indi-vidual variation in the germline Ig gene repertoire inferred from variable region gene rear-rangements," *J Immunol*, vol. 184, no. 12, 6986–6992, Jun. 2010.

Boyd, S.D., Marshall, E.L., Merker, J.D., Maniar, J.M., Zhang, L.N., Sahaf, B., et al. "Measure-ment and Clinical Monitoring of Human Lymphocyte Clonality by Massively Parallel V-D-J Pyrosequencing," *Science Translational Medicine*, vol. 1, no. 12, 12ra23–12ra23, Dec. 2009.

Campbell, P.J., Pleasance, E.D., Stephens, P.J., Dicks, E., Rance, R., Goodhead, I., et al. "Sub-clonal phylogenetic structures in cancer revealed by ultra-deep sequencing," *Proc Natl Acad Sci*, vol. 105, no. 35, 13081–13086, Sep. 2008.

Chang, B., Casali, P., "The CDR1 sequences of a major proportion of human germline Ig VH genes are inherently susceptible to amino acid replacement," *Immunol Today*, vol. 15, no. 8, 367–373, Aug. 1994.

Chen, Z., Collins, A.M., Wang, Y., Gaëta, B.A., "Clustering-based identification of clonally related immunoglobulin gene sequence sets," *Immunome research*, vol. 6 Suppl 1, p. S4, Jan. 2010.

Di Noia, J.M., Neuberger, M.S., "Molecular mechanisms of antibody somatic hypermutation," *Annual review of biochemistry*, vol. 76, 1–22, Jan. 2007.

Dörner, T., Foster, S.J., Farner, N.L., Lipsky, P.E., "Somatic hypermutation of human immu-noglobulin heavy chain genes: targeting of RGYW motifs on both DNA strands," *European journal of immunology*, vol. 28, no. 10, 3384–3396, Oct. 1998.

Dunn-Walters, D.K., Ademokun, A., "B cell repertoire and aging," *Curr Opin Immunol*, vol. 22, no. 4, 514–520, Aug. 2010.

Dunn-Walters, D.K., Belelovsky, A., Edelman, H., Banerjee, M., Mehr, R., "The dynamics of germinal center selection as measured by graph-theoretical analysis of mutational lineage trees," *Dev Immunol*, vol. 9, no. 4, 233–243, Dec. 2002.

Dunn-Walters, D.K., Spencer, J., "Strong intrinsic biases towards mutation and conservation of bases in human IgVH genes during somatic hypermutation prevent statistical analysis of antigen selection," *Immunology*, vol. 95, no. 3, 339–45, Nov. 1998.

Gaëta, B.A., Malming, H.R., Jackson, L., K.J., Bain, M.E., Wilson, P.C., Collins, A.M., "iHM-Mune-align: hidden Markov model-based alignment and identification of germline genes in rearranged immunoglobulin gene sequences," *Bioinformatics*, vol. 23, no. 13, 1580–1587, Jul. 2007.

Galan, M., Guivier, E., Caraux, G., Charbonnel, N., Cosson, J.-F. "A 454 multiplex sequencing method for rapid and reliable genotyping of highly polymorphic genes in large-scale studies," *BMC genomics*, vol. 11, 296–310, Jan. 2010.

Gibson, K.L., Wu, Y.-C., Barnett, Y., Duggan, O., Vaughan, R., Kondeatis, E., et al. "B-cell diversity decreases in old age and is correlated with poor health status," *Aging cell*, vol. 8, no. 1, 18–25, Feb. 2009.

Giudicelli, V., Chaume, D., Lefranc, M.-P. "IMGT/V-QUEST, an integrated software program for immunoglobulin and T cell receptor V-J and V-D-J rearrangement analysis," *Nucleic Acids Res*, vol. 32, no. Web Server issue, W435–40, Jul. 2004.

Hershberg, U., Uduman, M., Shlomchik, M.J., Kleinstein, S.H., "Improved methods for detecting selection by mutation analysis of Ig V region sequences," *International immunology*, vol. 20, no. 5, 683–694, May 2008.

Huse, S.M., Huber, J.A., Morrison, H.G., Sogin, M.L., Welch, D.M., "Accuracy and quality of massively parallel DNA pyrosequencing," *Genome Biol*, vol. 8, no. 7, R143–151, Jan. 2007.

Jukes, T.H., King, J.L., "Evolutionary nucleotide replacements in DNA," *Nature*, vol. 281, no. (5732): 605–606, Oct. 1979.

Larkin, M.A., Blackshields, G., Brown, N.P., Chenna, R., McGettigan, P.A., McWilliam, H., et al., "Clustal W and Clustal X version 2.0," *Bioinformatics Oxford, England.*, vol. 23, no. 21, 2947–2948, Nov. 2007.

Lossos, I.S., Tibshirani, R., Narasimhan, B., Levy, R., "The inference of antigen selection on Ig genes," *J Immunol*, vol. 165, no. 9, 5122–5126, Nov. 2000.

Margulies, M., Egholm, M., Altman, W.E., Attiya, S., Bader, J.S., Bemben, L.A., et al. "Genome sequencing in microfabricated high-density picoliter reactors," *Nature*, vol. 437, no. (7057): 376–380, Sep. 2005.

Mayorov, V.I., Rogozin, I.B., Adkison, L.R., Gearhart, P.J., "DNA polymerase eta contributes to strand bias of mutations of A versus T in immunoglobulin genes," *Journal of immunology Baltimore, Md. : 1950.*, vol. 174, no. 12, 7781–7786, Jun. 2005.

Michael, N., Martin, T.E., Nicolae, D., Kim, N., Padjen, K., Zhan, P., et al. "Effects of sequence and structure on the hypermutability of immunoglobulin genes," *Immunity*, vol. 16, no. 1, 123–134, Jan. 2002.

Michaeli, M., Barak, M., Hazanov, L., Noga, H., Mehr, R., "High-throughput sequencing and automated analysis of immunoglobulin genes: Life without a template," *Proceedings of the 2013 International Work-Conference on Bioinformatics and Biomedical Engineering IWB-BIO., Granada, Spain*, (2013):

Michaeli, M., Noga, H., Tabibian-Keissar, H., Barshack, I., Mehr, R., "Automated cleaning and preprocessing of immunoglobulin gene sequences from high-throughput sequencing," *Front. Immun.*, vol. 3, no. December, p. 386, (2012):

Munshaw, S., Kepler, T.B., "SoDA2: a Hidden Markov Model approach for identification of immunoglobulin rearrangements," *Bioinformatics*, vol. 26, no. 7, 867–872, Apr. 2010.

Neuberger, M.S., Di Noia, J.M., Beale, L., R.C., Williams, G.T., Yang, Z., Rada, C., "Somatic hypermutation at A.T pairs: polymerase error versus dUTP incorporation," *Nature reviews. Immunology*, vol. 5, no. 2, 171–178, Feb. 2005.

Neuberger, M.S., Rada, C., "Somatic hypermutation: activation-induced deaminase for C/G followed by polymerase eta for A/T," *The Journal of experimental medicine*, vol. 204, no. 1, 7–10, Jan. 2007.

Odegard, V.H., Schatz, D.G., "Targeting of somatic hypermutation," *Nat Rev Immunol*, vol. 6, no. 8, 573–583, Aug. 2006.

Quigley, M.F., Greenaway, H.Y., Venturi, V., Lindsay, R., Quinn, K.M., Seder, R.A., et al. "Convergent recombination shapes the clonotypic landscape of the naive T-cell repertoire," *Proceedings of the National Academy of Sciences of the United States of America*, vol. 107, no. 45, 19414–19419, Nov. 2010.

Rogozin, I.B., Diaz, M., "Cutting edge: DGYW/WRCH is a better predictor of mutability at G:C bases in Ig hypermutation than the widely accepted RGYW/WRCY motif and probably reflects a two-step activation-induced cytidine deaminase-triggered process," *Journal of immunology Baltimore, Md. : 1950.*, vol. 172, no. 6, 3382–3384, Mar. 2004.

Rogozin, I.B., Pavlov, Y.I., Bebenek, K., Matsuda, T., Kunkel, T.A., "Somatic mutation hotspots correlate with DNA polymerase eta error spectrum," *Nature immunology*, vol. 2, no. 6, 530–536, Jun. 2001.

Scheid, J.F., Mouquet, H., Feldhahn, N., Seaman, M.S., Velinzon, K., Pietzsch, J., et al. "Broad diversity of neutralizing antibodies isolated from memory B cells in HIV-infected individuals," *Nature*, vol. 458, no. (7238): 636–640, Apr. 2009.

Sievers, F., Wilm, A., Dineen, D., Gibson, T.J., Karplus, K., Li, W., et al. "Fast, scalable generation of high-quality protein multiple sequence alignments using Clustal Omega," *Molecular systems biology*, vol. 7, no. 539, p. 539, Jan. 2011.

Smith, D.S., Creadon, G., Jena, P.K., Portanova, J.P., Kotzin, B.L., Wysocki, L.J., "Di- and trinucleotide target preferences of somatic mutagenesis in normal and autoreactive B cells," *Journal of immunology Baltimore, Md. : 1950.*, vol. 156, no. 7, 2642–2652, Apr. 1996.

Souto-Carneiro, M.M., Longo, N.S., Russ, D.E., Sun, H., Lipsky, P.E., "Characterization of the human Ig heavy chain antigen binding complementarity determining region 3 using a newly developed software algorithm, JOINSOLVER," *Journal of immunology Baltimore, Md.: 1950.*, vol. 172, no. 11, 6790–6802, Jun. 2004.

Spencer, J., Dunn-Walters, D.K., "Hypermutation at A-T base pairs: the A nucleotide replacement spectrum is affected by adjacent nucleotides and there is no reverse complementarity of sequences flanking mutated A and T nucleotides," *J Immunol*, vol. 175, no. 8, 5170–5177, Oct. 2005.

Spencer, J., Dunn, M., Dunn-Walters, D.K., "Characteristics of sequences around individual nucleotide substitutions in IgVH genes suggest different GC and AT mutators," *Journal of immunology Baltimore, Md. : 1950.*, vol. 162, no. 11, 6596–6601, Jun. 1999.

Steiman-Shimony, A., Edelman, H., Hutzler, A., Barak, M., Zuckerman, N.S., Shahaf, G., et al. "Lineage tree analysis of immunoglobulin variable-region gene mutations in autoimmune diseases: chronic activation, normal selection," *Cell Immunol*, vol. 244, no. 2, 130–136, Dec. 2006.

Storb, U., "DNA polymerases in immunity: profiting from errors," *Nature immunology*, vol. 2, no. 6, 484–485, Jun. 2001.

Uduman, M., Yaari, G., Hershberg, U., Stern, J.A., Shlomchik, M.J., Kleinstein, S.H., "Detecting selection in immunoglobulin sequences," *Nucleic Acids Res*, vol. 39, no. Web Server issue, W499–504, Jul. 2011.

Venturi, V., Kedzierska, K., Price, D.A., Doherty, P.C., Douek, D.C., Turner, S.J., et al. "Sharing of T cell receptors in antigen-specific responses is driven by convergent recombination," *Proceedings of the National Academy of Sciences of the United States of America*, vol. 103, no. 49, 18691–18696, Dec. 2006.

Venturi, V., Quigley, M.F., Greenaway, H.Y., Ng, P.C., Ende, Z.S., McIntosh, T., et al. "A mechanism for TCR sharing between T cell subsets and individuals revealed by pyrosequencing," *Journal of immunology Baltimore, Md. : 1950.*, vol. 186, no. 7, 4285–4294, Apr. 2011.

Volpe, J.M., Cowell, L.G., Kepler, T.B., "SoDA: implementation of a 3D alignment algorithm for inference of antigen receptor recombinations," *Bioinformatics*, vol. 22, no. 4, 438–444, Feb. 2006.

Warren, R.L., Freeman, J.D., Zeng, T., Choe, G., Munro, S., Moore, R., et al. "Exhaustive T-cell repertoire sequencing of human peripheral blood samples reveals signatures of antigen selection and a directly measured repertoire size of at least 1 million clonotypes," *Genome research*, vol. 21, no. 5, 790–797, May 2011.

Weinstein, J.A., Jiang, N., White, R.A., Fisher, D.S., Quake, S.R., "High-throughput sequencing of the zebrafish antibody repertoire," *Science*, vol. 324, no. (5928): 807–810, May 2009.

Wu, Y.-C., Kipling, D., Leong, H.S., Martin, V., Ademokun, A., Dunn-Walters, D.K., "High-throughput immunoglobulin repertoire analysis distinguishes between human IgM memory and switched memory B-cell populations," *Blood*, vol. 116, no. 7, 1070–1078, Aug. 2010.

Yassai, M.B., Naumov, Y.N., Naumova, E.N., Gorski, J., "A clonotype nomenclature for T cell receptors," *Immunogenetics*, vol. 61, no. 7, 493–502, Jul. 2009.

Yu, D., Rao, S., Tsai, L.M., Lee, S.K., He, Y., Sutcliffe, E.L., et al. "The transcriptional repressor Bcl-6 directs T follicular helper cell lineage commitment," *Immunity*, vol. 31, no. 3, 457–468, Sep. 2009.

Zuckerman, N.S., Hazanov, H., Barak, M., Edelman, H., Hess, S., Shcolnik, H., et al. "Somatic hypermutation and antigen-driven selection of B cells are altered in autoimmune diseases," *J Autoimmun*, vol. 35, no. 4, 325–335, Aug. 2010.

Zuckerman, N.S., Howard, A., W., Bismuth, J., Gibson, K.L., Edelman, H., Berrih-Aknin, S., et al. "Ectopic GC in the thymus of myasthenia gravis patients show characteristics of normal GC," *European journal of immunology*, vol. 40, no. 4, 1150–1161, Apr. 2010.

Zuckerman, N.S., McCann, K.J., Ottensmeier, C.H., Barak, M., Shahaf, G., Edelman, H., et al. "Ig gene diversification and selection in follicular lymphoma, diffuse large B cell lymphoma and primary central nervous system lymphoma revealed by lineage tree and mutation analyzes," *Int Immunol*, vol. 22, no. 11, 875–887, Nov. 2010.

INDEX